Flexible Ureteroscopy

Guohua Zeng • Kandarp Parikh
Kemal Sarica
Editors

Flexible Ureteroscopy

Springer

Editors
Guohua Zeng
The Department of Urology
The First Affiliated hospital of
Guangzhou Medical University
Guangzhou, China

Kandarp Parikh
Urology
Shyam Urosurgical Hospital
Ahmedabad, India

Kemal Sarica
Department of Urology (UROLOGY)
Biruni University, Medical School
Istanbul, Turkey

ISBN 978-981-19-2938-0 ISBN 978-981-19-2936-6 (eBook)
https://doi.org/10.1007/978-981-19-2936-6

This Springer imprint is published by the registered company Springer Nature Singapore Pte Ltd.
The registered company address is: 152 Beach Road, #21-01/04 Gateway East, Singapore 189721, Singapore

Contents

History of Ureteroscopy

Kubilay Sabuncu and Kemal Sarica

Abstract

Seeing the inside of man has also been a mystery in the history of medicine and has been studied frequently. With the development of electricity and light bulb and the development of fiberoptic technology, it has been possible to reach even the body cavities that were previously unimaginable. Nowadays, especially in the field of urology, this situation has become such that there is almost no problem that cannot be solved endoscopically in the field of urology. When it is accepted that even cystoscopy is a great invention, entering into the kidney and intervening in kidney stones and tumors can be considered as a fully realized dream. It is an undeniable fact that one of the most important steps taken in this field is the integration of fiberoptic technology into endoscopy. Apart from this, the introduction of flexible devices, in particular, has made a breakthrough in the field of urology. Recently, with the introduction of digital products on the market, the comfort of the doctor has increased significantly. Infection complications that may develop in patients are prevented, and possible costs are minimized with disposable devices. With the advances in consumables, the ability of the urologist has increased enormously in the field of endourology.

Keywords

History · Ureterorenoscopy · URS · Endoscopy

K. Sabuncu (✉)
Department of Urology, Çam Sakura City Hospital, İstanbul, Turkey
e-mail: kubilay.sabuncu@saglik.gov.tr

K. Sarica
Department of Urology, Biruni University, Medical School, Istanbul, Turkey

The invention of fire and its control by human being were almost 1,000,000 years ago. It was a turning point in human history. The control of fire provided human warmth and enable to cook and to see even in the darkest nights. Until the nineteenth century, human used fire to illuminate. With the invention of electricity and light bulb, world history began to evolve at an unprecedented speed. With the implications of such technologies that were intended to make life easy in medicine, medicine also evolved inconceivably fast. The field of urology undeniably has its share of this.

As expected, the history of ureterorenoscope has evolved in parallel with the technology developed. It is fascinating to see how quickly is the technology implicated to ureteroscopy.

In Greek, endoscopy means to "watch inside." Actually, one of the most primitive examples of endoscopy is the speculum used by the Romans. In order to explicate the history of URS, it is

G. Zeng et al. (eds.), *Flexible Ureteroscopy*, https://doi.org/10.1007/978-981-19-2936-6_1

necessary to refer to the history of all inventions produced and developed for the purpose of performing endoscopy. Because there are similarities and getting ideas from each other between these technologies.

When we look at the history of endoscopy in urology, we can see the first examples of endoscopy in 1806 in the candlelight and thin cannulas used by Bozzini. This instrument was called "Lichtleiter" [1]. Daniel Colladon's conducted an experiment in London in 1841; it was shown how light can be directed by a curved water current, a phenomenon called internal reflection [2]. Babinet also used this phenomenon in 1840 to illuminate the inside of the mouth using bent glass rods [3]. Again, in the nineteenth century, with the extension of these experiments by the Irish scientist John Tyndall, optical fibers began to be used [4].

Anton J. Desmoreaux described an open tube endoscopy in Paris in 1867 using lenses that direct light to examine the male urethra [5]. After that, in 1879, modern cystoscope with warm light source was invented by Maximilian Nitze. It has a design flaw, and to cool the cystoscope, a water-cooling system was used [6]. However, this model has formed the basis of many endoscopes produced thereafter.

At the end of the nineteenth century, with the use of anesthesia in endoscopic procedures and the development of light, the age of endoscopy began to accelerate. Mignon bulbs, invented in New York, started to be used in cystoscopes. These small bulbs could be attached to the tip of the cystoscopes in order to provide imaging without getting too hot [7]. Light bulbs were first used in cystoscopes by Newman in Glasgow in 1883 followed by Nitze, Leiter, and Dittel at the same year 1887 [8].

In 1890, Tilden Brown cystoscope took its place in the market. In 1910, Buerger used Tilden Brown design and produced Brown–Buerger cystoscope which was long used [9].

Until 1927, no major progress was made, and only the light was transmitted from the fibers not the image. Baird in 1927 and Hansell in 1930 made it possible to transmit image through the fiber [3]. In 1957, Hirschowitz used flexible gastroscopy first clinically [10].

After briefly mentioning the history of cystoscopy and imaging systems, the first known ureteroscopy was done in 1912 by Hugh Hampton Young which was mentioned in a review in 1929. It was done using a pediatric cystoscope in a pediatric patient with posterior urethral valve. Ureteral orifices were severely dilated because of the posterior urethral valve, and it allowed cystoscope to pass into the ureter [11].

Flexible ureteroscope was first used by Marshall in 1964. This was an experimental surgery and was performed with forced diuresis since the system used had no irrigation and working channel [12]. But Takagi et al. developed 8 F 70 cm fiberoptic flexible ureteroscope with only passive deflection capability. They could use it for only diagnostic purposes because it was not possible to move the tip [13].

Goodman (1977) and Lyon (1978), two independent scientists, used small-diameter rigid cystoscopes as ureteroscopes in women, but the capabilities of these instruments were limited due to their short length and wide calibration [14, 15]. Lyon et al. in 1979 developed a 23 cm ureteroscope in partnership with Richard Wolf Instruments [16]. 13–16 F diameter ureteroscope allowed surgeons to reach distal ureters and with the use of working channel; this instrument also allowed manipulations. The width of the ureteroscope's diameter decreased the manipulation capacity and prevented access to the kidney. Later on, two different companies (Karl Storz Instruments and Richard Wolf Instruments) produced 40 cm 9–11 F ureteroscope at almost the same time. And this can be accepted as a breaking point in the history of ureteroscopy.

Ureteroscopes with working channels paved the way of using different instruments. The diameters of the ureteroscopes were reduced (6.9–9.5 F), and working channel calibers were increased (2–5.1 F).

Perez-Castro Ellendt and Martinez-Pineiro with Karl Storz Instruments Company produced ureteroscopes with different lengths and diameters. This development allowed to reach up to the level of renal calyceal system [17].

Still there were technical difficulties in reaching upper ureteral stones and renal stones especially in men. It was seen that an idea that was put on the shelf temporarily that had not lived long before came back to the agenda. In 1980 Olympus produced its first flexible ureteroscope, and it was a modification of its pediatric bronchoscope, but its deflection capacity was very limited [18].

Stone retrieval was one of the modes of treatment using ureteroscope, and Das (1981) performed the first basket retrieval of stone [19]. Until 1981, the main approach for ureteral stone disease was open surgery. However, an energy modality was still needed to break ureteral stones. To overcome this situation, Huffman et al. used first ultrasonic lithotripter in 1983 [20]. Although the electrohydraulic lithotripter was invented in 1955 by Yutkin, Green and Lytton, it was reported in 1985 [21].

Pneumatic lithotripsy was defined in 1990 by Languetin et al., and several studies about its use in flexible ureteroscope was done [22].

Ruby laser was invented by Theodore H. Maiman in 1960, and it was the first laser technology used for lithotripsy in 1968 even though it was for a bladder stone [23]. In fact, the first laser used in ureterolithotripsy was the pulsed dye laser. Holmium–YAG (Ho:YAG) laser was put into use in 1995 and has been maintaining its existence in this field ever since [24].

Nonflexible glass optical system containing ureteroscopes were named as rigid ureteroscopes. Fiberoptic bundles with bendable metallic sheath was released by ACMI with the name Rigiflex. While there are many successful semirigid ureterorenoscopes such as the MR-6, there has been no additional instrument with significant technology apart from the differences in length, caliber of the shafts, and caliber of the working channels of semirigid ureterorenoscopes.

Flexible URS, where the main revolutions in the history of ureterorenoscopy have been experienced very quickly, has been accelerated with the ACMI AUR, which is on the market with models capable of deflection. Although this device allows unidirectional deflection, it did not take much time for the AUR 7 model, which had bidirectional deflection. Flexible URS, which is fully used in clinical use, can be considered as cost-effective and whose derivatives are still widely used, was launched in 2012 by Karl Storz. Storz Flex X series allowed deflection of 220° in both directions.

As technology progressed, there were groundbreaking developments in illumination and imaging techniques, and these also found their place in ureterorenoscopy. Undoubtedly, one of the most striking among these breakthrough inventions was the digital transformation in camera systems. With the integration of these systems into ureterorenoscopy technology, digital ureterorenoscopes have found an undeniable place in the ureterorenoscopy market. The ureterorenoscopy industry, which has been dependent on fiberoptic technology for many years, has also gotten rid of this dependency and has gained more ergonomic, although still more expensive, ureterorenoscopes that are more cost-effective and with good images. With this development, which is called chip on the tip technology, it has been possible to produce thinner ureterorenoscopes thanks to the chips that shrink in size over time. With the widespread use of these chips and the reduction in costs, the concept of disposable ureterorenoscope has been formed. To name the chip on the tip technology, essentially two technologies CMOS (complementary metal-oxide semiconductor) and CCD (charge-coupled devices) chips have been used. In 2016, Boston Scientific produced a single-use digital flexible ureterorenoscope that was fully deflectable. After that, many brands from many countries produced similar products, and single-use ureterorenoscopes are still a rapidly developing and expanding market [25, 26].

References

1. Figdor PP, Figdor PP, Figdor PP. Philipp Bozzini: der Beginn der modernen Endoskopie: die Wiener und Frankfurter "Bozzini-Akte" und Publikationen der Jahre 1805 bis 1807 = Philipp Bozzini: the beginning of modern endoscopy: the "Bozzini files" from Vienna and Frankfurt and publications from 1805–1807. Tuttlingen: Endo-Press; 2002. p. 3.
2. Colladon D. On the reflections of a ray of light inside a parabolic liquid stream. Comptes Rendus. 1842;15:800–2.

3. Hecht J. City of light: the story of fiber optics. New York: Oxford University Press; 2004. p. 340.
4. Tyndall J. On some phenomena connected with the motion of liquids. Proc R Inst Great Britain. 1854;1:446.
5. Desmoreaux AJ. The endoscope and its application to the diagnosis and treatment of affections of the genitourinary passages. Chic Med J. 1867;24:177–94.
6. Nitze M. Eine neue Beleuchtungs und Untersuchungs method fur Harnrohre, Harnblase, und Rektum. Wiener Med Wochen. 1879;24:649.
7. Moran ME. The light bulb, cystoscopy and Thomas Alva Edison. J Endourol. 2010;24(9):1395–7.
8. Newell OK. The endoscopic instruments of Joseph Leiter of Vienna and the present development of endoscopy. Boston Med Surg J. 1887;117:528–30.
9. Buerger L. A new indirect irrigating observation and double catheterizing cystoscope. Ann Surg. 1909;49:225–37.
10. Hirschowitz BI, Curtiss LE, Peters CW. Gastroenterology PHM. In: Barlow DE, editor. Fiberoptic instrument technology. In: Small animal endoscopy. St. Louis: C.V. Mosby; 1958. p. 1.
11. Young HH, McKay R. Congenital valvular obstruction of the prostatic urethra. Surg Gynecol Obstet. 1929;48:509–12.
12. Marshall VF. Fiber optics in urology. J Urol. 1964;91(1):110–4.
13. Takayasu H, Aso Y. Recent development for pyeloureteroscopy: guide tube method for its introduction into the ureter. J Urol. 1974;112(2):176.
14. Goodman TM. Ureteroscopy with pediatric cystoscope in adults. Urology. 1977;9(4):394.
15. Lyon ES, Kyker JS, Schoenberg HW. Transurethral ureteroscopy in women: a ready addition to the urological armamentarium. J Urol. 1978;119(1):35–6.
16. Lyon ES, Banno JJ, Schoenberg HW. Transurethral ureteroscopy in men using juvenile cystoscopy equipment. J Urol. 1979;122(2):152–3.
17. Pérez-Castro Ellendt E, Martinez-Piñero JA. Ureteral and renal endoscopy. Eur Urol. 1982;8(2):117–20.
18. Vilardell F. Digestive endoscopy in the second millennium: from Lichleiter to endoscopy. Madrid: Thieme; 2006.
19. Das S. Transurethral ureteroscopy and stone manipulation under direct vision. J Urol. 1981;125(1):112–3.
20. Huffman JL, Bagley DH, Lyon ES. Treatment of distal ureteral calculi using rigid ureteroscope. Urology. 1982;20(6):574–7.
21. Green DF, Lytton B. Early experience with direct vision electrohydraulic lithotripsy of ureteral calculi. J Urol. 1985;133(5):767–70.
22. Languetin JM, Jichlinski P. The Swiss Lithoclast. J Urol. 1990;143:179.
23. Mulvaney WP, Beck CW. The laser beam in urology. J Urol. 1968;99(1):112–5.
24. Watson G, Murray S, Dretler SP, Parrish JA. The pulsed dye laser for fragmenting urinary calculi. J Urol. 1987;138(1):195–8.
25. Tom WR, Wolllin DA, Jiang R, Radvak D, Simmons WN, Preminger GM, et al. Next generation single use ureteroscopes: an in vitro comparison. J Endourol. 2017;12:1301–6.
26. Emiliani E, Traxer O. Single use and disposable flexible ureteroscopes. Curr Opin Urol. 2017;27:176–81.

Anatomical Considerations During Flexible Ureteroscopy

Amy E. Krambeck and Mark A. Assmus

Abstract

An understanding of the commonly encountered and variant anatomic urinary tract systems is crucial to achieving superior outcomes of endourologic procedures. Further understanding of the current endoscopic technologies and devices along with their physical anatomic restrictions can allow for optimal surgical planning and intraoperative troubleshooting for complex cases. In this chapter, we explore the normal urinary tract anatomy with respect to ureteroscopy and highlight unique anatomic situations including calyceal diverticulum, renal fusion anomalies (horseshoe kidneys, cross-fused ectopic kidneys), surgical anatomic disruptions (urinary diversions), and duplicated urinary systems.

Keywords

Endoscopic anatomy · Anomalous renal anatomy · Ureteroscopy · Urinary tract anatomy

A. E. Krambeck (✉) · M. A. Assmus
Department of Urology, Northwestern University, Chicago, IL, USA
e-mail: Amy.Krambeck@nm.org

1 Introduction

Technological advancements over the past two decades have resulted in ureteroscopy (URS) emerging as an invaluable minimally invasive surgical technique for both benign and malignant disease processes within the urinary tract. However, there are a number of anatomic considerations that influence the technique and success rates of URS which will be explored within this chapter. The vast majority of the academic literature on ureteroscopic management in the setting of anomalous anatomy focuses on urinary tract calculi; however, the principals and understanding gained from these described endourologic techniques are applicable to a wide array of clinical circumstances both benign and malignant. An understanding of the various ureteroscopes physical properties and capabilities is essential for urologists to problem solve difficult clinical scenarios. Furthermore, knowledge of normal and variant urinary tract anatomy equips the urologist with an armamentarium which is necessary to approach new endourologic conditions.

2 Urinary Tract Anatomy

Due to their location in the retroperitoneum, anterior (ventral) to the psoas and quadratus lumborum muscles, the orthotopic adult kidneys lay with an oblique longitudinal axis such that the upper poles are medial and posterior to the loca-

G. Zeng et al. (eds.), *Flexible Ureteroscopy*, https://doi.org/10.1007/978-981-19-2936-6_2

tion of the inferior poles [1]. The cranial and caudal boundaries of the kidneys usually extend from the 11 to 12th thoracic vertebrae to the 2–3rd lumbar vertebrae (Fig. 1) [2]. Greater than 100 years ago, Brodel first described that anterior renal calyces were more medial and posterior renal calyces were more lateral [3]. In contrast, Hodson et al. described that the anterior calyces were longer and extended more lateral than the posterior calyces [4]. In 1984, Kaye and Reinke examined CT scans of kidneys in order to ultimately determine that close to 70% of right kidneys follow the Brodel-described anatomy of the calyces while up to 80% of left kidneys follow the Hodson-described anatomical configuration (Fig. 2) [5, 6]. Overall, the majority (60–65%) of renal collecting systems feature two major calyces in which the midzone of the kidney drains via superior or inferior minor calyces while 35–40% of kidneys have a separate midzone calyx that drains directly to the renal pelvis. Most urinary tract systems contain 5–14 minor calyces in each kidney (with 70% of kidneys having 7–9 minor calyces) [1].

The normal anterior medial rotation of the kidneys is approximately 30° (Fig. 1) [8]; however, body positioning and respirations do affect the precise location of the kidneys. Respiratory effects on renal position have been shown to provide roughly 2–3 cm of caudal movement with inspiration as the diaphragm expands [2].

A detailed understanding of renal and ureteric vascular anatomy is valuable for many urologic surgeries with some specific URS considerations. One key example where vascular anatomy influences safety and success of endoscopic management occurs in the setting of ureteropelvic junction (UPJ) obstruction or proximal ureteric stricture. Ureteroscopic endopyelotomy outcomes for treating ureteropelvic junction obstructions (UPJO) identified that in the setting of a crossing vessel a lateral endoscopic ureteropelvic incision is the safest to minimize bleeding complications and ensure adequate ureteric blood supply [2]. Posterior, anterior, and medial incisions increase the risk of injury to the renal hilum, ureteropelvic vasculature, or aberrant crossing vessel itself. Emiliani et al. reported on the reasonably successful outcomes of an endoureterotomy approach to ureteral strictures (1.5 cm or less) in the absence of radiation [9]. Another key anatomic consideration is where the ureter passes anterior (ventrally) to the iliac vasculature. This is a common location where urinary tract calculi may obstruct the ureter or be unable to progress beyond due to the extrinsic effect of the iliac artery on the posterior wall of the ureter. Care should be taken to advance a semirigid uretero-

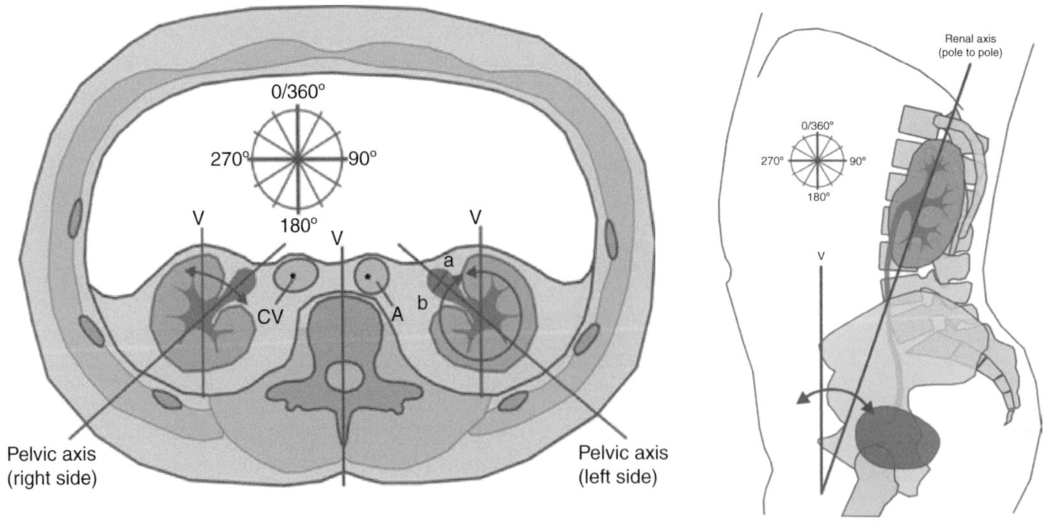

Fig. 1 Retroperitoneal location and angulation of the kidneys. 30° anterior rotation of the kidney from coronal plane. Sagittal view showing anterior lower pole displacement [7]

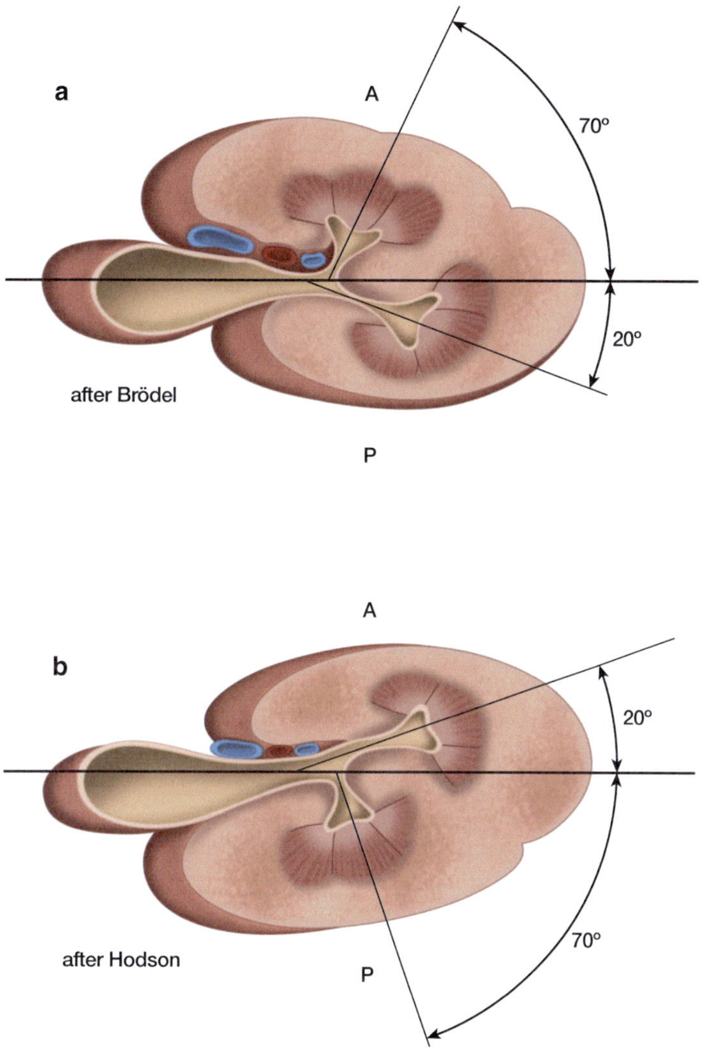

Fig. 2 Pyelocaliceal system after Brödel (**a**) and after Hodson (**b**) [5]

scope or ureteral access sheath against resistance in this location due to the class proximity of the adjacent iliac vasculature.

With respect to the renal collecting system, papillae drain urine into the most peripherally located minor calyces that are furthest from the renal pelvis. A single papilla draining into a single calyx is a simple calyx while two or more papillae that both drain into a single calyx is called a compound calyx. Compound calyces are most commonly located in the upper pole, followed by the lower pole, and rarely found in the middle pole calyces. Minor calyces funnel toward the renal pelvic and either join together with similarly located minor calyces to form a major calyx before inserting into the renal pelvis or directly join into the renal pelvis. The narrow channel by which minor or major calyces drain toward the renal pelvis is often termed the infundibulum.

The ureter is commonly divided into three segments. The proximal (cranial) ureter traverses from the renal pelvis to the upper border of the sacrum. The middle ureter is the segment from the upper to lower border of the sacrum. The distal (caudal) ureter runs from the lower border of the sacrum to the insertion into the bladder. Alternative nomenclature for the ureter has been suggested which includes an abdominal (renal pelvic to iliac vessels), pelvic (iliac vessels to bladder), and intramural ureter (within the urinary bladder). The intramural portion is commonly 1.5–2.5 cm in length [2]. Barrett et al. examined various approaches to determine ureteral length in an effort to improve intraoperative ureteric stent length selection [10]. They showed that coronal and axial computed tomography (CT) ureteral lengths were significantly associated with direct measurement; however, patient height, lumbar height, and surgeons' estimate of ureteral length were not. Average adult ureter length ranged from 22 to 30 cm with a diameter of 1.5–6 mm [10].

Moving in a caudal to cranial direction, the three historically taught most common anatomical narrowings along the length of the ureter are the ureterovesical junction (UVJ) which is where the ureter itself is the narrowest (3–4 mm) and travels intramurally through the wall of the urinary bladder to exit in a postero-lateral location. This segment may commonly require dilation prior to ureteroscope or access sheath placement [2]. The next potential anatomic narrowing of the ureter occurs over the iliac vessels as described above, and the third is the ureteropelvic junction. Some recent publications have challenged the dogma of three physiologic narrowings of the upper urinary tract with a review by Kamo et al. attributing significant advances in CT and MRI technologies along with their widespread use for renal colic evaluation in determining that the two commonly encountered physiologic narrowings are the UVJ and the upper ureter/UPJ [11]. With respect to the ureteral orifice itself, there is a wide range of size, shape, and locations that can exist (congenital or acquired). The angle that the ureter runs is roughly 90°–135° postero-laterally [5] away from the mid-line of the urinary bladder.

3 Anatomic Considerations Within Ureteroscope Technology

The invention and optimization of ureteral access sheaths, baskets, and laser fibers have drastically changed the approach to stone disease. Furthermore, scope advancements such as fiberoptics, charge-coupled device/digital scopes,

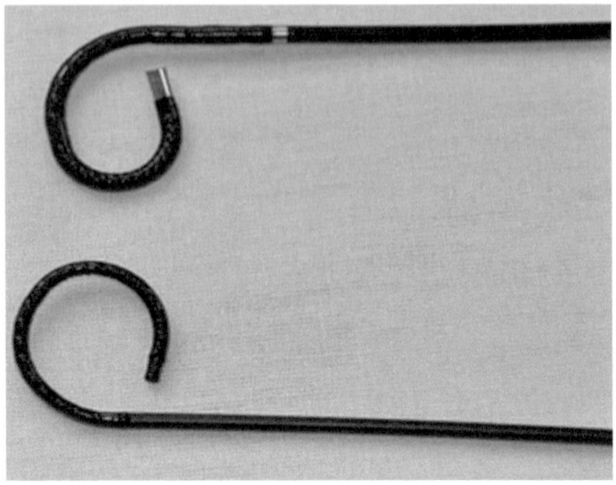

Fig. 3 Olympus URF-V (top) and KARL-STORZ Endoskope Flex-Xc (bottom) ureteroscopes. Photograph showing the distal working parts of these flexible ureteroscopes at maximum downwards deflection (275° and 270°, respectively). Both of these devices are fitted with digital optical systems. The instruments also both have a single channel of the same diameter (3.6 F), with the outer diameter of 9.9 F versus 8.5 F (tip diameters of 8.5 F and 7.8 F, respectively) [15]

digital chip processors, disposable ureteroscopes, decreasing size of flexible ureteroscopes (12–7.5 F), multichannel and flexible ureteroscopes with up to 270° of active deflection have helped to expand the surgical indications for ureteroscopy (Fig. 3). All these advancements taken together have drastically improved the utilization of URS in a variety of challenging anatomic situations [12].

Semirigid ureteroscopes often utilize a tapered distal tip (diameters ranging 4.5–9 F) that is narrower than the proximal shaft (6.5–15 F) [13]. This difference between the distal tip and proximal size ranges between 2 and 4 F depending on the scope. The working channels of most semirigid ureteroscopes are generally ≥3 F and can often times have two smaller individual working channels. Short and long semirigid ureteroscopes are available with common lengths of the shaft being roughly 30–33 cm or ≥40–43 cm, respectively. There is <10 (5°–12°) of angulation range for the tip of the semirigid ureteroscope with a field of view ranging between 61° and 95.1° [2].

Bagley et al. are credited with the introduction of the working channel, irrigation system, and active deflection in flexible ureteroscopes during the 1980s, marking a key turning point in the use of URS for the management of numerous urologic diseases [14]. Flexible ureteroscopes come in a variety of sizes with a range of length (54–85 cm) and distal tip size (4.5–11 F) with proximal shaft size ranging from 5.8 to 11 F [15–17]. With advances in scope design, the ability for distal tip deflection to 180° in either direction has been accomplished. Reaching this 180° deflection goal was driven by Bagley et al. who determined the average angle to be 140° and the maximum angle to be 175° in order to reach the lower pole in a retrograde manner when examining the ureteroinfundibular angle in 30 patients [14]. Interestingly, one anatomic study examining ureteral diameter found that 96% of patients had a native ureter ≤9 F [18] although this can often accommodate serial dilation or passive dilation secondary to interval ureteral stent placement if access to the upper tract was initially unsuccessful. Of note, when advancing a flexible ureteroscope through the UPJ in a retrograde manner, it is valuable to observe physiologic ureteral peristalsis in order to wait for relaxation before advancing the scope [2, 18]. Care should be taken to avoid advancing against the contracting ureter particularly at the UPJ which can lead to mucosal injury or ureteral perforation/avulsion injuries.

Flexible ureteroscopes are designed for both active and passive tip deflection. A European consensus statement on URS tricks and tips highlighted that an understanding of the three ways in which the provider can influence the position of the flexible ureteroscope tip is key in efficient and precise URS control [19]. The tip of the flexible ureteroscope itself can be advanced forward and backward (in and out), the tip can be deflected up and down, and the scope can be torqued to the left and the right. In order to gain additional deflection, particularly to access lower pole calyces, advancing the flexible ureteroscope against the wall of the renal pelvis or infundibulum to induce a passive deflection in addition to the active deflection may allow for access to otherwise inaccessible calyces. This passive deflection technique relies upon the anatomic configuration of the collecting system and infundibulum and may be obliterated in the setting of hydronephrosis.

The perceived decreased range of deflection in flexible URS with the insertion of laser fibers or retrieval baskets through the working channels has been explored within anomalous kidney patients. In the case of the Olympus P-5, the maximum active deflection is 180°s upward/270°s downward with a 90° field of view. Interestingly, with the insertion of a 200 μm laser fiber within the working channel, these maximum deflections were 180.4°/272.3°s and exchanging the laser fiber for a 2.2 F Cook basket resulted in 181.9°/280.6° maximum deflections [20, 21]. However, the maximum active deflection radius was significantly increased from 9.5 mm in the empty state to 11.3 mm and 11.4 mm in the laser and basket states, respectively [20, 21]. This increase in space required to reach the maximum deflection has been partly attributed to the perceived difficulty in accessing lower poles, particularly in small collecting systems or anomalous systems like horseshoe kidneys.

Novel flexible ureteroscope technologies are currently being explored and gaining widespread uptake. An example of such technologies include additional points of active deflection proximal to the ureteroscope tip with the added benefit of being able to lock this secondary deflection in a specific position. The locking secondary deflection mechanism allows for more controlled distal deflection into the hard-to-reach calyx. A similar concept is seen in the exaggerated deflection Flex-x flexible ureteroscope (Karl Storz Endoscopy, Tuttlingen, Germany) which provides >300° of primary deflection.

Upon introducing either a semirigid ureteroscope or a flexible ureteroscope into a urinary tract system, use of contrast opacification and fluoroscopy imaging can help map out the anatomic system that is to be explored. Examining all of the visible contrast filled areas of the urinary tract system in a systematic manner is essential in diagnosing or managing many urinary tract disease processes.

Available guidewires range from 80 to 260 cm in length and 0.018 to 0.038 in. in diameter. A segment, 1–15 cm, of the distal tip of these wires is flexible with varying degrees of stiffness proximal to this tip depending on the function desired. The wires can be straight, angled, or curved with a J hook to aid in specific anatomic access within the urinary tract. With respect to ureteral dilations, balloons, access sheaths, and stents, a wide range of sizes are available. Ureteral dilators often range from a 6 F tapered tip up to 12 F. Ureteroscopic balloon dilators which pass through the ureteroscope can be inflated under direct visualization ranging from 3 to 12 F. Large balloon dilators can be passed over a guidewire in the absence of a ureteroscope which can be inflated up to 30 F, although ureteric dilation beyond 15 F is rarely required. Although the rate of ureteral dilation is decreasing with miniaturization of scopes, historical URS series required dilation in 8–33% of cases in order to access the upper urinary tract [12, 22, 23].

4 Urinary Tract Angles and Lengths

Understanding urinary tract angles and lengths is critical in endourology in order to select the appropriate instruments to safely complete the minimally invasive procedure. Historically, renal collecting system anatomy and particularly the location of urinary tract calculi within the lower pole was of interest in shockwave lithotripsy management since success rates were much lower than for stones in other urinary tract locations. Over the last two decades, as URS utilization has increased, many studies have started to focus on the anatomic configuration of the urinary tract collecting system with respect to ureteroscopic access. More specifically, the lower pole infundibulopelvic angle (IPA), infundibular length (IL), and the infundibular width (IW) are considered important to URS success. Studies have determined that a wide lower pole IPA, short IL, and a broad IW are all individually and, in combination, associated with increased ability to access and remove urinary tract calculi [24].

Elbahasy et al. described IW to be the narrowest point measured in the axis of the lower infundibulum (Fig. 4). IL is measured as the distance

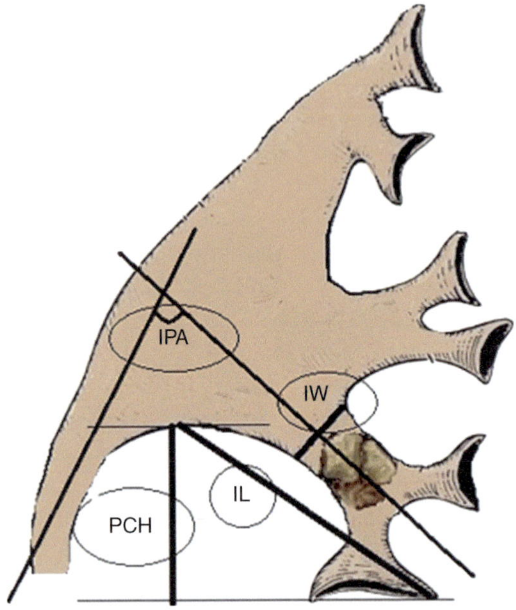

Fig. 4 IW, measured as the narrowest point in the axis of the lower infundibulum. IL, measured as distance between the most distal point of the calyx containing the calculi and the midpoint of the lower lip of the renal pelvis. PCH, measured as distance between the lower lip of the renal pelvic and the bottom of the lower calyx. IPA, determined by the intersection of infundibular axis (which is a line connecting the center of the pelvis with the bottom of the stone bearing calyx) and the ureteropelvic axis (which is a line connecting the center of the pelvis with a point in the upper ureter opposite the lower pole of the kidney) [24, 25]

between the most distal point of the calyx containing the calculi/tumor/foreign body and the midpoint of the lower lip of the renal pelvis. Pelvicalyceal height (PCH) is measured as the distance between the lower lip of the renal pelvis and the bottom of the lower most calyx. IPA is determined by the intersection of infundibular axis (which is a line connecting the center of the pelvis with the bottom of the stone/tumor/foreign body bearing calyx of interest) and the ureteropelvic axis (which is the line connecting the center of the renal pelvis with a point in the upper ureter opposite the lower pole of the kidney [24].

Various studies have examined particular angle and length cutoffs with some evidence to support that a lower pole IPA <70°, an IL >3 cm, and an IW ≤5 mm are individually unfavorable for ureteroscopic access and success of treatment. Corroborating these results, Resorlu et al.

found that an IPA >45° significantly predicts successful retrograde URS versus <45° [25]. Similarly, success rates for accessing a lower pole calyx via flexible URS was 87.5% (7/8 patients) with IPA >90°, 74.3% (26/35 patients) when IPA ranged between 30° and 90° and 0% (0/4 patients) when IPA <30° [26]. For patients with IPA between 30° and 90°, the length of the infundibulum further effected the success rate with an IL <3 cm having 88.2% access and only 61.1% success when ≥3 cm [26, 27].

In a recent 2020 publication, Dresner et al. examined the influence of IPA on lower pole urinary tract calculi treatment using a ureteroscopic approach [28]. They examined 745 total renal units undergoing flexible URS with laser lithotripsy with success defined as no residual fragments on KUB radiograph within 2 months postoperatively. The IPA was measured on intraoperative retrograde pyelograms [29]. The authors identified that postoperative residual fragments were associated with acute IPA <90° ($p < 0.001$) as well as lower pole stone location and large stone size. Similarly, IPA <90° and large stone size were associated with need for secondary surgery [28, 30]. A prospective study identified a cutoff of <41° for lower pole stones <2 cm as being significantly less successful for retrograde ureteroscopic treatment [30].

One interesting study examined the effect of patient positioning on the lower pole IPA during intravenous urography. A total of 46 kidneys across six different positions (supine level, supine 20° head down, supine 45° head up, prone level, prone 20° head down, and prone 45° head up) were examined. The authors determined that the broadest angle of entry to the lower pole infundibulum occurred with the patient in prone 20° head down positioning; however, the clinical utility of this position limits its use except in specific cases necessitating ureteroscopic lower pole management otherwise not accessible [31].

Pelvicocalyceal height can also affect outcomes at the time of URS. In a study of 67 patients undergoing URS for lower pole calculi, all had their IL, IW, IPA, as well as PCH determined on preoperative urographic imaging. Using a definition of residual fragments ≤3 mm in size at 2 month follow up to signify a successful URS, the mean IL and PCH of successful cases were larger than the unsuccessful cohort, although this did not meet statistical significance (IL 26.7 vs. 28.2 mm, $p = -0.14$; PCH 20.7 vs. 23.2 mm, $p = 0.072$) [25]. There was no impact on stone-free status based on IW. The only angle that met statistical significance for its impact on the stone-free rate was the IPA [25].

Although the vast majority of the literature has explored angles specific to retrograde access to the lower pole, there is a paucity of literature examining angles and lengths of middle and upper pole calyces. Generally the upper and mid calyces are readily accessible in most patients with high diagnostic and treatment success rates. However, it can be difficult to identify anteriorly located mid and upper calyces, and therefore, utilization of retrograde pyelograms and fluoroscopy can be beneficial in inspecting the entire kidney.

Beyond success of accessing the calyx, the effect of prolonged or extreme deflection on flexible ureteroscopes has been examined with respect to the IPA. A total of 381 flexible ureteroscopic procedures (68.24% for urinary tract calculi and 31.76% for diagnostic purposes) were performed with 9.9% of devices deemed to fail the postoperative assessment (deemed defective). Cases with postoperative defective flexible ureteroscopes were associated with more acute IPA (42.5° vs. 56°, $p < 0.001$). Additionally, more acute IPA was also associated with higher rate of Clavien–Dindo grade 2 or higher complications and longer hospitalization times [32]. There was no correlation between operative length and duration of fluoroscopy used during the cases.

5 Calyx Location

The two most commonly encountered upper pole configurations are three calyces followed by two calyces [2]. The interpolar region of the kidney may have 2–4 calyces most commonly while the lower pole usually has 2–3 calyces. There is a large range of variability in the configuration, size, and shape of the calyces with an additional variation in number of papilla encountered within each calyx [2]. In, total the average kidney contains 7–9 calyces (although this can vary between 4 and 19 or more calyces) [1, 2].

There have been numerous studies examining the optimal surgical modality [shock wave lithotripsy (SWL), URS, percutaneous nephrolithotomy (PCNL)] to manage varying sized urinary tract calculi found within different anatomic poles of the kidney collecting system. One early study examined the outcomes of SWL and URS for lower pole renal calculi that were ≤1 cm in size. This study found that radiographic stone-free rates were lower with URS (50%) with 7/35 cases experiencing an intraoperative complications (five failed access and two ureteral perforations) [33].

Subsequently, it has been well described that there are many advantages to relocation of a urinary tract calculi or fungal ball from a lower pole calyx into a mid or preferentially upper pole calyx. Relocation of the stone aids the efficiency of the procedure, improve stone-free rates, and minimize scope damage. Mapping of the collecting system with retrograde pyelogram contrast instillation under fluoroscopic imaging is useful in understanding the unique patient anatomy that may aid in ureteroscopic management.

In the vast majority of middle pole calyces, there is a paired anterior and posterior directed minor calyx which is often close to 90° from each other. Similarly, roughly 50% of lower pole systems contain both anterior and posteriorly paired minor calyces. Using a combination of fluoroscopic contrast enhancement mapping as well as direct visualization, comprehensive evaluation of the upper urinary tract can be confirmed, which is invaluable in the diagnostic evaluation for upper urinary tract urothelial cell carcinoma.

6 Variations in Calyceal Anatomy

The width and length of the calyceal infundibulum contribute to the degree of urine stasis, particularly in the case of a calyceal diverticulum (CD), with increased stasis found with more narrowed and longer infundibulum [2, 34–36]. Unilateral CD (97%) is more common than bilateral (3%) (with equal distribution seen between right and left side) with the following calyceal distribution: upper pole (48.9–70%), mid pole (12–29.7%), lower pole (10–21.4%) [37–40]. Additionally, posterior location is more common than anterior location. Historically, intravenous pyelogram (IVP) imaging was utilized to detect calyceal diverticulum (Fig. 5); however, CT urogram or even noncontrast CT scans with the presence of radio-opaque calyceal calculi are now commonly utilized imaging modalities (Fig. 6).

Embryologically, CD likely forms congenitally due to a lack of degeneration of small divisions of the ureteral bud [40, 41]. An additional proposed theory describes CD as an acquired condition due to recurrent infection, urinary obstruction, and subsequent infundibular fibrosis/stenosis [40]. Typically, CD is <1 cm in diameter although there is a wide range of width reported (4–75 mm). Stone analysis from CD has reported that the majority comprises calcium oxalate monohydrate, hydroxyapatite, or struvite [35]. Recurrent upper urinary tract infections may be associated with CD in 25% of cases with subsequent infundibulum obstruction leading to potential abscess formation, urosepsis, or hypertension. One study looking at 51 patients with CD identified that symptomatic diverticulum was more commonly upper pole versus middle or lower pole (52% vs. 38% vs. 10%, respectively, $p < 0.05$) [42].

Ureteroscopic treatment of CD was first reported in 1989 by David and Fuchs [44]. Advances in flexible ureteroscopes (improved deflection, larger working channels), ureteral access sheaths, wires, and laser fibers have all improved success rates and decreased surgical times of URS treatment of CD since the first. Long-term success of percutaneous, ureteroscopic, and laparoscopic minimally invasive approaches to managing CD has been reported [41, 45]. Posteriorly, percutaneous approaches have been well described while anteriorly the superior calyx is best approached in a ureteroscopic fashion and middle or lower pole anterior diverticulum may be approached laparoscopically or ureteroscopically [41]. Chong et al. rec-

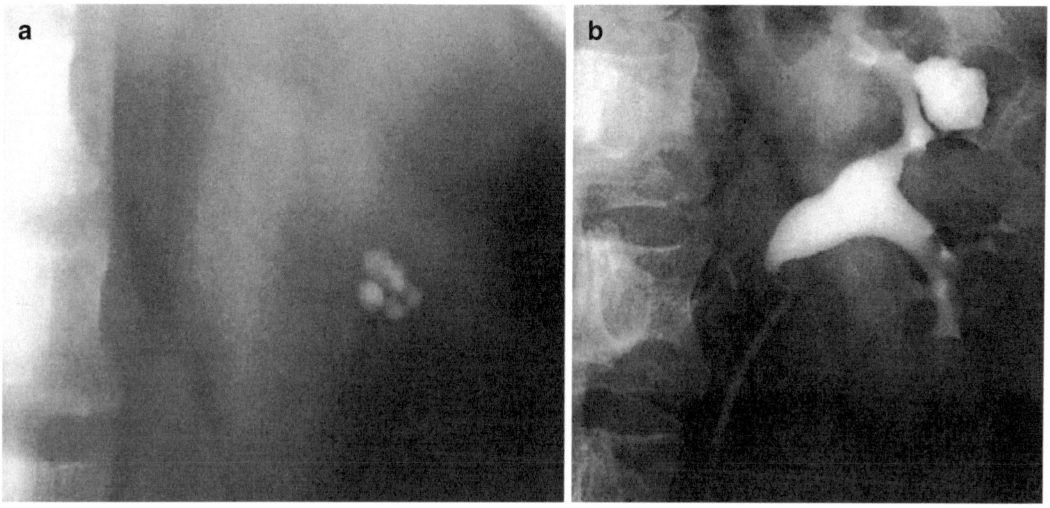

Fig. 5 Calculi (**a**) localizing to a calyceal diverticulum on intravenous pyelography (**b**) [41]

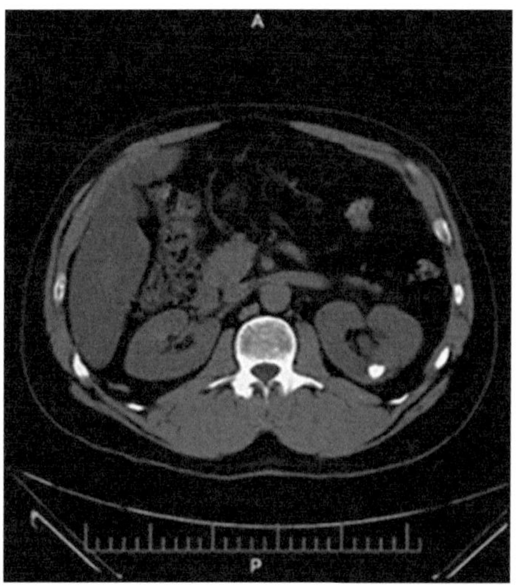

Fig. 6 Left calyceal diverticulum stone [43]

ommended URS management for upper and middle pole CD with stone burden 20 mm or less with consideration for lower pole CD management dependent upon the infundibulopelvic angle [29, 37].

Balloon dilation of CD has been described using many different 6–7 F balloon dilators, 3 F Bagley no tip dilating balloon or 3 F zero-tip dilating balloon (Microvasive) (Figs. 6 and 9). It is rare to require dilation of the infundibulum >12–15 F, so utilization of ureteroscopic balloon dilators allowing visualization can be used. Laser incision is an alternative approach with success for shorter length (<1 cm) infundibulum, while balloon dilation is preferred for longer length (>1 cm) infundibulum. Anatomically, CD and their infundibulum that are incised/dilated run in close proximity to interlobar renal vasculature which may lead to bleeding obscuring procedure progression. Care should be taken to minimize deep laser incisions and to ensure saved fluoroscopic images of the target calyx continue to be in line with laser progress. Grasso et al. described the use of injectable guide wires to pass through a diverticulum infundibulum and inject retrograde contrast into the CD prior to utilizing a balloon to dilate the neck [46].

Batter et al. described that >30% of CD were not identifiable on retrograde URS, particularly in the lower pole where scope deflection limitations may impede a comprehensive mapping. When examining URS success by CD location, 84% of middle or upper pole CD were accessible in contrast to 28.6% of lower pole diverticulum [47]. Similarly, in a retrospective cohort managed by URS, 24% of patients' ostium/infundibulum was not identifiable or could not be cannulated [48]. Subsequent publications have reported higher success with Chong et al. having 95% access success with retrograde URS in 96 patients with the only failures occurring in the lower pole [37].

Table 1 Summary of symptomatic (urinary tract calculi) calyceal diverticulum managed with retrograde ureteroscopic approach [39, 49]

Study primary author (year)	No. patients	Ureteroscopic access to diverticulum obtained (%)	Symptom-free rate at follow-up (%)	Postoperative follow-up duration (months)
Auge et al. [48] (2002)	17	76	35	1.5
Batter and Dretler [47] (1997)	26	69	100	45
Chong et al. [37] (2000)	96	96	NR	NR
Fuchs and David [44] (1989)	15	100	87	7.4
Grasso et al. [46] (1995)	3	67	100	5
Yang et al. [51] (2017)	26	84.6	84.6	11.5

An approach to CD based on objective anatomic findings was described by Canales et al. which supports ureteroscopic management of middle or upper pole, anterior or posterior CD that have thick parenchyma and are <1.5 cm in widest diameter [41]. Other additional clinical algorithms have been published with varying stone size cutoffs; however, none of these algorithms have been prospectively validated with respect to clinical outcomes [49]. The two notable anatomical classification systems published in the CD literature were published by Wulfson et al. and Dretler et al.; however, neither have gained significant clinical use [36, 50]. The anatomic classification proposed by Dretler classified type 1 diverticulum as an open mouth and short neck while type 2 has a closed mouth and short neck. Type 3 has a closed mouth and long neck while type 4 has an obliterated neck. The purpose of the classification was to aid in treatment selection and whether URS should be pursued versus an alternative approach (laparoscopic, PCNL).

Overall, there remains a paucity of detailed literature on anatomic findings of CD regarding their three-dimensional (3D) location (versus anterior–posterior), 3D size, and stone burdens. The systematic review by Ito et al. concludes that optimal treatment selection should be made by the surgical team. At this time, utilization of 3D data and use of strict anterior–posterior, upper–middle–lower pole CD location algorithms does not have strong supporting evidence (Table 1).

Although distinct from true calyceal diverticulum, the anatomic URS considerations and management of symptomatic hydrocalyces are similar in that a renal calyx outflow is obstructed by a narrow infundibulum that may restrict retrograde ureteroscopic access to that papilla/calyx. These may be congenital or acquired secondary to iatrogenic injury, trauma, or infections. Due to the continued production of urine within the dilated hydrocalyx, they often present with symptoms. In contrast, megacalycosis (idiopathic calyx dilation without infundibular narrowing) may be seen on imaging but rarely warrant intervention as many of these patients remain asymptomatic [52].

7 Duplicated Urinary Systems

A bifid appearing renal pelvis can occur in up to 10% of collecting systems, although complete ureteral duplication occurs in only 0.6–0.7% of the population [38, 53]. As opposed to many other renal anomalies, duplicated systems are unique in the potential variation of ureteric orifice location within the urinary bladder. The classically described Weigert–Meyer rule follows that the lower pole ureter drains into the cranial and lateral portion of the bladder. The upper pole ureter therefore opens into the bladder in a more caudal and medial location to that of the lower pole moiety [54]. Embryologically, the ureter develops when the ureteral bud branches off the mesonephric duct and extends toward the metanephric blastema. The process of a duplicated ureter occurs when the ureteral bud bifurcates prior to reaching the blastema and is one of the most common ureteral anomalies in population studies [53]. Rarely, trifurcation of the ureter may occur in which case the most common distal appearance is a single ureteral orifice entering the bladder. This single ureteral orifice can also occur in the case of a partial duplicated ureter, where there are two proximal ureters that join prior to the solitary urinary bladder orifice.

There are some variations in technique utilized during ureteroscopic management of duplicated systems depending on what disease process is being managed, and whether the primary target is renal or ureteric or whether the surgical team plans to utilize a ureteral access sheath (for example, in the case of dusting a large renal calculi). Care is first taken on cystoscopy of the urinary bladder to map out the trigone and identify the ureteral orifices. If preoperative imaging has identified a duplicated system, then all orifices should be identified; however, a study demonstrated that intraoperative detection of a duplicated systems did not negate a successful ureteroscopic approach [53]. Once the orifice/orifices are identified, a guidewire can be placed in a retrograde manner followed by a semirigid ureteroscope to the mid-ureter in males and proximal ureter in females for direct visualization of the lumen bifurcation. This allows for the placement of a secondary guidewire into the target collecting system with subsequent use of an access sheath or in some cases back loading the flexible ureteroscope over the correct guidewire and using that to advance the scope into the target collecting system. In many case reports of obstructing urinary tract calculi within duplicated ureters, the small caliber of the ureters necessitates interval placement of a double J ureteric stent for 10–14 days to allow passive dilation prior to URS [55].

Rana et al. and Ugurlu et al. both examined URS for stones in bifid pelvis/duplicated systems with 50–91.7% stone-free success rate, although multiple procedures were often required and varying definitions of stone-free rate were utilized [54, 56]. Chertack et al. compared URS outcomes in a matched cohort of 100 patients with and without ureteral duplication and found that although the cases with duplication required significantly longer average operative time (55 vs. 38.5 min, $p=0.022$), there was no difference in stone-free rates or need for secondary procedures. Additionally, Clavien–Dindo grade 4 or 5 complications occurred at equal rates between the cohorts (4 vs. 4%) [53]. Finally, when comparing partial duplication and complete duplication, there was no difference in operative times for urinary tract calculi management and no difference in the rate of secondary procedures (5% vs. 7%, $p = 0.754$) [53].

One interesting finding is that whether or not duplication is known preoperatively or identified intraoperatively did not affect operative time in the management of urinary tract calculi, stone-free rates, or need for secondary procedures. This study supports that in the setting of urinary tract calculi preoperative planning, the necessity of contrast-enhanced phases is not necessary to clearly delineate the presence or absence of duplications, and a non-contrast CT abdomen-pelvis is adequate for surgical planning.

Distinct from duplicated urinary systems, supernumerary kidneys can exist in which there are >2 kidneys within a single patient. This additional kidney is usually smaller than the two orthotopic kidneys and commonly displays either a bifid or duplicated ureter. Supernumerary kidney is a particularly rare anomaly with only around 100 cases reported in the literature, and no defined true incidence rate is known [57, 58]. Within the small body of literature, supernumerary kidneys have been noted to be more common on the left side with 60% located caudal to the ipsilateral dominant orthotopic kidney and very rarely has occurred bilaterally [59, 60].

8 Alternative Renal Anatomy

Without complete cranial migration due to a fused isthmus, the horseshoe kidney has a more caudal location on each side with malrotation, resulting in renal pelvises having a more anterior position and calyces having a more posterior position (Fig. 7) [7]. One study examining fusion kidneys identified that 97.1% of cases had the renal pelvis oriented ventral (anterior) to the renal parenchyma [7]. The isthmus of a

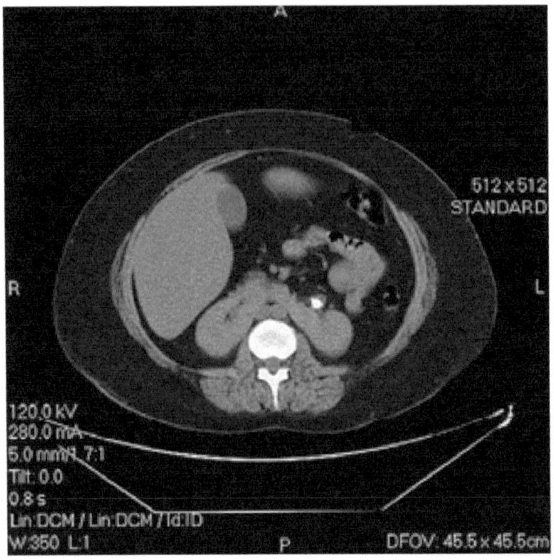

Fig. 7 Patient with a horseshoe kidney. Note the anterior displacement of the kidney and long shock wave path [64]

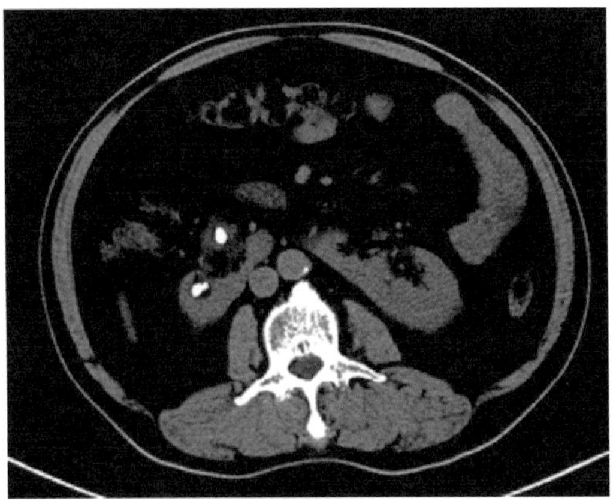

Fig. 8 CT scan of renal stones in a horseshoe kidney [20]. (Open Access distributed under Creative Commons Attribution. CC-BY. Ding J. et al. 2015 Brazilian Society of Urology http://creativecommons.org/licenses/by/4.0/)

horseshoe kidney is typically anterior to the aorta and inferior vena cava and caudal to the inferior mesenteric artery with isthmic calyces seen to enter the pelvis at acute angles—making ureteroscopic access to this location very challenging [61]. Additionally, similar to other ectopic kidneys, there is an increased rate of ureteropelvic junction obstruction with hydronephrosis seen in up to 15–35% of horseshoe kidneys (Fig. 8) [62, 63].

Use of a ureteral access sheath along with a Trendelenburg (15°–30° head down) supine position can help improve success of accessing the upper tract collecting system with the ureteroscope despite these anatomic differences in horseshoe kidneys [20]. In these cases, the ureteral access sheath can be positioned distal to the UPJ and the flexible ureteroscope advanced through the sheath and subsequently through the UPJ into the collecting system by riding over an additional guidewire placed retrograde through the ureteroscope.

Stone relocation in horseshoe kidneys has been shown to improve stone-free rates and minimize scope damage by minimizing duration of deflection [20, 65]. Some groups have published on the use of slight Trendelenburg positioning in order to help facilitate urinary tract calculi to reposition to the upper pole calyx [66]. Use of semirigid ureteroscope and ureteral access sheath placement has been effective in these patients.

Another unique anatomic finding in many horseshoe kidneys is that the renal pelvis has a narrowed cranial-caudal size. This narrow intrarenal space increases the difficulty of utilizing passive deflection along with active deflection into the lower pole calyces, particularly if a laser or basket is required within the working channels. In horseshoe kidneys, there is also a high insertion of the ureter into the renal pelvis along with an increased acuity of the IPA, which decreases stone-free rate and increases the risk of secondary URS compared to non-horseshoe kidney urinary tract calculi (Fig. 9) [67]. Despite these anatomic considerations, two large retrospective series examining urinary tract calculi management in horseshoe kidneys achieved satisfactory stone-free rates after a single URS (Table 2) [66, 68]. SFR when examining patients with stones located within the lower pole was 80% while the SFR was 93% without the presence of a lower pole calculi, further supporting the difficult lower pole deflection in horseshoe kidneys and that the anatomic changes in these collecting systems influence ureteroscope success [68].

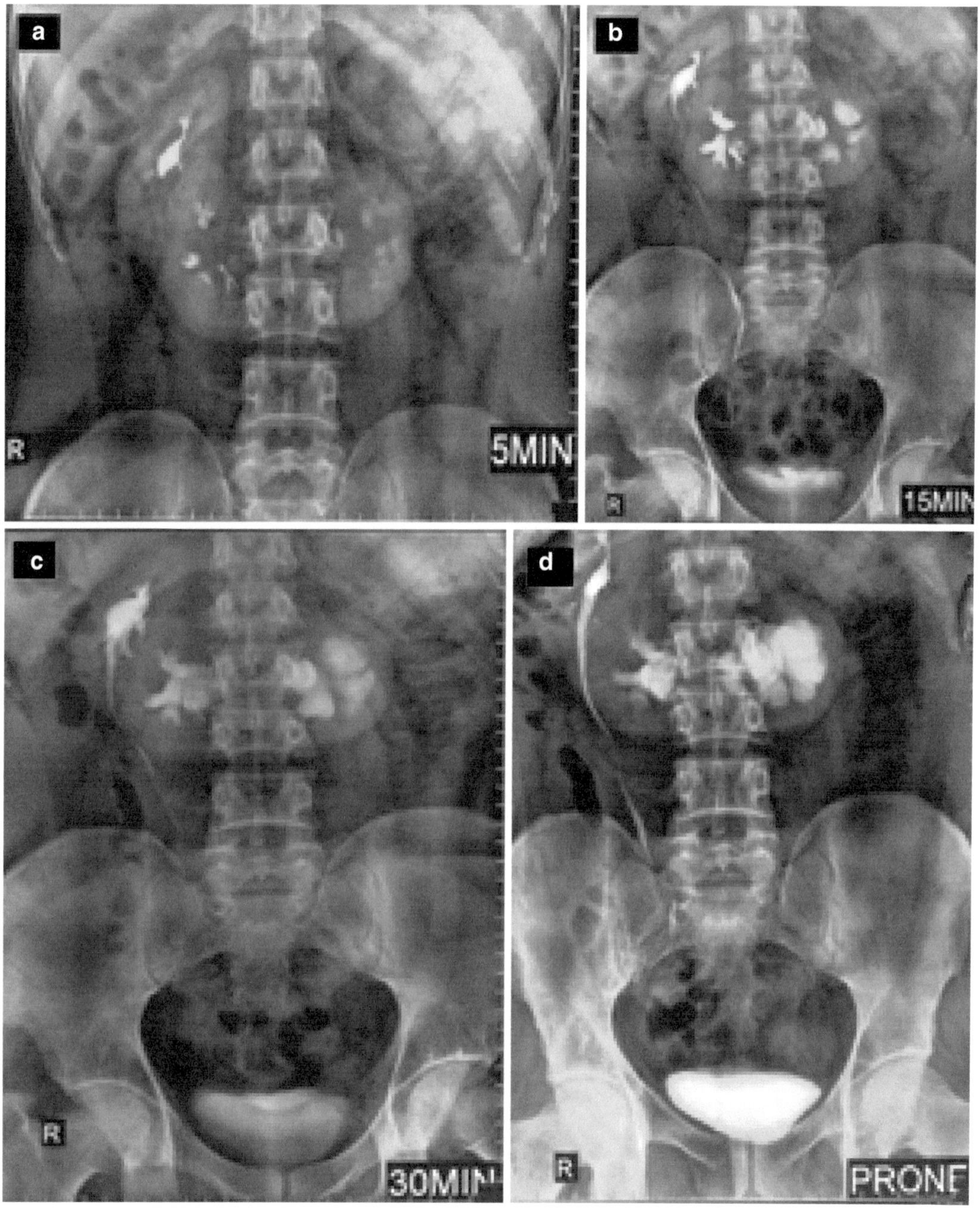

Fig. 9 Intravenous urography shows a horseshoe kidney and a malrotated supernumerary kidney cephalad to and fused with the right renal moiety (**a**, **b**). Horseshoe kidney shows delayed excretion and moderate hydronephrosis of left moiety as well as mild pyelocaliceal dilation on the right (**c**, **d**) [58]

Table 2 Summary of urinary tract calculi in horseshoe kidneys managed with ureteroscopy [49, 71] (Adapted from Open Access distributed under Creative Commons Attribution. CC-BY. Lavan et al. 2019. Springer Nature http://creativecommons.org/licenses/by/4.0/)

Study primary author (year)	No. patients with horseshoe kidneys	Preop stent placement (%)	Use of ureteral access sheath (%)	Primary outcome success	Overall success rate (%)	Clavien–Dindo 3+ complication (*N*)
Molimard et al. [69] (2010)	17	23.5	100	RF ≤3 mm	88.2	0
Ding et al. [20] (2015)	16	NR	100	NR	87.5	0
Blackburn et al. [68] (2016)	20	NR	NR	RF <4 mm	84	NR
Gokce et al. [66] (2016)	23	NR	100	RF <3 mm	73.9	0
Astolfi et al. [70] (2017)	8	84.6	NR	RF <2 mm	75	0

9 Ectopic Kidneys

Anomalous kidneys are due to variable abnormalities that occur in the normal embryologic development of the kidneys and urinary tract system. The interruption in the normal sequence of development can lead to incomplete ascent of the kidneys, fusion of the kidneys, rotational abnormalities, or a combination of all of these. Due to the anatomic variation, the drainage of these renal systems may be impaired, leading to increased urinary stasis and subsequent risk for symptom development—particularly urinary tract calculi. Over the past decade, there has been an increase in publications examining URS outcomes in anomalous kidneys, although the vast majority are retrospective. One group recommended the stepwise practice guidance for managing anomalous kidneys using URS depicted in Fig. 10.

Often the abnormal location of an ectopic kidney results in a tortuous ureter with resultant difficulty in gaining upper tract access. In such cases, the ability to utilize a ureteral access sheath to attempt to straighten out the tortuous ureter is valuable, and in many described cases, patients are pre-stented prior to surgery to optimize the ability to place the ureteral access sheath. The majority of ectopic kidneys have a pelvic location (55%), laying deep within the pelvis below the aortic bifurcation [72] although they can be found iliac (lumbar), abdominal, thoracic, or crossed/crossed-fused (Fig. 11). Ectopic kidneys often have some aspects of malrotation depending on their final position, with the majority of renal pelvises having a more anterior position.

From an anatomic perspective, some groups advocate that in anomalous kidneys, particularly pelvic ectopic, ureteral access sheaths should be positioned in the mid or distal ureter to allow for unrestricted ureteroscope flexion/deflection within the collecting system [45]. Placement of the ureteral access sheath into the proximal ureter or renal collecting system in these pelvic ectopic kidneys has been shown to restrict ureteroscope flexion and limit access to lower pole calyces [73].

In contrast, some recommend avoiding ureteral access sheaths in pelvic ectopic kidneys due to the short and tortuous ureter which may experience increase in trauma from attempted sheath placement. Success with advancing a flexible ureteroscope over a guidewire without the use of

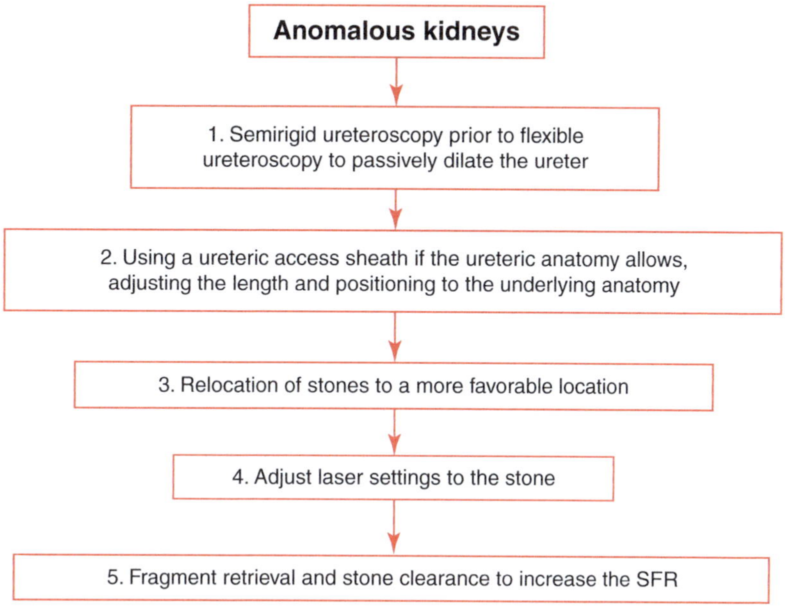

Fig. 10 Tips and practical guidance for management [71]. (Open Access distributed under Creative Commons Attribution. CC-BY. Lavan et al. 2019. Springer Nature http://creativecommons.org/licenses/by/4.0/)

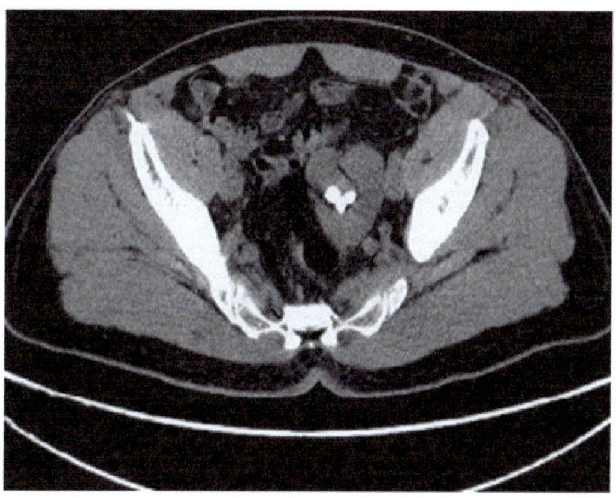

Fig. 11 Patient with pelvic kidney and staghorn calculus. Note the intervening bowel loops and bony pelvis, precluding safe SWL [64]

an access sheath has been reported (Fig. 12). One study identified that ureteroscopy failure in pelvic kidneys was a result of unfavorable infundibulopelvic anatomy [74].

Crossed renal ectopia can occur in roughly 1/800–1000 individuals [38, 70]. In crossed fused ectopia, one kidney crosses over the midline and fuses with the opposite kidney. Typically, the kidney in the more caudal location will drain via a ureter that crosses midline and inserts into the urinary bladder in the orthotopic position; however, there are many variations that have been reported (Fig. 13). URS outcomes for these cases are rarely reported in the literature with very small patient numbers in most series. In the series of anomalous kidney stone treatment by Ugurlu et al., one case of crossed ectopy underwent ureteroscope with the use of a ureteral access sheath for an 85 mm upper pole calculi. The case lasted 65 min, and they were unable to access the stone solely with the ureteroscope [54]. One study examining 209 patients with fused kidneys determined that crossed fused ectopia kidneys, when compared to horseshoe kidneys are more caudal, have greater axial rotation as well as a smaller pelvic width [7].

Beyond horseshoe kidneys or ectopic kidneys, isolated malrotation is rare with no definite series identifying the incidence. Overall, rotational

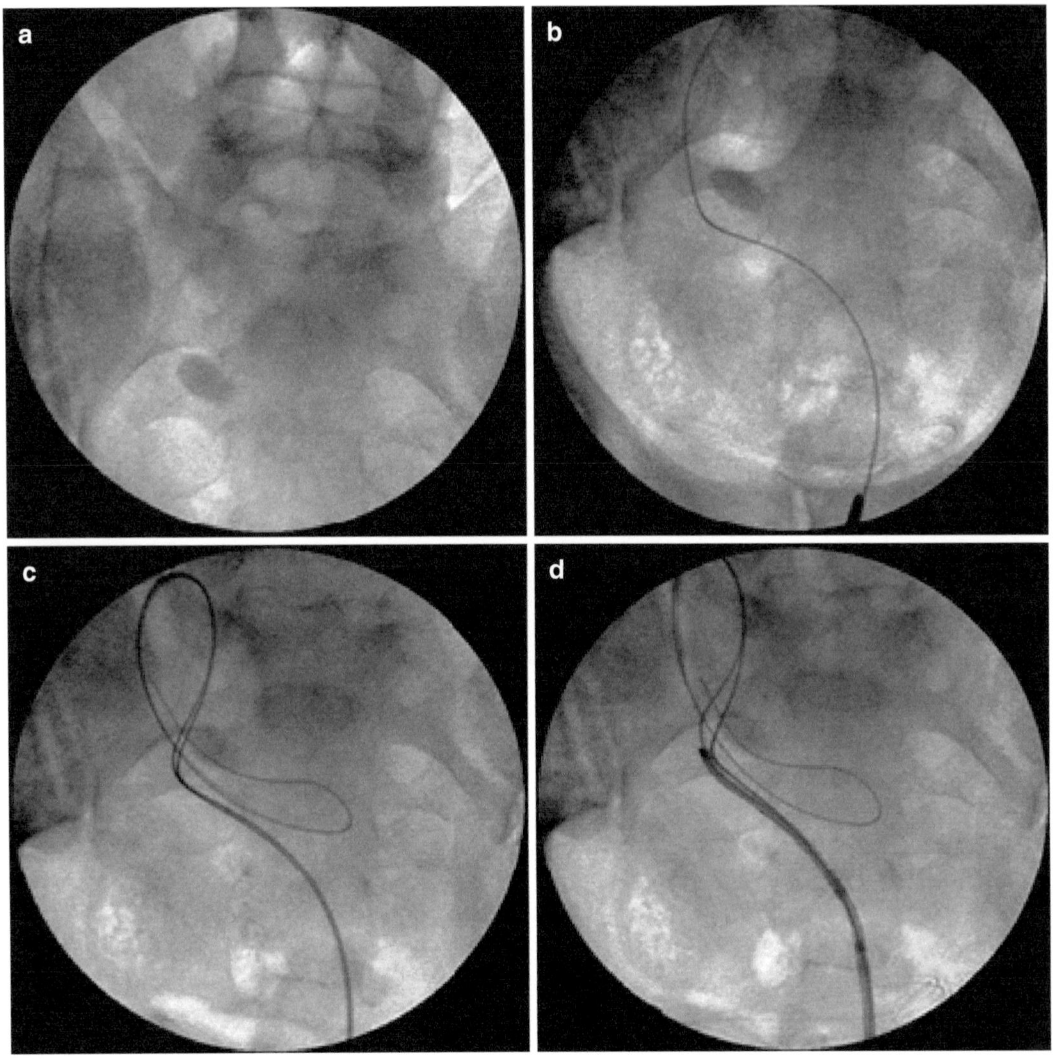

Fig. 12 The placement of guidewires into a right pelvic ectopic kidney (**a–c**) with advancement of flexible ureteroscope (**d**) over the guidewire without aid of an access sheath [74]

abnormalities with or without additional urinary tract variations occur at an incidence of roughly 1/500 individuals [38]. The radiographic hallmark of malrotated kidneys is the centrally located renal pelvis with some calyces located medial to the renal pelvis [2]. Ergin et al. and Oguz et al. examined SFR in specifically isolated renal rotational anomalies and after flexible URS found a 75% SFR after a single procedure [76, 77]. After secondary procedures, this increased to 83.3%.

Normal renal rotation during development starts from a ventral position at the sixth week of gestation. Subsequently, a 90° rotation toward midline occurs as the renal units migrate to the renal fossa. Finally, before the ninth week of gestation, the renal units rotate such that calyces are lateral, and the renal pelvis is medial. Various descriptions and definitions of malrotation have been proposed with some using a strict definition of the kidneys that remain in the ventral position

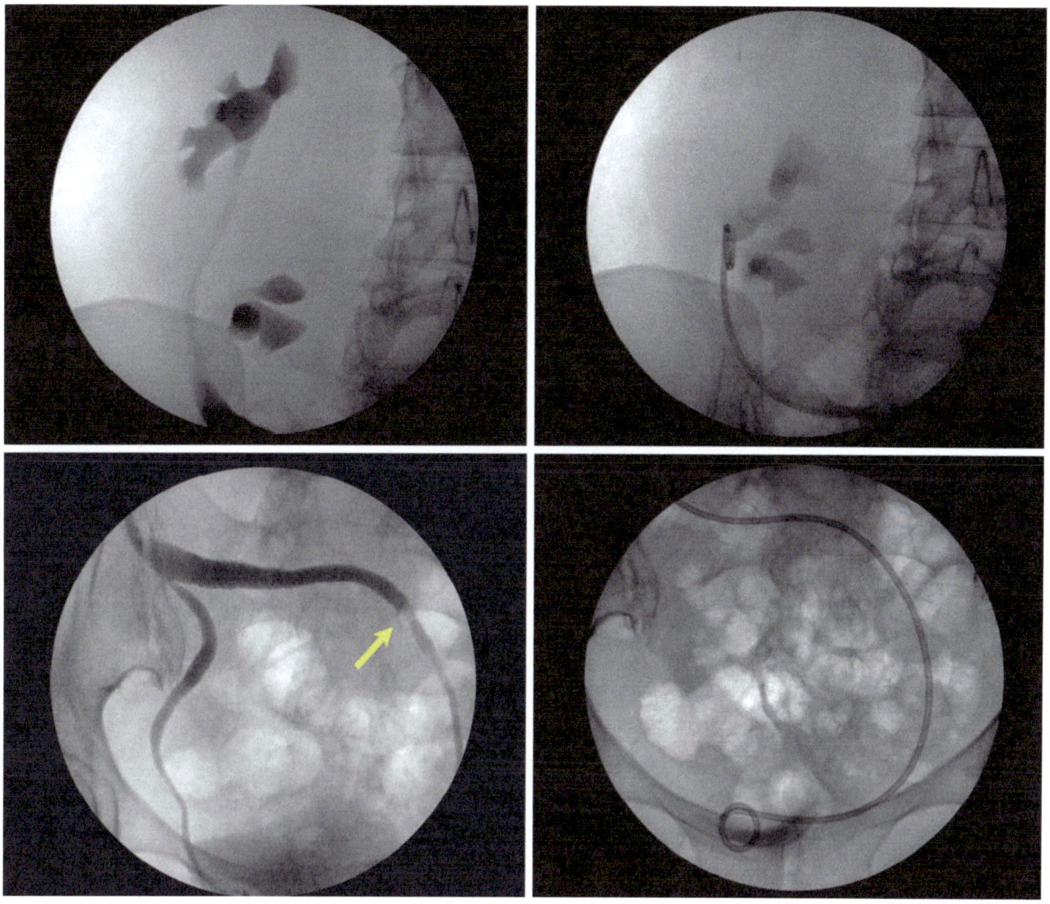

Fig. 13 Double J stent placement in crossed fused ectopia after mid ureteric calculi treatment with URS [75]. (Open Access distributed under Creative Commons Attribution. CC-BY 4.0. Toussi et al. 2018. Mary Ann Liebert http://creativecommons.org/licenses/by/4.0/)

(Fig. 14) [77]. This ventral renal positioning is the most common malrotation anomaly.

Apart from urinary tract calculi, ectopic kidneys (Fig. 15) often are associated with UPJO in up to 22% of cases [72]. Care should be taken to perform renal scans, through retrograde pyelograms or in some cases a Whitaker test to definitively ensure that hydronephrosis of these anomalous kidneys warrants surgical intervention, as up to a quarter of ectopic kidneys may have nonobstructive, nonrefluxing hydronephrosis on imaging (Fig. 16). There does remain a paucity of evidence on the outcomes of endoscopic proximal ureteral stricture/UPJO treatment in anomalous kidneys due to the rarity of these cases. Jabbour et al. reported on antegrade

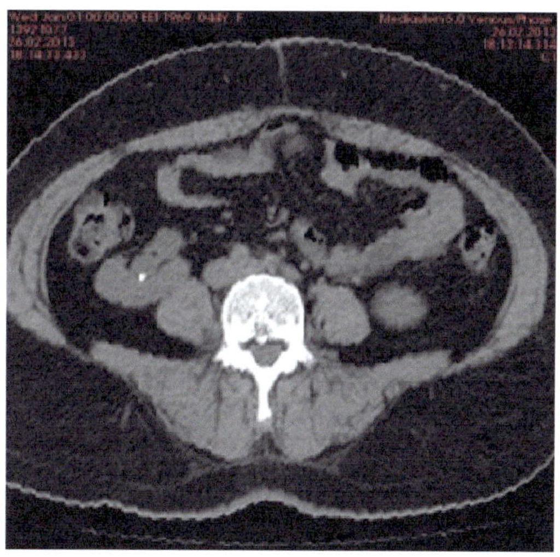

Fig. 14 Isolated anomaly of right kidney malrotation with a urinary tract calculi [77]

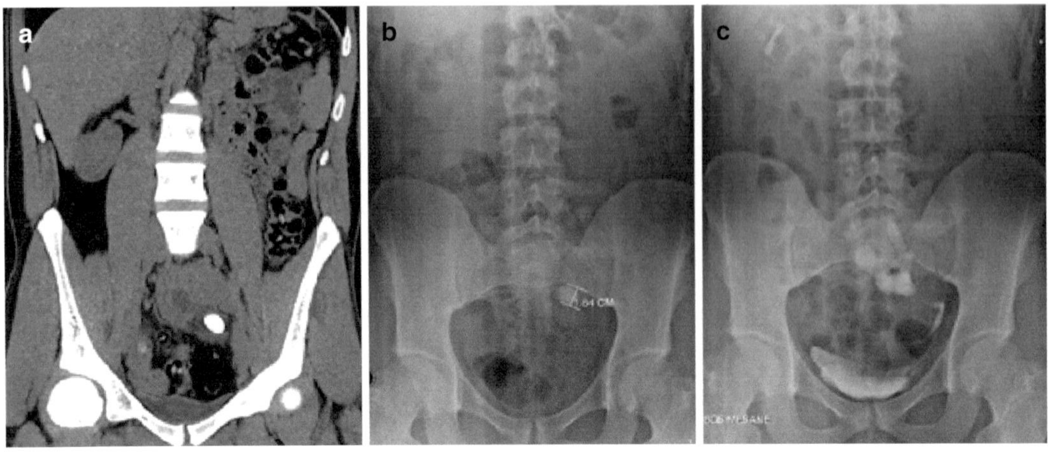

Fig. 15 Computed tomography with (**a**) intravenous urography (**b**, **c**) of a patient with a 1.84 cm calculi within a left pelvic ectopic kidney [74]

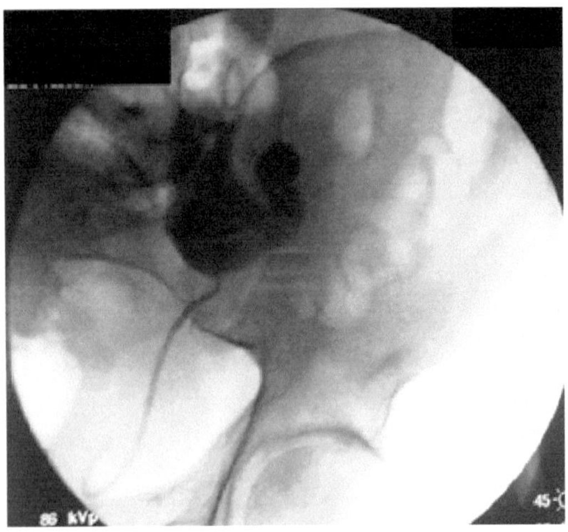

Fig. 16 Retrograde pyelogram in patient with pelvic kidney associated with renal stones and UPJ obstruction [64]

endopyelotomy outcomes in four patients with horseshoe kidneys and five patients with ectopic kidneys in 1998 [72]. Retrograde endopyelotomy for ectopic kidneys has been associated with high rates of ureteral strictures. Overall success rates of endoscopic UPJO or proximal ureteral strictures <2 cm have been reported in the 55–78% range [72].

Bas et al. examined complication rates in 1571 retrograde flexible URS cases and found that only three factors influenced complication rate, one of which was congenital renal abnormalities [78], which remainder the only significant factor on multivariate analysis ($p = 0.02$). Such findings further highlight that ureteroscopic management of disease processes in anomalous kidneys is challenging. Within their series of 1395 patients with 1411 renal units that underwent 1571 URS interventions, the overall rate of anomalous kidney anatomy was 2.99% with one bifid pelvis, nine complete ureteral duplications, 18 calyceal diverticulum, 15 horseshoe kidneys, two pelvic ectopic kidneys, and two solitary malrotation anomalies [78]. Giusti et al. performed a review of URS in anomalous kidney stone surgery and found that on average 1.17 procedures per patient obtained a 70–99% stone-free rate with a 2.7% major complication rate [79].

The anatomic variations highlighted above influence the prevalence of stone formation within the urinary tract of these patients. For malrotated kidneys, SFR for renal and ureteral stones was 71% and 88%, respectively [80]. With regard to stone location, in 20 cases of horseshoe kidneys with ureteral stones, the stones were found in distal ureter (35%), mid ureter (30%), proximal ureter (30%), and multiple locations (5%) [80]. In another study, renal stone location in 23 horseshoe kidneys was distributed as follows: lower pole (52%), middle pole (4.3%), upper pole (0%), renal pelvis (4.3%), and multiple locations (39.4%). Looking at stone location in ectopic kidneys, the ureteral stone distribution in 17 patients was distal ureter (35%), mid ureter

(41%), proximal ureter (24%), and no cases of multiple ureteric calculi. Renal stone location in 10 ectopic kidneys was lower pole (30%), middle pole (20%), upper pole (20%), renal pelvis (10%), and multiple locations (20%). Finally, looking at malrotated kidneys, ureteric stone location was distal ureter (37.5%), mid ureter (25%), and proximal ureter (37.5%). Renal calculi in malrotated kidneys were lower pole (37.5%), middle pole (0%), upper pole (0%), real pelvis (12.5%), and multiple locations (50%) [80].

10 Surgical Anatomic Variations

One particularly unique set of anatomic considerations for URS occurs in the setting of acquired surgical changes to the urinary tract. Many unique reconstructive techniques are available and evolving in order to manage both benign and malignant conditions; however, in this chapter, we will focus primarily on anatomic considerations of urinary diversions (in particular, incontinence urinary diversions like ileal conduits), transureteroureterostomies, and various ureteral reimplants that may be encountered.

A variety of surgical techniques are used for ureteral reimplant (ureteroneocystotomy) in both pediatric and adult cases, which are most often performed for vesicoureteral reflux (VUR) or traumatic injury, respectively. Each reimplant technique has their own advantages and disadvantages which may lead to their utilization, so understanding the relevant anatomic considerations for these techniques is important prior to any planned URS. In extravesical techniques, the ureteral orifice will be in an orthotopic position, whereas in transvesical cases, the two most commonly encountered techniques include the Cohen cross-trigonal and the Politano–Leadbetter reimplant. Additionally, the Glenn–Anderson technique may commonly be used in which the ureteral orifice is advanced distal to the orthotopic location.

The Cohen cross-trigonal ureteral reimplant has classically posed a significant challenge in retrograde ureteroscopic access to the upper urinary tract as the ureter crossed to insert with the orifice on the contralateral side of the trigone to that renal moiety [81]. Wallis et al. described a unique approach to gaining access in these patients [82]. They described using a 4 F curved tip angiographic glide catheter via the working channel of a rigid cystoscope while it is directed in line with the ureteral orifice. A number of potential angled catheters are used now, which allow for 360° provider manipulation of the distal tip in order to orient and support retrograde placement of a 0.035 in. angle tipped or straight tipped glide wire. Additional use of a torque device can allow for 360° fine manipulation of the wire as well. The combination of the curved catheter and the angled glide wire allows up to 120° angulation from the tip of the cystoscope [82]. Systematic advancement of the wire and catheter can allow for proximal placement and subsequent exchange to an Amplatz super stiff guide wire to straighten out the ureter permitting rigid or flexible ureteroscope access. In their early series consisting of four pediatric patients that had undergone Cohen cross-trigonal reimplant, they successfully gained retrograde upper tract access in all cases. Another series examining nine patients with Cohen cross-trigonal reimplants failed to provide retrograde access in two patients (22.2%) [81]. Access to the ureter in 15 Glenn–Anderson reimplants was successful in all cases.

One of the most commonly utilized incontinent urinary diversion is the creation of an ileal conduit. This is seen in both management of benign (e.g., refractory stress urinary incontinence) and malignant (e.g., urothelial cell carcinoma of the urinary bladder) disease processes. It is well described that patients who undergo creation of ileal conduit urinary diversions may proceed to a number of upper tract diseases or complications at a higher incidence then the general public. Some of such diseases warranting ureteroscopic management include, but are not limited to, urinary tract calculi, recurrent urinary tract infections, and anastomotic strictures. The largest cited reason for failed ureteric access was long, tortuous conduit with inability to localize orifice [83].

One series examining retrograde URS in continent urinary diversions found that the overall success in accessing the desired renal units was 59% with the etiology of failure attributed to inability to identify the afferent limb or ureteral orifice (20%), afferent limb tortuosity (40%), angulation (20%), and length of the afferent limb (20%). A loopogram can be valuable in providing anatomic information about the total length, angles, and tortuosity of diversion afferent limbs. If ureteric stenting is required at the conclusion of the case, care should be taken to select a long ureteral stent that will extend through the afferent limb with its distal most end near the bladder neck for ease of outpatient cystoscopy stent removal.

A unique management option for ureteral obstruction is the transureteroureterostomy [84]. A classic contraindication for performing this repair is a patient with known urinary tract calculi who may require ureteroscopic management after the transureteroureterostomy (TUU). However, the potential development of new onset stone disease or urinary drainage-related complications, signs or symptoms that necessitate retrograde URS of the upper urinary tract may still occur in patients who undergo this procedure. In some ways, the approach to gaining access is similar to that in partially duplicated ureteric systems, although the absolute length and angles required to reach the upper urinary tract system may prevent flexible URS access depending on the location of the stone/stricture/tumor. Iwaszko et al. followed 63 patients who underwent TUU for a mean duration of 5.8 years (ranging from 0.1 to 22.2 years) and found that 3.6% of patients developed obstruction and 12.7% developed urinary tract calculi requiring intervention [84]. They did report successful URS management in one patient; however, the stone was located distal to the TUU anastomosis. All proximal urinary tract calculi that did not pass spontaneously required PCNL intervention due to the difficulty in cannulating and advancing a flexible ureteroscope to the level of the proximal ureter or renal pelvis.

11 Summary

In this chapter, we examined how improvements in URS technology along with increased understanding of normal and commonly encountered anomalous urinary tract anatomy have led to minimally invasive management of multiple different conditions. Knowledge of the various physical properties and capabilities of ureteroscopes along with normal and variant urinary tract anatomy equips the urologist with an armamentarium from which they can draw upon in order to adapt to solving a new endourologic problem. Combining this understanding of the urinary tract anatomy, along with its variations, helps us continue to improve the efficiency and safety of endourology.

References

1. Sampaio FJ, Mandarim-De-Lacerda CA. Dimensional and radiological pelviocaliceal anatomy for endourology. J Urol. 1988;140:1352–5.
2. Partin AW, Wein AJ, Kavoussi LR, Peters CA, Dmochowski RR. Campbell-Walsh Wein urology. 12th ed. Amsterdam: Elsevier; 2020.
3. Brodel M. The intrinsic blood vessels of the kidney and their significance in nephrotomy. Bull Johns Hopkins Hosp. 1901;12:10.
4. Hodson J. The lobar structure of the kidney. Br J Urol. 1972;44:246.
5. Shnorhavorian M, Anderson KR. Anatomic and physiologic considerations in ureteroscopy. Urol Clin N Am. 2004;31(1):15–20.
6. Kaye K, Reinke D. Detailed caliceal anatomy for endourology. J Urol. 1984;132:1085–8.
7. Glodny B, Petersen J, Hofmann KJ, Schenk C, Herwig R, Trieb T, et al. Kidney fusion anomalies revisited: clinical and radiological analysis of 209 cases of crossed fused ectopia and horseshoe kidney. BJU Int. 2009;103(2):224–35.
8. Wein AJ, Kavoussi LR, Novick AC, Partin AW, Peters CA. Campbell-Walsh urology. 11th ed. Philadelphia: Saunders; 2015.
9. Emiliani E, Breda A. Laser endoureterotomy and endopyelotomy: an update. World J Urol. 2015;33:583–7.
10. Barrett K, Ghiculete D, Sowerby RJ, Farcas M, Pace KT, Honey RJD. Intraoperative radiographic determination of ureteral length as a method of determining ideal stent length. J Endourol. 2017;31(S1):S101–S5.

11. Kamo M, Nozaki T, Horiuchi S, Muraishi N, Yamamura J, Akita K. There are no three physiological narrowings in the upper urinary tract: a new concept of the retroperitoneal anatomy around the ureter. Jpn J Radiol. 2021;39(5):407–13.
12. de La Rosette J, Denstedt J, Geavlete P, Keeley F, Matsuda T, Perale M, Preminger G, Traxer O. The clinical research office of the Endourological Society Ureteroscopy Global Study: indications, complications, and outcomes in 11,885 patients. J Endourol. 2014;28(2):131–9.
13. Le CQ, Segura JW. Surgical atlas ureterorenoscopy. BJU Int. 2006;98(1):235–45.
14. Bagley DH, Huffman JL, Lyon E. Flexible ureteropyeloscopy: diagnosis and treatment in the upper urinary tract. J Urol. 1987;138:280–5.
15. Geavlete P, Multescu R, Geavlete B. Pushing the boundaries of ureteroscopy: current status and future perspectives. Nat Rev Urol. 2014;11(7):373–82.
16. Keller EX, De Coninck V, Traxer O. Next-generation fiberoptic and digital ureteroscopes. Urol Clin N Am. 2019;46(2):147–63.
17. Geavlete P, Multescu R, Geavlete B. Retrograde flexible ureteroscopic approach of upper urinary tract pathology: what is the status in 2014? Int J Urol. 2014;21(11):1076–84.
18. Andonian S, Okeke Z, Smith AD. Digital ureteroscopy: the next step. J Endourol. 2008;22:603–6.
19. Rukin N, Somani B, Patterson J, Grey B, Finch W, McClinton S, Parys B, Young G, Syed H, Myatt A, Samsudin A, Inglis J, Smith D. Tips and tricks of ureteroscopy: consensus statement. Part II. Advanced ureteroscopy. Cent Eur J Urol. 2016;69:98–104.
20. Ding J, Huang Y, Gu S, Chen Y, Peng J, Bai Q, et al. Flexible ureteroscopic management of horseshoe kidney renal calculi. Int Braz J Urol. 2015;41(4):683–9.
21. Paffen M, Keizer J, de Winter G, Arends A, Hendrikx A. A comparison of the physical properties of four new generation flexible ureteroscopes: (de)flection, flow properties, torsion stiffness, and optical characteristics. J Endourol. 2008;22:2227–34.
22. Elashry OM, Elbahnasy AM, Rao G, et al. Flexible ureteroscopy: Washington University experience with the 9.3 F and 7.5 F flexible ureteroscopes. J Urol. 1997;157:2074–80.
23. Grasso M, Bagley D. Small diameter, actively deflectable, flexible ureteropyeloscopy. J Urol. 1998;160:1648–53.
24. Elbahnasy A, Shalhav A, Hoenig D, Elashry O, Smith D, McDougall E, Clayman R. Lower caliceal stone clearance after shock wave lithotripsy or ureteroscopy: the impact of lower pole radiographic anatomy. J Urol. 1998;159:676–82.
25. Resorlu B, Oguz U, Resorlu EB, Oztuna D, Unsal A. The impact of pelvicaliceal anatomy on the success of retrograde intrarenal surgery in patients with lower pole renal stones. Urology. 2012;79(1):61–6.
26. Geavlete P, Multescu R, Geavlete B. Influence of pyelocaliceal anatomy on the success of flexible ureteroscopic approach. J Endourol. 2008;22(10):2235–9.
27. Inoue T, Murota T, Okada S, Hamamoto S, Muguruma K, Kinoshita H, et al. Influence of pelvicaliceal anatomy on stone clearance after flexible ureteroscopy and holmium laser lithotripsy for large renal stones. J Endourol. 2015;29(9):998–1005.
28. Dresner SI, Iremashvili V, Best S, Hedican S, Nakada S. Influence of lower pole infundibulopelvic angle on success of retrograde flexible ureteroscopy and laser lithotripsy for the treatment of renal stones. J Endourol. 2020;34(6):655–60.
29. Elbahnasy A, Clayman R, Shalhav A, Hoenig D, Chandhoke P, Lingeman J, Denstedt J, Kahn R, Assimos D, Nakada S. Lower-pole caliceal stone clearance after shockwave lithotripsy, percutaneous nephrolithotomy, and flexible ureteroscopy: impact of radiographic spatial anatomy. J Endourol. 1998;12:113–9.
30. Danilovic A, Rocha BA, Torricelli FCM, Marchini GS, Batagello C, Vicentini FC, et al. Size is not everything that matters: preoperative CT predictors of stone free after RIRS. Urology. 2019;132:63–8.
31. Bercowsky E, Shalhav AL, Elbahnasy AM, Owens E, Clayman RV. The effect of patient position on intrarenal anatomy. J Endourol. 1999;13(4):257–60.
32. Ozimek T, Cordes J, Wiessmeyer JR, Schneider MH, Hupe MC, Gilbert N, et al. Steep infundibulopelvic angle as a new risk factor for flexible ureteroscope damage and complicated postoperative course. J Endourol. 2018;32(7):597–602.
33. Pearle MS, Lingeman JE, Leveillee R, Kuo R, Preminger GM, Nadler RB, et al. Prospective randomized trial comparing shock wave lithotripsy and ureteroscopy for lower pole caliceal calculi 1 cm or less. J Urol. 2008;179(5 Suppl):S69–73.
34. Prather G. Calyceal diverticulum. J Urol. 1941;45:55.
35. Monga M, Smith R, Ferral H, Thomas R. Percutaneous ablation of caliceal diverticulum: long-term followup. J Urol. 2000;163:28–32.
36. Wulfsohn M. Pyelocaliceal diverticula. J Urol. 1980;123:1.
37. Chong T, Bui M, Fuchs G. Calyceal diverticula ureteroscopic management. Urol Clin N Am. 2000;27(4):647–54.
38. Gross AH, Herrmann T. Management of stones in calyceal diverticulum. Curr Opin Urol. 2007;17:136–40.
39. Waingankar N, Hayek S, Smith A, Okeke Z. Cayceal diverticula: a comprehensive review. Rev Urol. 2014;16:29–43.
40. Timmons J, Malek R, Hattery R, Deweerd J. Caliceal diverticulum. J Urol. 1975;114:6–9.
41. Canales B, Monga M. Surgical management of the calyceal diverticulum. Curr Opin Urol. 2003;13:255–60.
42. Parkhomenko E, Tran T, Thai J, Blum K, Gupta M. Percutaneous management of stone containing calyceal diverticula: associated factors and outcomes. J Urol. 2017;198(4):864–8.

43. Tan YK, Cha DY, Gupta M. Management of stones in abnormal situations. Urol Clin N Am. 2013;40(1):79–97.
44. Fuchs G, David R. Flexible ureterorenoscopy, dilation of the narrow calyceal neck and extracorporeal shock wave lithotripsy: a new, minimally invasive approach to stones in calcyeal diverticula. J Endourol. 1989;3:255–63.
45. Duvdevani M, Sfoungaristos S, Bensalah K, Peyronnet B, Krambeck A, Khadji S, et al. Stones in special situations. World J Urol. 2017;35(9):1381–93.
46. Grasso M, Lang G, Loisides P, Bagley D, Taylor F. Endoscopic management of the symptomatic caliceal diverticular calculus. J Urol. 1995;153:1878–81.
47. Batter S, Dretler S. Ureterorenoscopic approach to the symptomatic caliceal diverticulum. J Urol. 1997;158:709–13.
48. Auge BK, Munver R, Kourambas J, Newman GE, Preminger GM. Endoscopic management of symptomatic caliceal diverticula: a retrospective comparison of percutaneous nephrolithotripsy and ureteroscopy. J Endourol. 2002;16(8):557–63.
49. Ito H, Aboumarzouk OM, Abushamma F, Keeley FX Jr. Systematic review of caliceal diverticulum. J Endourol. 2018;32(10):961–72.
50. Dretler S. A new useful endourologic classification of calyceal diverticula. J Endourol. 1992;6:81.
51. Yang H, Yao X, Tang C, Shan Y, Weng G. Flexible ureterorenoscopy management of calcyeal diverticular calculi. Urol J. 2019;16:12–5.
52. Kieran K, Nelson C, Wolf S. Ureteroscopy for symptomatic hydrocalices: a case series. J Endourol. 2006;20:413–7.
53. Chertack N, Jain R, Monga M, Noble M, Sivalingam S. Two are no different than one: ureteral duplication appears to have no effect on ureteroscopy outcomes. J Endourol. 2018;32(8):692–7.
54. Ugurlu IM, Akman T, Binbay M, Tekinarslan E, Yazici O, Akbulut MF, et al. Outcomes of retrograde flexible ureteroscopy and laser lithotripsy for stone disease in patients with anomalous kidneys. Urolithiasis. 2015;43(1):77–82.
55. Nyanhongo DK, Antil S, Nasir S. Pitfalls of the duplex system: the mystery of the missing stone. BMJ Case Rep. 2017;2017:220198.
56. Rana A, Bhojwani AP. Percutaneous nephrolithotomy in renal anomalies of fusion, ectopia, rotation, hypoplasia, and pelvicalyceal aberration: uniformity inhetergeneity. J Endourol. 2009;23:609–14.
57. Houat AP, Guimaraes CTS, Takahashi MS, Rodi GP, Gasparetto TPD, Blasbalg R, et al. Congenital anomalies of the upper urinary tract: a comprehensive review. Radiographics. 2021;41(2):462–86.
58. Jamshidian H, Tavakoli K, Salahshour F, Nabighadim A, Amini E. Supernumerary kidney associated with horseshoe malformation: a case report and review of literature. Urol Case Rep. 2017;11:57–9.
59. Oto A, Kerimoğlu U, Eskicorapci S, et al. Bilateral supernumerary kidney: imaging findings. JBR-BTR. 2002;85:300–3.
60. N'Guessan G, Stephens F. Supernumerary kidney. J Urol. 1983;130:649–53.
61. Al-Otaibi K, Hosking DH. Percutaneous stone removal in horseshoe kidneys. J Urol. 1999;162(3 Pt 1):674–7.
62. Stein R, Desai M. Management of urolithiasis in the congenitally abnormal kidney (horseshoe and ectopic). Curr Opin Urol. 2007;17:125–31.
63. Lampel A, Hohenfellner M, Schultz-Lampel D, Lazica M, Bohnen K, Thuroff J. Urolithiasis in horseshoe kidneys: therapeutic management. Urology. 1996;47:182–6.
64. Gupta M, Lee MW. Treatment of stones associated with complex or anomalous renal anatomy. Urol Clin N Am. 2007;34(3):431–41.
65. Ganpule AP, Desai MR. Urolithiasis in kidneys with abnormal lie, rotation or form. Curr Opin Urol. 2011;21(2):145–53.
66. Gokce MI, Tokatli Z, Suer E, Hajiyev P, Akinci A, Esen B. Comparison of shock wave lithotripsy (SWL) and retrograde intrarenal surgery (RIRS) for treatment of stone disease in horseshoe kidney patients. Int Braz J Urol. 2016;42(1):96–100.
67. Jessen JP, Honeck P, Knoll T, Wendt-Nordahl G. Flexible ureterorenoscopy for lower pole stones: influence of the collecting system's anatomy. J Endourol. 2014;28(2):146–51.
68. Blackburne AT, Rivera ME, Gettman MT, Patterson DE, Krambeck AE. Endoscopic management of urolithiasis in the horseshoe kidney. Urology. 2016;90:45–9.
69. Molimard B, Al-Qahtani S, Lakmichi A, Sejiny M, Gil-Diez de Medina S, Carpentier X, et al. Flexible ureterorenoscopy with holmium laser in horseshoe kidneys. Urology. 2010;76(6):1334–7.
70. Astolfi RH, Freschi G, Berti FF, Gattas N, Molina WRJ, Meller A. Flexible ureterorenoscopy in position or fusion anomaly: is it feasible? Rev Assoc Med Bras. 2017;63(8):685–8.
71. Lavan L, Herrmann T, Netsch C, Becker B, Somani BK. Outcomes of ureteroscopy for stone disease in anomalous kidneys: a systematic review. World J Urol. 2020;38(5):1135–46.
72. Jabbour M, Goldfischer E, Stravodimos K, Klima W, Smith A. Endopyelotomy for horseshoe and ectopic kidneys. J Urol. 1998;160:694–7.
73. Singh AG, Jairath A, Balaji SS, Tak G, Ganpule AP, Vijayakumar M, et al. Changing trends in the endourological management of urolithiasis in anomalous kidneys. BJU Int. 2019;123(2):318–27.
74. Bozkurt OF, Tepeler A, Sninsky B, Ozyuvali E, Ziypak T, Atis G, et al. Flexible ureterorenoscopy for the treatment of kidney stone within pelvic ectopic kidney. Urology. 2014;84(6):1285–9.
75. Toussi A, Boswell T, Potretzke A. Ureteroscopic stone extraction in cross-fused renal ectopia. J Endourol Case Rep. 2018;4(1):195–7.
76. Ergin G, Kirac M, Unsal A, Kopru B, Yordam M, Biri H. Surgical management of urinary stones with abnormal kidney anatomy. Kaohsiung J Med Sci. 2017;33:207–11.

77. Oguz U, Balci M, Atis G, Bozkurt OF, Tuncel A, Halis F, et al. Retrograde intrarenal surgery in patients with isolated anomaly of kidney rotation. Urolithiasis. 2014;42(2):141–7.
78. Bas O, Tuygun C, Dede O, Sari S, Cakici MC, Ozturk U, et al. Factors affecting complication rates of retrograde flexible ureterorenoscopy: analysis of 1571 procedures—a single-center experience. World J Urol. 2017;35(5):819–26.
79. Giusti G, Proietti S, Peschechera R, Taverna G, Sortino G, Cindolo L, et al. Sky is no limit for ureteroscopy: extending the indications and special circumstances. World J Urol. 2015;33(2):257–73.
80. Legemate JD, Baseskioglu B, Dobruch J, Gutierrez-Aceves J, Negrete O, Rioja Sanz C, et al. Ureteroscopic urinary stone treatment among patients with renal anomalies: patient characteristics and treatment outcomes. Urology. 2017;110:56–62.
81. Krambeck AE, Gettman MT, BaniHani AH, Husmann DA, Kramer SA, Segura JW. Management of nephrolithiasis after Cohen cross-trigonal and Glenn–Anderson advancement ureteroneocystostomy. J Urol. 2007;177(1):174–8.
82. Wallis MC, Brown DH, Jayanthi VR, Koff SA. A novel technique for ureteral catheterization and/or retrograde ureteroscopy after cross-trigonal ureteral reimplantation. J Urol. 2003;170(4 Pt 2):1664–6. discussion 6
83. Hertzig LL, Iwaszko MR, Rangel LJ, Patterson DE, Gettman MT, Krambeck AE. Urolithiasis after ileal conduit urinary diversion: a comparison of minimally invasive therapies. J Urol. 2013;189(6):2152–7.
84. Iwaszko MR, Krambeck AE, Chow GK, Gettman MT. Transureteroureterostomy revisited: long-term surgical outcomes. J Urol. 2010;183(3):1055–9.

Armamentarium and Endoscopes

Sven Lahme

Abstract

Flexible ureterorenoscopy is a highly technical procedure in urology that requires a wide range of different technical items and disposables. Only the optimally combined devices enable a good treatment result. With the introduction of chip-on-the-tip endoscopes and, more recently, the manufacture of single-use endoscopes, flexible ureterorenoscopy is subject to constant progress. In addition to the endoscopes, the selection of disposables for access to the ureter, for the disintegration and removal of urinary stones, and the question of irrigation are of particular importance. The present chapter summarizes the essential aspects of the armamentarium for flexible ureterorenoscopy.

Keywords

Flexible ureterorenoscopy · Chip-on-the-tip endoscopes · Disposable endoscopes · Ureteral access sheath · Tipless baskets · Irrigation

S. Lahme (✉)
Goldstadt Private Clinic, Special Clinic for Minimally Invasive Urological Surgery and Da Vinci Robotics, Pforzheim, Germany
e-mail: lahme@goldstadt-privatklinik.com

1 Introduction

Meanwhile flexible ureterorenoscopy is a standard treatment in upper urinary tract calculi [1]. Flexible ureterorenoscopy for the therapy of stones of the upper urinary tract is a treatment modality that requires a lot of special technical equipment. It is not only about the endoscopes used but also about access to the ureter through an ureteral access sheath, the disintegration of the stones, and the disposables used for removing stone fragments. Hardly any other topic in urology is so affected by changes and advances in technology as endourology. Practically, every year, new instruments and single-use items are presented which further perfect the technique of flexible ureterorenoscopy. For some years now, the trend toward single-use endoscopes has continued, and nowadays, it is practically impossible to imagine everyday clinical practice without them. The quality of the video image and the usability of these new instruments are in no way inferior to the reusable instruments. Knowledge of the armamentarium and the endoscopes is an important prerequisite for the successful performance of flexible ureterorenoscopy. It is really very important to precisely choose the best equipment for flexible ureterorenoscopy in order to achieve the best treatment results.

G. Zeng et al. (eds.), *Flexible Ureteroscopy*, https://doi.org/10.1007/978-981-19-2936-6_3

2 Access to the Ureter

Before getting access to the upper urinary tract in flexible ureterorenoscopy, it is recommended to perform a retrograde pyelography. Conventional ureteral catheters are suitable devices to perform a retrograde pyelography. Then either access to the ureter by advancing the flexible endoscope over a guidewire or the use of an ureteral access sheath is possible.

The use of the ureteral access sheath ensures a low-pressure situation in the upper urinary tract, because there is sufficient space between the endoscope and the inner wall of the ureteral access sheath for the backflow of the irrigation. The use of ureteral access sheaths reduces the risk of febrile pyelonephritis. In addition, the use of ureteral access sheaths leads to an increase in the stone-free rate. For this reason, the use of a ureteral access sheath can be generally recommended for the treatment of urinary stones of the upper urinary tract [2].

Only in case of a diagnostic flexible ureterorenoscopy, it is advisable not to use a ureteral access sheath. Here the flexible ureterorenoscope is advanced into the ureter via a guidewire. When doing this, it must be taken into consideration that the irrigation flow into the renal calyceal system via the endoscope can lead to an increase of the pressure in the renal calyceal system. It is therefore important to ensure that the drainage of the renal calyceal system is sufficient and that the irrigation flow is reduced to a minimum.

3 General Information on Ureteral Access Sheaths

A plastic tube that is placed over a guidewire under radiological control to the upper urinary tract is called a ureteral access sheath. The ureteral access sheath consists of two parts: an outer tube and a solid inner part, which is a little longer and shows a conically shaped tip (Fig. 1a–c).

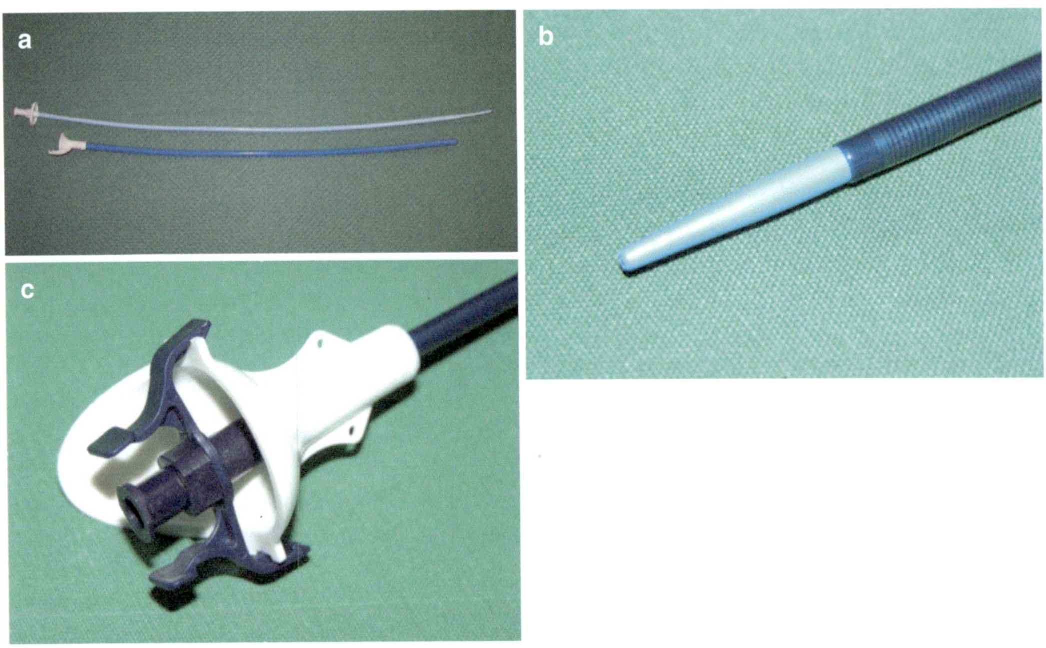

Fig. 1 Ureteral access sheath (12/14 F, Cook Medical, Bloomington, Indiana, USA). (**a**) Inner and outer part of the ureteral access sheath. (**b**) Inner part of the ureteral access sheath shows a conically shaped tip, in order to facilitate the dilation of the orifice. (**c**) Fixation of the inner to the outer part of the ureteral access sheath

3.1 Insertion of the Ureteral Access Sheath

The surface of the ureteral access sheath is nowadays usually hydrophilic. This means that the surface of the outer and inner part of the ureteral access sheath must be made wet with sterile water before insertion. The ureteral access sheath is then inserted over a guidewire. It has been proven useful to use a more rigid guidewire that makes it easier to advance the ureteral access sheath. The ureteral access sheath is usually advanced below the ureteropelvic junction (Fig. 2a, b). If there is a wide ureter, e.g., after a preoperative DJ insertion, the ureteral access sheath can be advanced into the renal pelvis. In this case, the removal of the disintegrated stones is easier. However, the ureteropelvic junction is a fragile part of the ureter, so that any forced insertion of a ureteral access sheath should be avoided here.

3.2 Different Diameters of the Ureteral Access Sheaths

Ureteral access sheaths are available in various diameters. The specification is made as a combination of the inside and outside diameters. Common diameters are: 10/12 F, 12/14 F, and 14/16 F.

The small-caliber ureteral access sheaths are usually easy to insert. However, the small sizes of the ureteral access sheath are not suitable for all flexible endoscopes. As an example, it should be mentioned here that the flexible ureterorenoscope "Boa Vision" from the Richard Wolf company fits through a 10/12 F ureteral access sheath, but the flexible ureterorenoscope "Cobra Vision" from the same manufacturer does not fit [3].

Larger ureteral access sheaths have the advantage that all types of flexible ureterorenoscopes can be used. In addition, larger ureteral access sheaths allow removal of larger stone fragments.

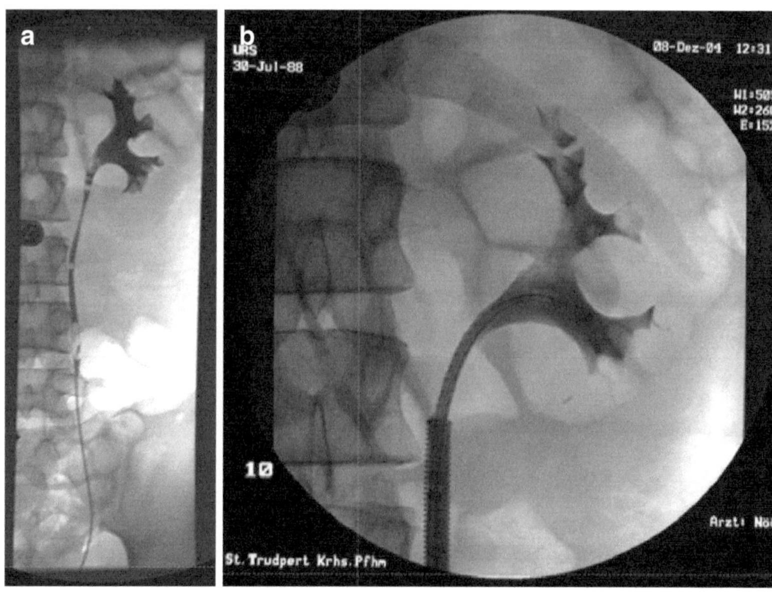

Fig. 2 Placement of ureteral access sheath. (**a**) Retrograde pyelography. (**b**) Position of the ureteral access sheath after insertion

This can reduce the operating time. The disadvantage of the larger ureteral access sheaths is the greater risk of causing a lesion of the ureter when the shaft is inserted. It is therefore advisable to use the largest ureteral entry shafts with a diameter of 14/16 F only in the case of wide ureters, preferably only after the ureter has been presented by a DJ catheter.

3.3 Types of Ureteral Access Sheaths

Ureteral access sheaths are offered as simple ureteral access sheaths or as ureteral access sheaths with a second lumen for inserting an additional guidewire. There are also ureteral access sheaths which, after the shaft has been inserted, allow a guidewire to be placed outside the ureteral access sheaths. In principle, it is a good idea to have a dedicated channel for the guidewire. However, it must not be forgotten that each additional channel of a ureteral access sheath reduces the usable cross section of the shaft, which has a significant effect on the usable internal cross section and the removal of urinary stones. The placement of the guidewire outside the ureteral access sheath also has disadvantages, since the guidewire placed in this way has an unfavorable influence on the visibility due to hematuria. For this reason, many surgeons prefer not to use the guidewire while using the flexible ureterorenoscope and only reinsert it over the ureteral access sheath when the procedure is to be completed and a ureteral stent has to be inserted [4].

4 General Information on Flexible Ureterorenoscopes

Flexible ureterorenoscopes that allow flexion of 270° in both directions have existed for about 20 years. Only the development of these endoscopes made it possible to reach every part of the renal calyceal system (Fig. 3a, b).

The first generation of these flexible ureterorenoscopes were fiber-optic instruments that transfer the optical image to the eyepiece via glass fibers. The instrument could then be inserted

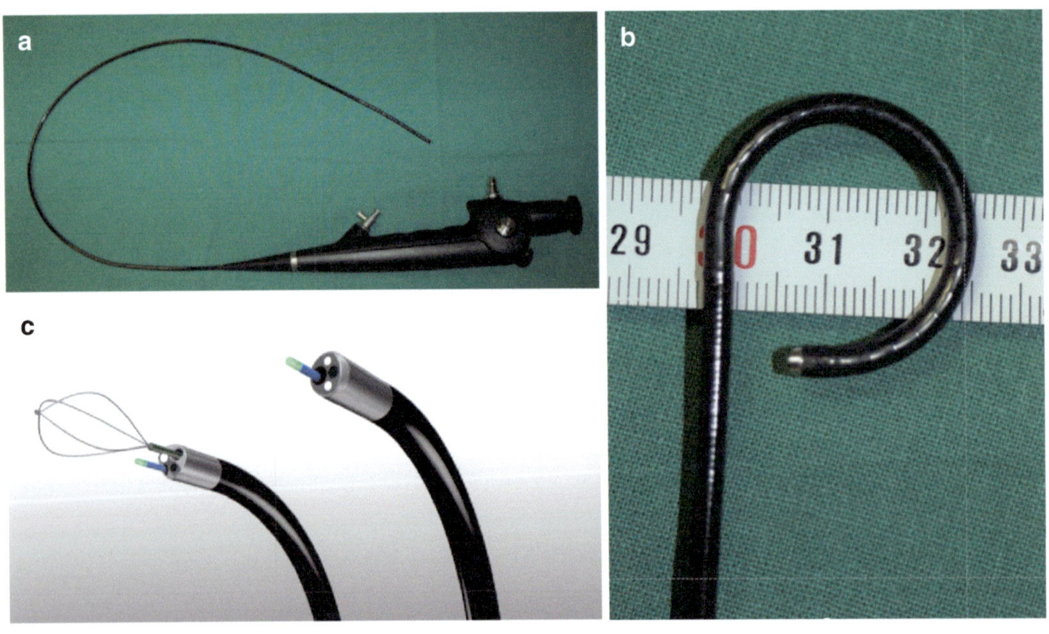

Fig. 3 Flexible ureterorenoscopes with 270° deflexion (Richard Wolf, Knittlingen, Germany). (**a**) Flexible fiber-optic scope (Viper). (**b**) 270° deflexion (Viper). (**c**) Comparison of dual channel digital scopes: (left: Cobra-Vision) and single channel (right: Boa-Vision)

either with a direct view into the endoscope or by attaching an external video camera.

Flexible ureterorenoscopes with a built-in video camera at the tip of the endoscope have been manufactured for about 10 years. This is called the "chip-on-the-tip" technology. This design has the advantage that a defect in the flexible ureterorenoscope due to fiber breakage is avoided. In addition, with the "chip-on-the-tip" endoscopes, the rasterization of the image, which resulted from the use of fiber-optic bundles with fiber-optic ureterorenoscopes, is eliminated. Overall, the "chip-on-the-tip" endoscopes offer a more brilliant and sharper image. A concern about "chip-on-the-tip" endoscopes is that due to the video chip construction, in the event of hematuria and the strong red color of the urine, a poor endoscopic imaging can result.

Another important technical innovation is the development of single-use endoscopes. The image quality is comparable to reusable scopes, and the single-use ureterorenoscopes do not require any repairs or the entire reprocessing process.

4.1 Reusable Flexible Ureterorenoscope

Reusable flexible ureterorenoscopes are available from all renowned endoscope manufacturers. The individual models differ in some technical details. What they have in common is that the flexion angle is approximately 270° in both directions and that all endoscopes have a working channel with a diameter of 3.6 F. The design and construction of the conventional reusable flexible ureterorenoscopes is practically the same for all manufacturers. In all flexible ureterorenoscopes, the flexion of the tip of the ureterorenoscope is done with the thumb.

Reusable ureteroscopes require careful handling during the procedure, but also during the reprocessing process. Especially in the flexible tip of the ureterorenoscope, there is a great risk that the use of a laser fiber will damage the working channel. This damage leads to the penetration of water into the instrument and its destruction. Repairs of this damage usually mean replacing the flexible ureteroscope. This means that the cost of the repair replacement is approximately €10,000. According to the literature, around 30% of damage to flexible ureterorenoscopes occurs during reprocessing. For economic reasons, semiskilled workers, who often do not sufficiently take into account the fragility of flexible endoscopes, are doing the reprocessing in particular. The damage to the flexible ureterorenoscopes and the often necessary replacement of the scopes lead to costs around €500 per use of the flexible ureterorenoscope.

The reprocessing of the flexible ureteroscope is a challenge because of the long and very small-caliber working channel and the materials used in instrument construction. Apart from the microbiological situation, sterilization processes are also used that are not available in every hospital, e.g., plasma sterilization. The cost of reprocessing per flexible ureterorenoscope is currently around €180.

Richard Wolf, Knittlingen, Germany, offers a flexible ureterorenoscope that has two working channels. In addition to the usual working channel, a second working channel allows the simultaneous insertion of a laser fiber. The laser fiber can be locked in the working channel and, if necessary, extended out of the working channel with the so-called laser shifter and then draw back again. In this way, a basket can be used to remove stones at the same time as the laser is inserted (Fig. 3c).

Olympus offers flexible ureteroscopes with a handle that can be rotated 120°. In addition, these endoscopes have a special shape of the tip that allows the ureteral orifice easily to be passed.

The Karl Storz company was the first manufacturer of ureterorenoscopes (Flex-X) that can be deflexed 270°. The endoscopes are characterized by a more filigree construction, which allows the use of small ureteral access sheaths.

All manufacturers mentioned above continue to offer their endoscopes either with fiber optic or "chip-on-the-tip" design.

4.2 Disposable Ureteroscopes

Flexible ureterorenoscopes that are intended for single use have been available since 2015 (Lithovue, Boston Scientific, USA). Since then, a large number of other manufacturers of single-use endoscopes have established themselves on the market (e.g., Pusen). The well-known endoscope manufacturers of reusable ureterorenoscopes also have a single-use ureterorenoscope in their portfolio or are actively working on this topic (Fig. 4a, b).

Disposable endoscopes are supplied sterile and ready for use by the manufacturer. The setup time for endoscopic surgery is significantly reduced. Another advantage of the single-use endoscope is the lack of repairs. On the basis of previous scientific studies, the image quality of the single-use endoscopes is comparable with the image quality of the reusable endoscopes. The environmental balance is also no less favorable with the single-use ureteroscopes than with the reusable endoscopes [5].

The question of whether and, if so, in which situation a single-use ureteroscopic scopes should be used depends on several influencing factors [6–8]. Due to the respective instrument specifications, single-use and reusable ureteroscopes could be used for the same indications. With respect to the cost-effectiveness of the intervention, however, there are further aspects that cannot be answered simply and globally in view of the different cost reimbursement systems around the world [9]. So far, it has been recommended to carry out an individual local assessment of the cost-effectiveness based on the national reimbursement situation and the number of possible repairs of reusable ureterorenoscopes. It is recommended to use single-use ureterorenoscopes only for certain indications with a high risk of damage to the instrument.

The manufacturing of single-use endoscopes in particular is subject to constant change: smaller instrument cross sections, higher video resolution, and lower costs due to increased quantities. For this reason, the significance of the single-use endoscopes can only be assessed provisionally at this point and requires regular reassessment.

5 General Information on Disposables for the Removal of Urinary Stones

In flexible ureterorenoscopy, various aids are used for active stone removal: tipless baskets, forceps, grasper. All disposables must be sufficiently flexible so that the flexion of the ureterorenoscope is not unnecessarily impaired. For this reason, the diameter of the disposables should be small and the material made of nitinol.

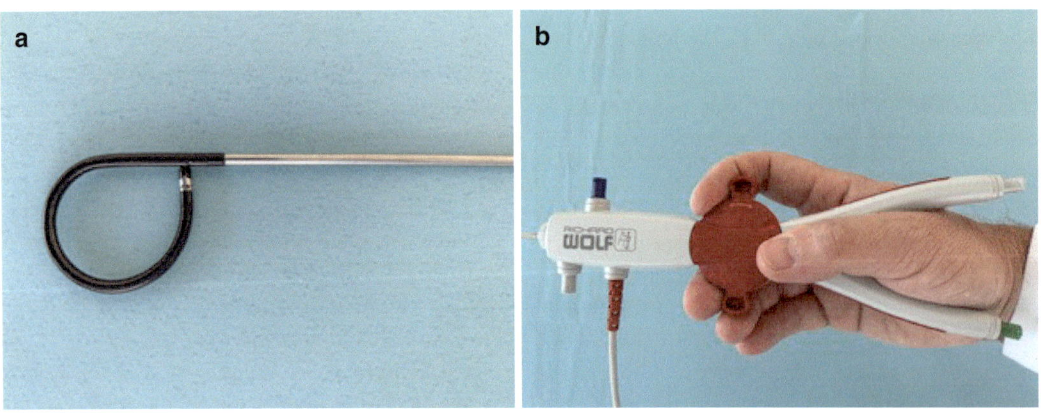

Fig. 4 Modern disposable ureterorenoscopes (Richard Wolf, Knittlingen, Germany). (**a**) Rigid shaft with 270° flexible tip. (**b**) Modified handgrip with operation by two fingers

5.1 Tipless Baskets

Removal of kidney stones requires different characteristics of a basket in comparison to the use in the ureter. Since the upper urinary tract stones are usually located at the wall of the calyx or pelvis, flexible ureteroscopy requires baskets that do not have any tip (Fig. 5a). These baskets, known as tipless baskets, are made with three or more wires. The diameters of the baskets start at 1.2 F. Smaller diameters of the basket provide a better irrigation flow and a better view.

In recent years, manufacturers have also been offering modified tipless baskets that have a different mechanism (e.g., N-Gage, Cook Medical) (Fig. 5b). To what extent a better removal of the urinary stone fragments is possible is not yet clear and usually depends on the personal preference of the surgeon.

Occasionally it happens that a stone trapped in the basket cannot be removed from the basket in the renal calyceal system of the kidney. In such cases, the use of detachable baskets is recommended. After removing the flexible endoscope, the previously disconnected basket can be reconnected to the handpiece and be used again (Fig. 5c).

5.2 Graspers

Graspers also have indications in flexible ureteroscopy in certain situations. Since a grasper always pulls something out, it is not the tool of choice for removing urinary stones. However, a grasper can be used very well for removing broken laser fibers. In this respect, a grasper should not be missing in an endourologist's armamentarium.

5.3 Forceps

Conventional, reusable forceps have no place in modern flexible ureterorenoscopes. Reusable for-

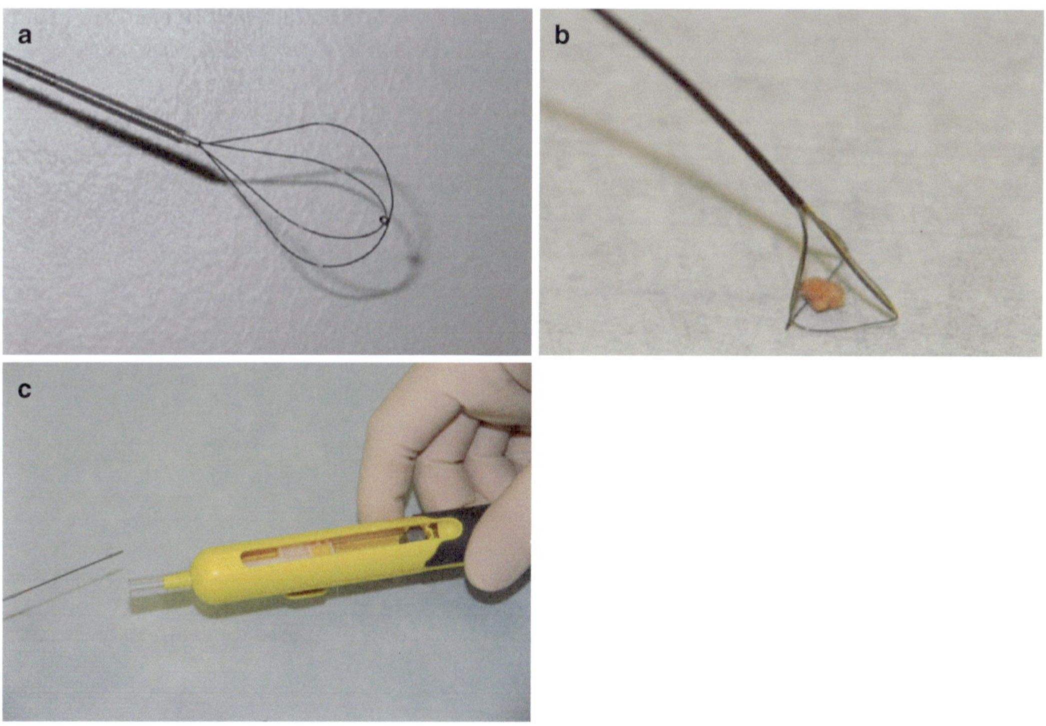

Fig. 5 Different types of tipless baskets. (**a**) Conventional tipless basket (Cook Medical, Bloomington, Indiana, USA). (**b**) Modified type of tipless basket (Cook Medical, Bloomington, Indiana, USA). (**c**) Disconnectable tipless basket (Mediglobe, Achenmühle, Germany)

ceps have a too large cross section and reduce the irrigation flow so much that there is an insufficient visibility in the renal calyceal system.

5.4 Biopsy Forceps

In the case of an oncological diagnosis, it may be necessary to take a sample biopsy from the renal calyceal system. Specially developed biopsy forceps have proven successful for this purpose. It is important that a sufficiently large and representative biopsy can be taken with the biopsy forceps. A sufficient size of the biopsy mouth is required for this. The size of the biopsy mouth is then larger than the cross section of the working channel. This means that appropriate biopsy forceps have to be inserted from the tip of the instrument through the working channel and then pushed in front of the ureterorenoscope during the endoscopy (Bigopsie®, Cook Medical). This requires the surgeon to have appropriate experience in order not to injure the ureter [10].

5.5 Guidewires

Various guidewires are available for performing flexible ureterorenoscopy. The guidewire in flexible ureterorenoscopy is used either to insert the ureteral access sheath or to insert the flexible ureterorenoscope directly.

The guidewires are basically differentiated according to their material and surface characteristics as well as their stiffness. While conventional PTFE-coated guidewires have the advantage of being sufficiently rigid when inserting ureteral access sheaths, hydrophilic guidewires have the advantage of being able to pass any kinking in the case of an unfavorable morphology of the ureter (Fig. 6a, b). In everyday flexible ureterorenoscopy, the combination of both the guidewires has often proven successful.

If possible, a rigid guidewire should be used when inserting a ureteral access sheath. A more rigid guidewire reduces the risk of injuring the ureter, and the ureteral access sheath can be more easily advanced in the ureter.

Hydrophilic guidewires are suitable for establishing access to the upper urinary tract in the case of unfavorable ureteral conditions. After temporarily using a ureteral catheter, the hydrophilic guidewire can then be exchanged for a rigid PTFE-coated guidewire.

Recent developments combine a rigid mid part of the guidewire with a hydrophilic, very flexible, tip (Fig. 6c).

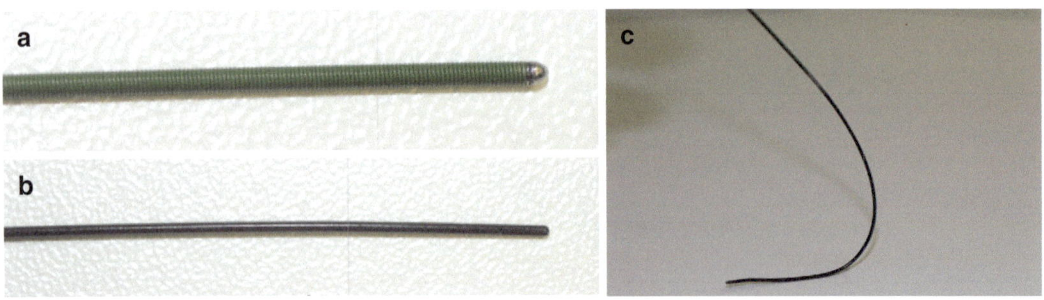

Fig. 6 Different types of guidewires. (**a**) PTFE-coated guidewire. (**b**) Hydrophillic guidewire. (**c**) PTFE-coated guidewire with hydrophilic tip

5.6 Irrigation

Irrigation is always required to perform flexible ureterorenoscopy. It can be generated either by gravity or by a so-called active irrigation with a pump. It is crucial that the flush should be as strong as necessary but as little as possible. In this context, the hydrostatic pressure that arises in the renal calyceal system as a result of the irrigation used plays an important role. If the hydrostatic pressure in the renal calyceal system increases in an uncontrolled manner, there is an increased risk of a febrile urinary tract infection and rupture of the renal calyceal system. Cases of urosepsis have also been reported. For this reason, in addition to irrigation, the drainage of the irrigation fluid is an essential factor that influences the hydrostatic pressure in the renal calyceal system. In this context, the use of ureteral access sheaths plays an important role. Because there is a sufficient space in the ureteral access sheath for the drainage of irrigation fluid, the use of an ureteral access sheath for flexible ureterorenoscopy is preferred, particularly with respect to the reduction of the hydrostatic pressure in the renal calyceal system [11]. If the flexible ureterorenoscope is used without an ureteral access sheath, the visibility is less favorable and the hydrostatic pressure in the calyceal system of the kidney is higher. For this reason, the renouncement of the use of a ureter access sheath should only be reserved for situations in which only a diagnosis of the renal calyceal system is carried out in the case of flexible ureterorenoscopy.

In order to improve the endoscopic visibilty in the renal calyceal system, there are special devices available to flush.

For example, a hand pump (Coloplast, France) which leads to flushing in the renal calyceal system can thus improve visibility (Fig. 7a). However, with this device, there is a great risk that an excessive increase in pressure can lead to a rupture of the renal calyceal system and, in individual cases, not only a febrile urinary tract infection, but also urosepsis.

Another possibility to enhance the irrigation is the use of a suitable foot pump (Peditrol®, Wismed, South Africa). A 2-ml syringe is used here via a foot pump to improve the flushing. This device has the advantage that the foot, which is rarely used in endourology, can also be used during the operation. In addition, the volume of the syringe used is so small that damage to the renal pelvis calyx system is less likely (Fig. 7b).

The easiest way to improve the irrigation is to use a 20-ml syringe, which is filled with saline and attached to the handpiece of the endoscope via a T-adapter.

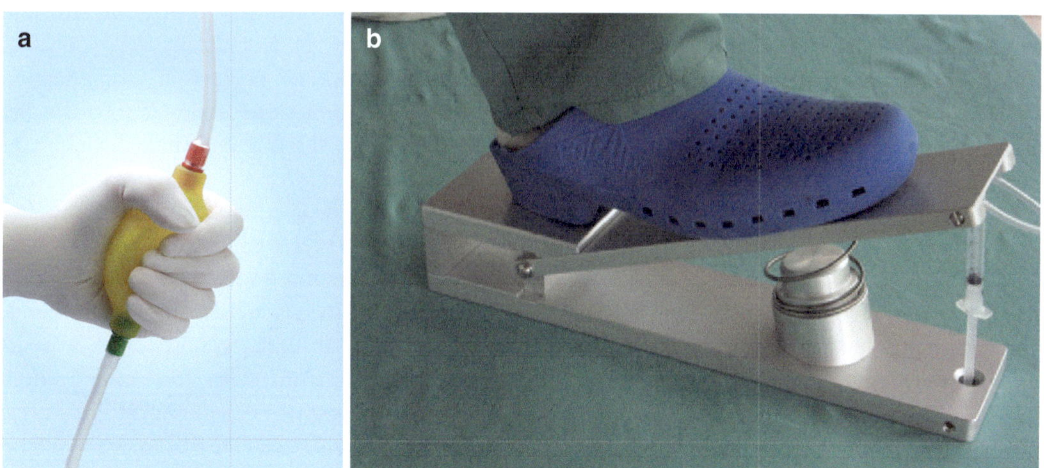

Fig. 7 Disposables for flushing during ureterorenoscopy. (**a**) Hand pump (Coloplast, France). (**b**) Peditrol® (Wismed, South Africa)

5.7 Suction

In principle, the use of suction in retrograde flexible ureterorenoscopy is also possible. For this you need either an endoscope with two working channels or a combination of flexible ureterorenoscope and ureteral access sheath. The problem is that the strength of the suction must be related to the inflow of the irrigation in order to ensure good visibility in the renal calyceal system. For this reason, the active suction in retrograde flexible ureterorenoscopy has not yet proven its worth.

6 General Information on Lithotripsy in Flexible Ureterorenoscopy

When choosing lithotripsy in flexible ureterorenoscopy, only lithotripsy procedures that do not or only slightly impair the flexion of the endoscope are used. This is the reason why only laser lithotripsy is used in flexible ureterorenoscopy. Ballistic lithotripsy and ultrasound disintegration play no role in flexible ureterorenoscopy.

6.1 Holmium Laser

The lithotripsy of choice in flexible ureterorenoscopy is the holmium laser. For this purpose, small-caliber probes are available that do not impair the flexion of the endoscope or only slightly impair them. The use of laser fibers with a diameter of 250 μm or 375 μm is common.

By modifying the frequency and energy of the transmitted laser pulses, the type of disintegration in flexible ureterorenoscopy can be varied. Low frequency and high energy lead to fragmentation of the calculi. High frequency and low energy lead to the disintegration of the urinary stones into the smallest, often dust-like particles. This is called dusting. If a high frequency is combined with a high energy, the so-called popcorn effect occurs. The tip of the laser fiber is held fixed in the lumen of the renal calyceal system and the stone fragments automatically move toward the tip of the laser fiber due to the impact of the laser pulses. This leads to constant movement and disintegration of the urinary stones.

6.2 Thulium Fiber Laser

The thulium fiber laser has recently been introduced. This technology allows a significant increase of the frequency of the laser and thus leads to faster disintegration of the urinary stones. In addition, the risk of propulsion of the stone fragments is lower. To what extent the thulium fiber laser will replace the holmium laser in the disintegration of upper urinary tract stones remains to be seen [12, 13].

7 Summary

In summary, the retrograde flexible ureterorenoscopy is a high-tech procedure in which the selection of the instruments and the additional devices used is very important.

To successfully carry out a retrograde flexible ureterorenoscopy, it is necessary to optimally combine the endoscope used with the additionally required disposable items. If the armamentarium is well selected, retrograde flexible ureterorenoscopy is technically very feasible. With the appropriate equipment, complication rate in flexible ureterorenoscopy is low. But the risk of damaging the fragile technical equipment is rather high. This is one of the reasons why single-use endoscopes are increasingly being used for flexible ureterorenoscopy.

The challenge of retrograde flexible ureterorenoscopy is still its cost effectiveness. In general, retrograde flexible ureterorenoscopy is a treatment modality with poor cost effectiveness because of the expensive equipment. However, the cost effectiveness can only be assessed on the basis of the respective national cost reimbursement system.

References

1. Türk C, Petřík A, Sarica K, Seitz C, Skolarikos A, Straub M, Knoll T. EAU guidelines on diagnosis and conservative management of urolithiasis. Eur Urol. 2016;69(3):468–74. https://doi.org/10.1016/j.eururo.2015.07.040.
2. Osther PJS. Risks of flexible ureterorenoscopy: pathophysiology and prevention. Urolithiasis. 2018;46(1):59–67. https://doi.org/10.1007/s00240-017-1018-6.
3. Al-Qahtani SM, Letendre J, Thomas A, Natalin R, Saussez T, Traxer O. Which ureteral access sheath is compatible with your flexible ureteroscope? J Endourol. 2014;28(3):286–90. https://doi.org/10.1089/end.2013.0375.
4. Traxer O, Wendt-Nordahl G, Sodha H, Rassweiler J, Meretyk S, Tefekli A, Coz F, de la Rosette JJ. Differences in renal stone treatment and outcomes for patients treated either with or without the support of a ureteral access sheath: The Clinical Research Office of the Endourological Society Ureteroscopy Global Study. World J Urol. 2015;33(12):2137–44. https://doi.org/10.1007/s00345-015-1582-8.
5. Davis NF, McGrath S, Quinlan M, Jack G, Lawrentschuk N, Bolton DM. Carbon footprint in flexible ureteroscopy: a comparative study on the environmental impact of reusable and single-use ureteroscopes. J Endourol. 2018;32(3):214–7. https://doi.org/10.1089/end.2018.0001.
6. Bourdoumis A, El Howairis MEF, Stephen B, Buchholz N. Ex vivo comparison of 2 disposable versus a state-of-the-art reusable ureterorenoscope. Urol Int. 2020;104(5–6):437–44. https://doi.org/10.1159/000502759.
7. Shin RH, Lipkin ME, Preminger GM. Disposable devices for RIRS: where do we stand in 2013? What do we need in the future? World J Urol. 2015;33(2):241–6. https://doi.org/10.1007/s00345-014-1368-4.
8. Moore B, Proietti S, Giusti G, Eisner BH. Single-use ureteroscopes. Urol Clin N Am. 2019;46(2):165–74. https://doi.org/10.1016/j.ucl.2018.12.002.
9. Martin CJ, McAdams SB, Abdul-Muhsin H, Lim VM, Nunez-Nateras R, Tyson MD, Humphreys MR. The economic implications of a reusable flexible digital ureteroscope: a cost-benefit analysis. J Urol. 2017;197(3 Pt 1):730–5. https://doi.org/10.1016/j.juro.2016.09.085.
10. Breda A, Territo A, Sanguedolce F, Basile G, Subiela JD, Reyes HV, Ferrer OM, Gaya JM, Palou J. Comparison of biopsy devices in upper tract urothelial carcinoma. World J Urol. 2019;37(9):1899–905. https://doi.org/10.1007/s00345-018-2586-y.
11. Wright A, Williams K, Somani B, Rukin N. Intrarenal pressure and irrigation flow with commonly used ureteric access sheaths and instruments. Cent Eur J Urol. 2015;68(4):434–8. https://doi.org/10.5173/ceju.2015.604.
12. Traxer O, Keller EX. Thulium fiber laser: the new player for kidney stone treatment? A comparison with Holmium:YAG laser. World J Urol. 2020;38(8):1883–94. https://doi.org/10.1007/s00345-019-02654-5.
13. Kronenberg P, Traxer O. The laser of the future: reality and expectations about the new thulium fiber laser—a systematic review. Transl Androl Urol. 2019;8(Suppl 4):S398–417. https://doi.org/10.21037/tau.2019.08.01.

Accessories, Sterilization, and Instrument Care in Flexible Ureteroscopy

Yuyi Yeow, Silvia Proietti, Mario Basulto-Martinez, Maria Pia Pavia, and Guido Giusti

Abstract

Flexible ureteroscopes are versatile instruments that allow a wide range of diagnostic and therapeutic procedures to be performed in the upper urinary tract. The ureteroscope allows visualization of the tract, while accessories and tools allow diagnostic and therapeutic procedures to be performed, such as biopsy or lithotripsy. This chapter will discuss some of these accessories to facilitate ureteroscopic surgery, as well as the procedures involved in reprocessing and sterilization of these instruments.

Keywords

Guidewire · Access sheath · Basket · Forceps · Sterilization · Disinfection · Durability

1 Guidewires

Guidewires remain the backbone of many endourological procedures. In 1978, Hepperlen et al. first described the insertion of a ureteric stent over a Teflon guidewire [1]. Today, guidewires are used in many procedures, and there are different types of guidewires for every situation. The ideal guidewire is one that is flexible enough to negotiate obstructions without perforation, and yet stiff enough to resist kinking from passage of instruments and devices. It should also be hydrophilic for insertion, but not too much so as to prevent displacement during manipulation.

Guidewires range in diameter from 0.018 to 0.038 in., although the most often used are 0.035 and 0.038 in. The tip of the guidewire is usually flexible in the last 3–5 cm to reduce the risk of tissue injury, while the shaft is usually stiffer to facilitate passage of other devices over it. The tip could be straight or angled, with varying degrees of tip angulation.

Most modern guidewires are manufactured with a stainless steel or nitinol core. Nitinol is an acronym that stands for a metal alloy of *NI*ckel and *TI*tanium developed at *N*aval *O*rdinance *L*aboratory back in 1962 [2]. The most important feature of nitinol is its kink-resistance due to a significant shape memory. This makes kinking almost impossible even when high forces are applied. The surface of the guidewire is then coated with lubricious material such as polytetrafluoroethylene (PTFE) to facilitate smooth insertion. Alternatively, hydrophilic polymers may be used to significantly increase its lubricity such as "M" polymer introduced by Terumo more than two decades ago. The guidewire should also be able to transmit torque from the proximal operator end to the distal tip, allowing good control of rotation particularly when using

Y. Yeow · S. Proietti · M. Basulto-Martinez · M. P. Pavia · G. Giusti (✉)
Department of Urology, European Training Center in Endourology, San Raffaele Hospital, IRCCS, Milan, Italy
e-mail: giusti.guido@hsr.it

G. Zeng et al. (eds.), *Flexible Ureteroscopy*, https://doi.org/10.1007/978-981-19-2936-6_4

angled-tip guidewires. Hydrophilic guidewires come with two different stiffness (standard and stiff) according to the percentage of nitinol within the core: regarding different content of nitinol in 0.035 and 0.038 guidewire, stiff type contains 51% and 42% more nitinol, respectively (Fig. 1).

Hybrid guidewires were made to combine the advantages of both a flexible and hydrophilic tip with a stiff shaft. This in theory could reduce the number of guidewires used or the need for guidewire exchange during a urological procedure. Some examples of these hybrid guidewires include the Sensor (Boston Scientific, Natick, MA) and the Solo Plus (Bard Urological, Covington, GA).

For situations when strong kink-resistance is desired, such as stent insertion in a tightly strictured ureter, super stiff stainless steel guidewires such as the Amplatz Superstiff (Boston Scientific) are available. They have been also commonly used in procedures such as PCNL where serial dilatation requires resistance to kinking. These guidewires can also be useful in tortuous or redundant ureters as they can straighten out the kinks to facilitate coaxial placement of stents or catheters. Due to the widespread advent of nitinol especially in Europe, these guidewires are much less utilized in clinical practice than in the past.

Within one subset of guidewires, the characteristics could be different for wires from different manufacturers. An in vitro evaluation of hybrid and hydrophilic guidewires for tip and shaft bending, friction, and tip puncture force showed statistically different results even within each guidewire type [3]. Therefore, it is difficult to recommend any one guidewire over another. Rather, other factors such as individual experience, preference, and availability may guide selection of the appropriate wire instead [4]. This also means that failure of access with one guidewire does not imply failure with another guidewire of the same type but different manufacturer.

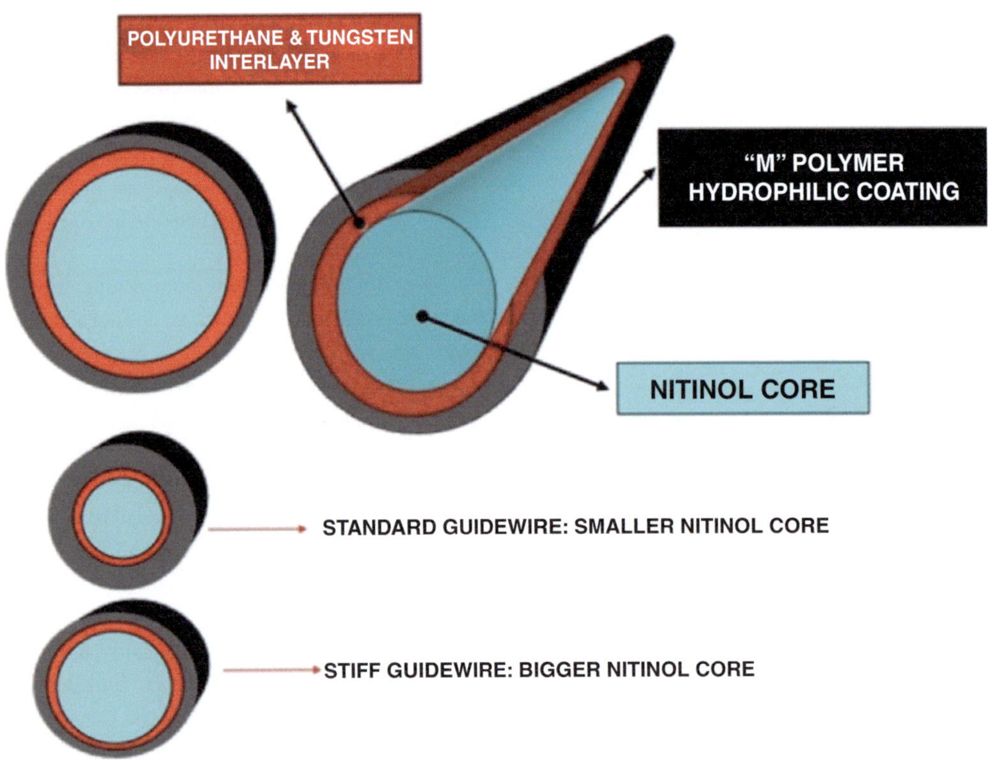

Fig. 1 Anatomy of a hydrophilic guidewire

In personal practice, the authors prefer to use stiff hydrophilic or hybrid guidewires as the first guidewire, particularly if the stone is located within the ureter rather than the renal pelvis. This reduces the risk of ureteral injury and allows for some guidewire manipulation past the stone with less concern for potential ureteral perforation. Where there is an impacted ureteral calculus preventing the passage of standard guidewires, a hydrophilic guidewire may perform better [5]. In the absence of ureteral pathology, a PTFE guidewire with a floppy tip could be used first, simply due to the lower cost compared to hybrid guidewires [6]. Stiff type is strongly recommended because the stability of the standard type may not be enough to allow placement of different endourological devices such as ureteral catheters, stents, and ureteral access sheaths (UAS).

It remains a matter of debate whether a safety guidewire is required during flexible ureteroscopy. A recent survey of endourologists reported a 84.5% use of safety guidewires [7]. However, a previous retrospective study by Dickstein et al. concluded that the majority of cases performed without a UAS on uncomplicated stones in the kidney or ureteropelvic junction did not require a safety guidewire [8].

The authors' personal practice is to use a safety guidewire in all cases of flexible ureteroscopy as we treat the safety wire like a safety belt in a motor vehicle—rarely required, but lifesaving when it works as planned.

2 Ureteral Access Sheath

The ureteral access sheath (UAS) was first introduced back in 1974 by Takayasu to enable the passage of a passive flexible ureteroscope [9]. Over time, numerous improvements were made, resulting in the current form of the UAS as we know it [10].

The UAS generally comes in two parts, consisting of the outer sheath and the inner dilator with an interlocking hub so that both the parts can be passed into the ureter as a single unit. The tip of the dilator is tapered, and the sheath is usually coated with a hydrophilic material that significantly reduces friction, thus facilitating its introduction into the ureter. To accommodate different ureter characteristics and ureteroscope sizes, the UAS comes in a variety of diameters and lengths.

Some manufacturers have developed proprietary features in their UAS that may theoretically confer certain advantages. For example, there are UAS such as the Retrace (Coloplast, Humlebaek, Denmark) (Fig. 2) and the Flexor Parallel (Cook Medical, Bloomington, IN) which have a slit on the dilator that allows the guidewire to remain parallel to the sheath after withdrawal of the dilator. This allows the use of one single guidewire instead of two as is the usual case if a safety guidewire is desired.

The use of a UAS is to primarily facilitate the repeated insertion and removal of the ureteroscope. Without the UAS, every time the ureteroscope is removed, a second guidewire would be used for reinsertion. Alternatively, direct visualization and cannulation of the ureteral orifice can be performed with the flexible ureteroscope, but this could be challenging at times.

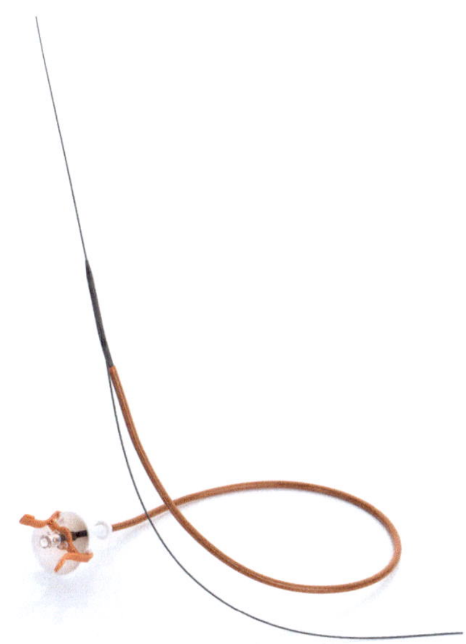

Fig. 2 Coloplast retrace UAS. (Courtesy of Coloplast, Humlebaek, Denmark)

During flexible ureteroscopy, vision is ensured by irrigation fluid. In order to reduce intra-renal pressure and potential urinary backflow into the blood stream during the procedure, there should be outflow of such fluid from the ureter. The presence of an appropriately sized UAS allows constant outflow of irrigation fluid in the space between the ureteroscope and UAS. This improves visualization and reduces intra-renal pressure and therefore reduces the risk of infection, renal damage, or inadvertent tissue injury from poor vision.

The decision to use a UAS depends on a variety of factors. This could be made prior to the procedure as part of planning, or during the procedure should clinical circumstances change. For example, in the treatment of significant stone load where a prolonged procedure is to be expected, with multiple attempts at basket retrieval of calculi fragments, then the use of a UAS would greatly facilitate surgery and decrease operative time. In another situation with a lower stone load, with the presence of a high-powered holmium laser where the operative time is expected to be short and the stone almost completely pulverized, then a UAS may not be used.

2.1 Size and Length

UAS of many different diameters and lengths are available commercially. Traditional nomenclature has the diameter of the UAS stated using two numbers (e.g., 12/14) using the French scale. The smaller number refers to the inner diameter, while the larger number refers to the outer diameter.

The size of the UAS usually ranges from 9.5 to 14 F for the inner diameter, and an outer diameter ranging from 11.5 to 16 F. A UAS with a 12 F internal diameter will fit all current flexible ureteroscopes available on the market [11]. However, for the smaller UAS sizes, in particular the 9.5/11.5 F, it is important to be familiar with the specifications of the ureteroscopes in your own practice as not all ureteroscopes will fit. With improvements in technology and miniaturization, it is expected that ureteroscopes will be thinner, and therefore, the minimum required size for a UAS will be smaller as well in future.

2.2 Innovations in UAS Design

Although the UAS facilitates repeated basket extraction of calculi, the process remains time-consuming and tedious. By utilizing dusting as a technique, tiny stone fragments are generated, with the thinking that these would pass with time. Zeng et al. described a modified UAS with a size of 12/14 F, with a side-port for continuous suction evacuation of stone fragments [12] (Fig. 3). The median operative time in this study was 27.3 min with a stone-free rate of 97.3% in the immediate postoperative period. Another group led by Zhu et al. studied the differences between

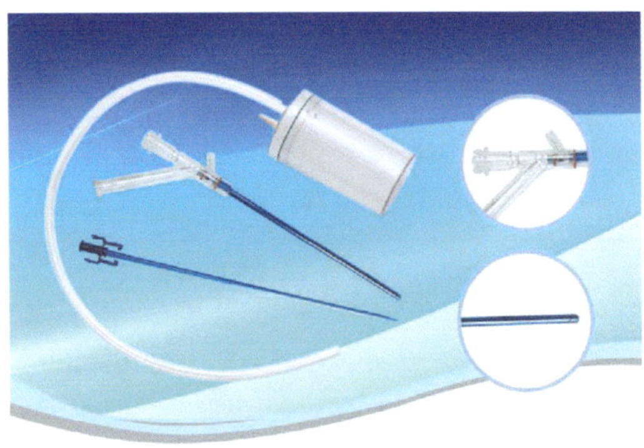

Fig. 3 ClearPetra™ suction ureteral access sheath. (Courtesy of Prof GH Zeng)

their suction UAS which has suction and vent ports for calibrating the suction force, and a traditional UAS. They found that using the suction UAS resulted in a shorter operating time, higher immediate stone-free rate, and lower total complication rate, in particular infectious complications [13]. That being said, robust scientific evidence of these advantages is not available yet.

2.3 Advantages of Using a UAS

Theoretically, the placement of a UAS would facilitate multiple removal and reinsertions of the ureteroscope. It could also reduce the risk of ureteroscope buckling in the bladder when attempting to advance beyond narrow parts of the ureter [10]. Unfortunately, good quality data to support this hypothesis is lacking and conflicting. Traxer et al. reviewed 2239 patients treated with and without UAS use and found that those who had UAS placement had a longer operative time of 80 vs. 65 min [14]. However, the patients were not randomized, and those who had UAS placement had a higher stone burden.

In cases where there is significant stone load, the UAS also provides a straight, open channel for stone retrieval using baskets. The size of stone fragments that can be removed is limited by the internal diameter of the access sheath used. The larger the access sheath, the larger the maximum single stone volume that can be removed. In fact, a small increase in the internal diameter of the access sheath from 10 to 12 F theoretically results in almost double the spherical stone volume that can be removed (from 19 to 34 mm^3).

Even in cases where a stone fragment is too large to fit entirely within the UAS, a technique has been described to extract the fragment with the UAS as a single unit alongside a safety guidewire [15]. For this to happen, the stone should be able to be wedged into the UAS opening, the stone surface exposed to the ureter should be smooth, and the stone should not be embedded within the ureteral mucosa. The UAS can be reintroduced after the stone fragment is removed, over a second guidewire or over the same one in case innovative UAS are available (Coloplast Retrace or Cook Flexor Parallel). Notably, in our opinion, this practice is suggested only in prestented patients and in experienced hands.

The impact of UAS use on stone-free rates is still controversial. Traxer et al. found that in patients with smaller stones below 10 mm, the use of a UAS had a higher stone-free rate (73 vs. 59%). However, for larger stones above 10 mm, the use of a UAS was associated with lower stone-free rate (81 vs. 85%) [14].

Fluid irrigation is key during flexible ureteroscopy for clear visualization of tissue and pathology. By increasing inflow, vision is enhanced. This naturally increases the intra-pelvic pressure, which can increase the risk of complications such as bleeding, sepsis, and postoperative pain. Jung et al. studied intrapelvic pressures during flexible ureterorenoscopy without a UAS. Intrapelvic pressures were highest during holmium laser use, and during forced irrigation, reaching up to 328 and 288 mmHg, respectively [16]. According to this concept, the use of common irrigation systems can often generate excessive pressure especially with an unoccupied working channel of the ureteroscope. Depending on the strength of force applied, very high pressure can be generated by most irrigation devices irrespective of whether the scope is occupied or not [17]. Our personal preference is for T-flow irrigation system (Rocamed, Monaco) (Fig. 4).

That being said, it is of utmost importance for the surgeon to be aware of the irrigation enhancement device properties in conjunction with the

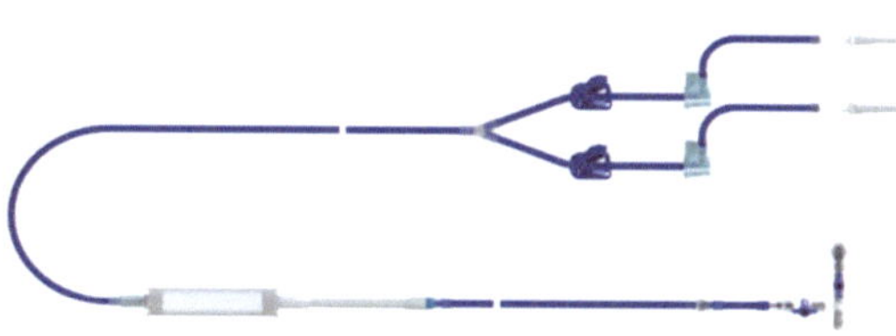

Fig. 4 TraxerFlow device. (Courtesy of Rocamed, Monaco)

experience and physical strength of their assistant: all devices may become very dangerous if not utilized properly. As such, training, education, teamwork, and awareness are essential to work in full safety.

The intrapelvic pressure is a function of irrigation inflow and outflow. Inflow is controlled by the surgeon and/or the assistant, and the pressure can be controlled by gravity, a pressure-controlled pump, or manual irrigation. The outflow itself would depend on two main factors—the size of the ureteroscope and the UAS. The difference in size between the two would be the space in the UAS that allows for irrigation outflow. In a study performed comparing varying ureteroscopes with varying UAS sizes, it was found that the combination of a large ureteroscope (Olympus URV-V) with a diameter of 9.6 F, and a small UAS with a 11/13 F diameter, the intrapelvic pressures rose above 30 mmHg beyond an irrigation pressure of 200 cmH_2O. However for other combinations studied, the intrarenal pressures did not exceed the threshold of 30 mmHg even up to an irrigation pressure of 500 cmH_2O [18]. When using a UAS of 10/12 F or above with a 7.5 F ureteroscope, intrapelvic pressures remain below 30 mmHg even at an irrigation pressure of 200 cmH_2O [19].

When exposed to high pressures for prolonged periods of time, this could lead to renal damage and parenchymal scarring. To prevent this from happening, intrapelvic pressures should be kept below 30 mmHg as far as possible. Therefore, when using the smallest flexible ureteroscope possible, it would result in the best outflow through the UAS and the lowest intrapelvic pressure.

The placement of the UAS should be at the optimal position as close to the tip of the ureteroscope as possible to reduce intrapelvic pressure. Therefore, the appropriate length should be chosen to allow the tip of the UAS to lie at the pelvic–ureteral junction. Depending on the population where the urologist practices, most urologists would use a 36 cm length for female patients and a 36 or 46 cm length for male patients [20].

2.4 Disadvantages of Using a UAS

Primary insertion of a UAS in a nonstented ureter is sometimes not possible. The failure rates in such a situation ranges from 16 to 42% [21–23]. Prestenting the ureter increases the success rate of UAS insertion significantly. A recent study found that prestenting significantly decreased the need for balloon dilatation of the ureter, as well as increased the rate of successful placement of the UAS [24]. Prestenting was also found to decrease the incidence of severe ureteral injury from UAS placement significantly [25]. However, the disadvantages of requiring prestenting are mainly the need for two separate procedures, as well as morbidity arising from the indwelling stent.

An alternative to prestenting would be active dilatation of the ureter, which could be with a semirigid ureteroscope, balloon dilators, or coaxial serial dilators. Some authors have used the semirigid ureteroscope to assess the ureteral compliance in order to select the appropriate size for the UAS [26]. Others have used the inner dilator first, prior to inserting the sheath together [27]. No high-level evidence exists recommending one approach over the other.

Also, pretreatment with tamsulosin for 1 week might facilitate UAS insertion, in particular for the larger 16 F size [28]. This increased the success rate from 43 to 87%.

The European Association guidelines [29] leave it to the surgeons' preference for the use of UAS, whereas the American Urological Association guidelines [30] recommend UAS use in situations of high stone load and patients who are on anticoagulation, in order to minimize intrarenal pressure and complications of bleeding.

A recent survey of Endourology Society members revealed that 46% of respondents used a

UAS routinely for ureteral stones, with the number increasing to 75.7% for renal stones. The most commonly used access sheath size is the 12/14 F. Over 90% believed that prestenting is not mandatory prior to UAS use [31].

Another major concern with UAS use is iatrogenic trauma to the ureter. Early experiences from the 1980s reported a ureteral perforation rate of 19%, with two-thirds of cases caused by the dilator [32]. With subsequent improvements to the design of the sheath as well as the addition of the hydrophilic coating, such complications have thankfully become less common. A recent study comparing two different brands of 12/14 F UAS reported an overall ureteral perforation rate of 10.4%, with lower injury grades of 61.2% [33]. Based on the Post Ureteroscopic Lesion Score, the majority of injuries can be treated conservatively by placement of a stent postoperatively, with the exception of a complete avulsion injury [34].

Despite previous reports about ureteral ischemia and inflammatory changes reported in animal studies [35], the significance of this in long-term ureteral injury rates in humans has not been well studied. A previous study reviewing correlation of stricture and UAS use found no relation between the two [36].

2.5 Conclusion

UAS use facilitates flexible ureteroscopy, especially in cases of significant stone load where a prolonged procedural time is to be expected. Pressure measurements have confirmed a reduced intrapelvic pressure with UAS use, which could lead to lower complication rates such as hemorrhage, renal damage, and infection. However, placement of the UAS could be potentially difficult in non-prestented ureters. Besides the choice of appropriate length and diameter, it is not possible to recommend any one particular UAS over another, in view of subjective opinions among practicing endourologists. Achieve the aims of patient safety, stone clearance, and minimal complications with whatever makes you comfortable [37].

3 Baskets and Biopsy Devices

3.1 Baskets

Fragmentation and dusting are the two main methods for laser lithotripsy in the treatment of renal calculi. The pros and cons of either technique is not within the scope of this chapter. While both the techniques each have their own proponents, the ability to manipulate and extract stones, or obtain tissue samples in the case of biopsies, remains essential during flexible ureteroscopy.

The first urological basket was described in Italy by Dormia et al. back in 1961 [38]. Baskets were traditionally made of steel, although modern baskets are now mainly made of nitinol. Flatwire baskets are not in common use currently, as they were previously shown to restrict scope deflection more and were associated with higher risk of renal papilla injury [39]. The two major basket designs are tipless (four-wire) and tipless (end-engaging) with a frontal mechanism of stone catching.

The tipless four-wire baskets have been the mainstay of endourology in recent years. The advantages include a relatively atraumatic design due to the lack of a tip and ability to ensnare stones beyond the reach of the endoscope tip.

A comparison of different nitinol stone baskets with sizes ranging from 1.5 to 2.2 F was performed by Patel et al. in 2016. The perforation force measured for the basket tip to perforate a piece of aluminum foil was highest for the Sacred Heart 1.5 F basket and lowest for the Coloplast 2.2 F basket [40]. Another study comparing 11 nitinol baskets found significant correlation between basket size and decrease in irrigant flow, as well as limitation of deflection. Among the baskets studied, the average irrig-

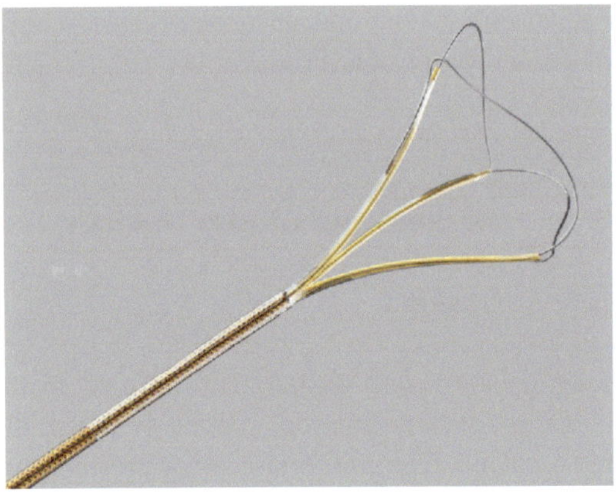

Fig. 5 NGage nitinol stone extractor (Courtesy of Cook Medical, USA)

ant flow decreased by 78.5% even with the smallest baskets used (Microvasive 1.9 and Cook 2.2 F). Deflection was decreased by 2°–6° for the same two smallest baskets. For the same sized baskets across different brands, the alteration of irrigant flow and deflection were also different, suggesting differences resulting from other factors like materials and manufacturing process [41].

A recent study comparing two end-engaging baskets NGage (Cook Medical, Bloomington, IN) (Fig. 5) and Dakota (Boston Scientific, Natick, MA) found that the Dakota basket was more effective in the capture and release of stone models above 7 mm in size [42]. Of note, this feature of the Dakota basket does not make significant difference as 7 mm is significantly larger than the diameter of most UAS in use. Notably, other baskets with similar features have been recently commercialized by other companies such as Dormia-Front (Coloplast, Humlebaek, Denmark) and Kobot MITT (Rocamed, Monaco) with similar outcomes.

When deciding on the optimal basket for use during a procedure, the main factors of basket design, opening diameter, and sheath diameter should be taken into consideration. Particularly so when planning for the re-positioning of lower pole calculi into the mid or upper pole calyces, what is initially visible on ureteroscopy may subsequently become inaccessible after the insertion of a basket. Therefore, the smallest available basket that can effectively grasp the stone while limiting ureteroscope deflection to a minimum would be the instrument of choice. Of course, personal preferences may also play a role in the choice.

3.2 Biopsy Forceps

For the evaluation of suspected upper tract urothelial carcinoma, obtaining an adequate tissue sample is key to diagnosis. The most commonly used devices for biopsy would be the nitinol basket, 3 F cup biopsy forceps such as the Piranha (Boston Scientific), and 6 F backloaded cup biopsy forceps (Bigopsy, Cook Medical) [43].

A comparison of five different biopsy forceps in the ex vivo setting by Ritter et al. compared various characteristics of these devices, including irrigation flow, scope deflection, field of view, as well as tissue sample quality. The flow rates and angle of deflection were least affected by the Bigopsy forceps (Cook), although the field of view was most decreased by the same [44] (Fig. 6).

A retrospective analysis performed of 182 biopsies using these three different devices showed that the biopsy size and presence of intact urothelium in the specimen was significantly higher when using both the nitinol basket and backloaded cup forceps, compared to the standard 3 F cup forceps [45].

Another study recommended the use of the nitinol basket for the biopsy of exophytic papillary lesions as it was associated with higher rates of successful diagnosis [46]. For non-papillary or sessile lesions, use of the backloaded cup forceps was recommended for the same reasons. The main drawback of using the larger cup forceps was limitation of scope deflection, which was therefore associated with difficulty in the biopsy of lesions in the lower pole.

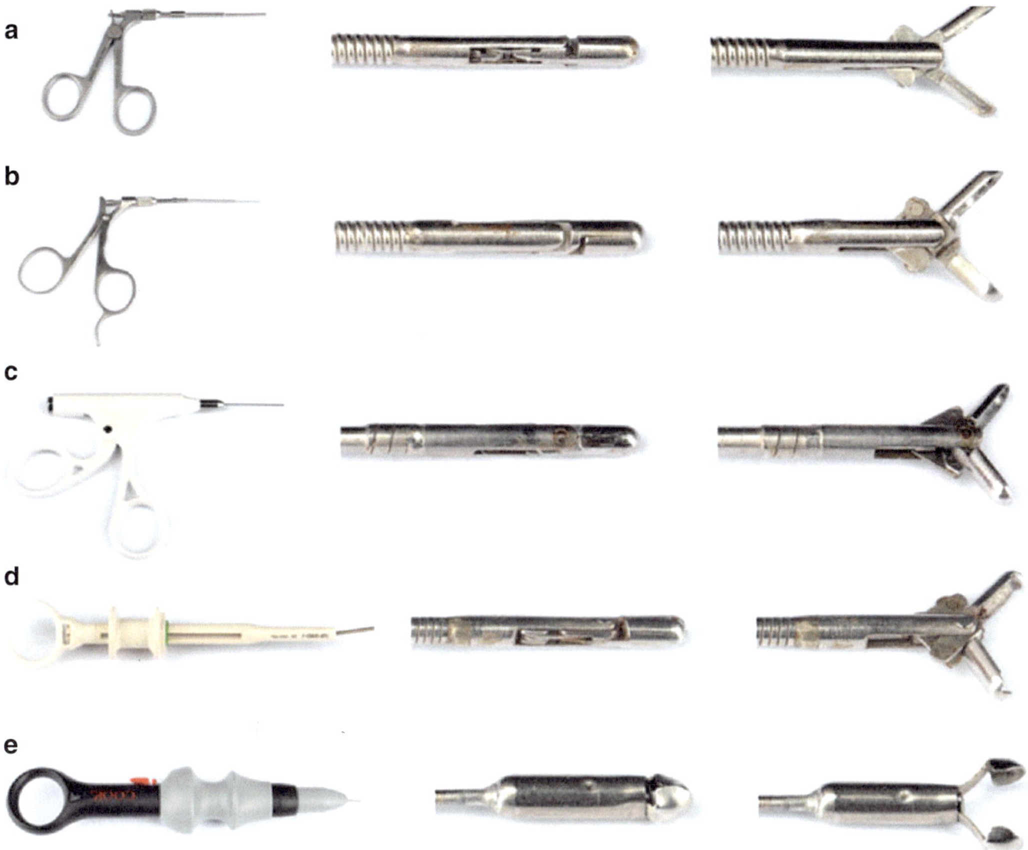

Fig. 6 Biopsy devices (reused with permission from Ritter et al., 2013): (**a**) Storz, (**b**) Wolf, (**c**) Boston Scientific, (**d**) Olympus, (**e**) Cook Medical

4 Endoscopic Sterilization and Care

Ureteroscopes are cleaned after each procedure using high-level disinfection (HLD) or sterilization or a combination of both. Each institution would generally have their own guidelines for reprocessing of endoscopes after use. Beyond disinfection and sterilization, other commonly performed actions as part of protocols include leak testing, manual cleaning, and drying [47, 48].

There are two main concerns with the cleaning and sterilization process: ensuring thorough decontamination and reducing risk of damage to the endoscope.

4.1 Decontamination Efficacy

HLD typically involves soaking the ureteroscope in a chemical disinfectant, while sterilization can involve low-temperature hydrogen peroxide gas plasma (STERRAD NX) or peroxy-acetic acid (STERIS).

A study by Chang et al. noted contamination of a semirigid ureteroscope with *E. cloacae* that failed to be eliminated by HLD alone [49]. After the addition of ethylene oxide to the reprocessing protocol, the pathogen was no longer detected.

Another study showed that there was a concerning level of ureteroscope contamination at two different sites, with varying reprocessing practices [47]. Of note, new ureteroscopes that initially tested negative subsequently tested positive after reprocessing despite not being clinically used. This suggests some contamination of new clean ureteroscopes by the reprocessing process. In the study, meticulous manual cleaning and bedside precleaning were cited as possible reasons for better sterilization results.

Previous data from gastroscopes and colonoscopes suggest that HLD may not be effective in removing contamination even when guidelines are strongly adhered to [50]. Therefore, a sterilization technique should be added to HLD to minimize ureteroscope contamination, since it can be argued that ureteroscopes should be held to a higher standard of decontamination than gastroscopes or colonoscopes.

4.2 Effect on Ureteroscope Durability

Flexible ureteroscopes are fragile and easily damaged. Although many cases of damage occur intra-operatively during surgery, some instances of damage also occur away from the operating room during reprocessing [51, 52]. Carey et al. reported that 7.7% of damage occurred during reprocessing [51].

A study by Abraham et al. compared two fiber-optic ureteroscopes that underwent either Steris (peroxy-acetic acid) or Cidex OPA (*ortho*-phthalaldehyde) HLD [53]. After 100 cycles, the ureteroscope that underwent Steris had a 12 mm shaft tear and 297 damaged fibers. The ureteroscope that underwent HLD with Cidex had 10 damaged fibers at the end of 100 cycles with no visible external damage. Of note, both scopes passed the leak test at the end of the study despite the damage observed.

In an attempt to reduce repair costs and ureteroscope damage, Semins et al. reported their experience of retraining urology nursing staff for scope reprocessing. They found that the average number of cases between repair had increased from 10.8 to 28.1. This resulted in a reduction in amortized repair costs from $418.29 per use to $120.63 per use [54]. These are certainly promising results, although it may be difficult to implement in many institutions due to the need for staff retraining and equipment purchase to allow reprocessing outside centralized areas.

5 Conclusion

While there is no good guideline or consensus on the optimal method for ureteroscope reprocessing, it is evident that the choice of method and adherence to institutional protocols may have significant impact on sterilization efficacy and possibly scope durability. It is therefore important to be familiar with the protocols at your institution and ensure that staff are well-trained to perform these procedures safely.

References

1. Mardis HK, Hepperlen TW, Kammandel H. Double pigtail ureteral stent. Urology. 1979;14(1):23–6. https://doi.org/10.1016/0090-4295(79)90205-X.
2. Civjan S, Huget EF, Desimon LB. Potential applications of certain nickel–titanium (nitinol) alloys. J Dent Res. 1975;54(1):89–96. https://doi.org/10.1177/00220345750540014301.
3. Sarkissian C, Korman E, Hendlin K, Monga M. Systematic evaluation of hybrid guidewires: shaft stiffness, lubricity, and tip configuration. Urology. 2012;79:513–7.
4. Liguori G, Antoniolli F, Trombetta C, Biasotto M, Amodeo A, Pomara G, Bucci S, Belgrano E. Comparative experimental evaluation of guidewire use in urology. Urology. 2008;72(2):286–9. https://doi.org/10.1016/j.urology.2007.12.098.
5. Amasyali AS, Groegler J, Hajiha M, Shah M, Alsyouf M, Stokes P, Belay R, Maldonado J, Baldwin DD. What guidewire is the best for bypassing an impacted ureteral stone? J Endourol. 2020;34:629–36.
6. Clayman M, Uribe CA, Eichel L, Gordon Z, McDougall EM, Clayman RV. Comparison of guide wires in urology. Which, when and why? J Urol. 2004;171:2146–50.
7. Pietropaolo A, Bres-Niewada E, Skolarikos A, et al. Worldwide survey of flexible ureteroscopy practice: a survey from European Association of Urology sections of young academic urologists and uro-technology groups. Cent Eur J Urol. 2019;72(4):393. https://doi.org/10.5173/ceju.2019.0041.
8. Dickstein RJ, Kreshover JE, Babayan RK, Wang DS. Is a safety wire necessary during routine flex-

ible ureteroscopy? J Endourol. 2010;24(10):1589–92. https://doi.org/10.1089/end.2010.0145.
9. Takayasu H, Aso Y. Recent development for pyelo-ureteroscopy: guide tube method for its introduction into the ureter. J Urol. 1974;112(2):176–8. https://doi.org/10.1016/S0022-5347(17)59675-5.
10. Monga M, Bhayai S, Landman J, Conradie M, Sundaram C, Clayman R. Ureteral access for upper urinary tract disease: the access sheath. J Endourol. 2001;15:831–4.
11. Al-Qahtani SM, Letendre J, Thomas A, Natalin R, Saussez T, Traxer O. Which ureteral access sheath is compatible with your flexible ureteroscope? J Endourol. 2014;28:286–90.
12. Zeng G, Wang D, Zhang T, Wan SP. Modified access sheath for continuous flow ureteroscopic lithotripsy: a preliminary report of a novel concept and technique. J Endourol. 2016;30(9):992–6. https://doi.org/10.1089/end.2016.0411.
13. Zhu Z, Cui Y, Zeng F, Li Y, Chen Z, Hequn C. Comparison of suctioning and traditional ureteral access sheath during flexible ureteroscopy in the treatment of renal stones. World J Urol. 2019;37(5):921–9. https://doi.org/10.1007/s00345-018-2455-8.
14. Traxer O, Wendt-Nordahl G, Sodha H, Rassweiler J, Meretyk S, Tefekli A, Coz F, de la Rosette JJ. Differences in renal stone treatment and outcomes for patients treated either with or without the support of a ureteral access sheath: The Clinical Research Office of the Endourological Society Ureteroscopy Global Study. World J Urol. 2015;33:2137–44.
15. Gur U, Holland R, Lask DM, Livne PM, Lifshitz DA. Expanding use of ureteral access sheath for stones larger than access sheath's internal diameter. Urology. 2007;69:170–2.
16. Jung HU, Frimodt-Møller PC, Osther PJ, Mortensen J. Pharmacological effect on pyeloureteric dynamics with a clinical perspective: a review of the literature. Urol Res. 2006;34:341–50.
17. Proietti S, Dragos L, Somani B, Buttìcè S, Talso M, Emiliani E, Baghdadi M, Giusti G, Traxer O. In vitro comparison of maximum pressure developed by irrigation systems in a kidney model. J Endourol. 2017;31(5):522–7. https://doi.org/10.1089/end.2017.0005.
18. Fang L, Xie G, Zheng Z, Liu W, Zhu J, Huang T, Lu Y, Cheng Y. The effect of ratio of endoscope-sheath diameter on intrapelvic pressure during flexible ureteroscopic lasertripsy. J Endourol. 2019;33:132–9.
19. Sener TE, Cloutier J, Villa L, Marson F, Buttìcè S, Doizi S, Traxer O. Can we provide low intrarenal pressures with good irrigation flow by decreasing the size of ureteral access sheaths? J Endourol. 2016;30:49–55.
20. Kaplan AG, Lipkin ME, Scales CD, Preminger GM. Use of ureteral access sheaths in ureteroscopy. Nat Rev Urol. 2016;13:135–40.
21. Viers BR, Viers LD, Hull NC, Hanson TJ, Mehta RA, Bergstralh EJ, Vrtiska TJ, Krambeck AE. The difficult ureter: clinical and radiographic characteristics associated with upper urinary tract access at the time of ureteroscopic stone treatment. Urology. 2015;86(5):878–84. https://doi.org/10.1016/j.urology.2015.08.007.
22. Mogilevkin Y, Sofer M, Margel D, Greenstein A, Lifshitz D. Predicting an effective ureteral access sheath insertion: a bicenter prospective study. J Endourol. 2014;28:1414–7.
23. Doizi S, Knoll T, Scoffone CM, Breda A, Brehmer M, Liatsikos E, Cornu JN, Traxer O. First clinical evaluation of a new innovative ureteral access sheath (Re-Trace™): a European study. World J Urol. 2014;32:143–7.
24. Navetta AF, Elmekresh A, Doersch K, Durdin T, MacHen G, Cohen A, Lowry P, el Tayeb M. Preoperative ureteral stenting prior to ureteroscopy for management of urolithiasis does not impact the postoperative return for unplanned care. Urol Ann. 2019;11:282–6.
25. Traxer O, Thomas A. Prospective evaluation and classification of ureteral wall injuries resulting from insertion of a ureteral access sheath during retrograde intrarenal surgery. J Urol. 2013;189:580–4.
26. Boulalas I, de Dominicis M, Defidio L. Semirigid ureteroscopy prior retrograde intrarenal surgery (RIRS) helps to select the right ureteral access sheath. Arch Ital Urol Androl. 2018;90:20–4.
27. L'Esperance JO, Ekeruo WO, Scales CD, Marguet CG, Springhart WP, Maloney ME, Albala DM, Preminger GM. Effect of ureteral access sheath on stone-free rates in patients undergoing ureteroscopic management of renal calculi. Urology. 2005;66:252–5.
28. Kaler KS, Safiullah S, Lama DJ, Parkhomenko E, Okhunov Z, Ko YH, Huynh L, Patel RM, Landman J, Clayman RV. Medical impulsive therapy (MIT): the impact of 1 week of preoperative tamsulosin on deployment of 16-French ureteral access sheaths without preoperative ureteral stent placement. World J Urol. 2018;36(12):2065–71. https://doi.org/10.1007/s00345-018-2336-1.
29. Turk C, Neisius A, Petrik A, Seitz C, Skolarikos A, Thomas K. EAU guidelines on urolithiasis. In: Presented at the EAU Annual Congress Amsterdam 2020.
30. Assimos D, Krambeck A, Miller NL, et al. Surgical management of stones: American Urological Association/Endourological Society Guideline, Part I. J Urol. 2016;196(4):1153–60. https://doi.org/10.1016/j.juro.2016.05.090.
31. Zilberman DE, Lazarovich A, Winkler H, Kleinmann N. Practice patterns of ureteral access sheath during ureteroscopy for nephrolithiasis: a survey among endourologists worldwide. BMC Urol. 2019;19(1):1–5. https://doi.org/10.1186/s12894-019-0489-x.
32. Newman RC, Hunter PT, Hawkins IF, Finlayson B. The ureteral access system: a review of the immediate results in 43 cases. J Urol. 1987;137(3):380–3. https://doi.org/10.1016/S0022-5347(17)44039-0.

33. Loftus CJ, Ganesan V, Traxer O, Schold JD, Noble M, Sivalingam S, Muruve N, Monga M. Ureteral wall injury with ureteral access sheaths: a randomized prospective trial. J Endourol. 2020;34(9):932–6. https://doi.org/10.1089/end.2018.0603.
34. Schoenthaler M, Wilhelm K, Kuehhas FE, Farin E, Bach C, Buchholz N, Miernik A. Postureteroscopic lesion scale: a new management modified organ injury scale-evaluation in 435 ureteroscopic patients. J Endourol. 2012;26:1425–30.
35. Lildal SK, Nørregaard R, Andreassen KH, Christiansen FE, Jung H, Pedersen MR, Osther PJS. Ureteral access sheath influence on the ureteral wall evaluated by cyclooxygenase-2 and tumor necrosis factor-α in a porcine model. J Endourol. 2017;31(3):307–13. https://doi.org/10.1089/end.2016.0773.
36. Delvecchio FC, Auge BK, Brizuela RM, Weizer AZ, Silverstein AD, Lallas CD, Pietrow PK, Albala DM, Preminger GM. Assessment of stricture formation with the ureteral access sheath. Urology. 2003;61(3):518–22. https://doi.org/10.1016/S0090-4295(02)02433-0.
37. Sofer M, Giusti G. Editorial Comment on: "Ureteral Wall Injury with Ureteral Access Sheaths: A Randomized Prospective Trial" by Loftus et al. J Endourol. 2020;34:937–8.
38. Dormia E, Gallivanone A, Bossi R. Remote results of endoscopic therapy of ureteral calculosis with the Dormia catheter. Arch Ital Urol. 1961;34:443–51.
39. Honey RJDA. Assessment of a new tipless nitinol stone basket and comparison with an existing flat-wire basket. J Endourol. 1998;12(6):529–31. https://doi.org/10.1089/end.1998.12.529.
40. Patel N, Akhavein A, Hinck B, Jain R, Monga M. Tipless nitinol stone baskets: comparison of penetration force, radial dilation force, opening dynamics, and deflection. Urology. 2017;103:256–60. https://doi.org/10.1016/j.urology.2017.01.010.
41. Ames CD, Perrone JM, Weld KJ, Foyil KV, Yan Y, Venkatesh R, Landman J. Alteration in irrigant flow and deflection of flexible ureteroscopes with nitinol baskets. J Endourol. 2006;20(1):74–7. https://doi.org/10.1089/end.2006.20.74.
42. Bechis SK, Abbott JE, Sur RL. In vitro head-to-head comparison of the durability, versatility and efficacy of the NGage and novel Dakota stone retrieval baskets. Transl Androl Urol. 2017;6(6):1144. https://doi.org/10.21037/tau.2017.11.30.
43. Wason SEL, Seigne JD, Schned AR, Pais VM. Ureteroscopic biopsy of upper tract urothelial carcinoma using a novel ureteroscopic biopsy forceps. Can J Urol. 2012;19(6):6560–5.
44. Ritter M, Bolenz C, Bach T, Ströbel P, Häcker A. Standardized ex vivo comparison of different upper urinary tract biopsy devices: impact on ureterorenoscopes and tissue quality. World J Urol. 2013;31(4):907–12. https://doi.org/10.1007/s00345-012-0854-9.
45. Lama DJ, Safiullah S, Patel RM, et al. Multi-institutional evaluation of upper urinary tract biopsy using backloaded cup biopsy forceps, a nitinol basket, and standard cup biopsy forceps. Urology. 2018;117:89–94. https://doi.org/10.1016/j.urology.2018.03.040.
46. Breda A, Territo A, Sanguedolce F, Basile G, Subiela JD, Reyes HV, Ferrer OM, Gaya JM, Palou J. Comparison of biopsy devices in upper tract urothelial carcinoma. World J Urol. 2019;37(9):1899–905. https://doi.org/10.1007/s00345-018-2586-y.
47. Ofstead CL, Heymann OL, Quick MR, Johnson EA, Eiland JE, Wetzler HP. The effectiveness of sterilization for flexible ureteroscopes: a real-world study. Am J Infect Control. 2017;45(8):888–95. https://doi.org/10.1016/j.ajic.2017.03.016.
48. Bashaw MA. Guideline implementation: processing flexible endoscopes. AORN J. 2016;104(3):225–36. https://doi.org/10.1016/j.aorn.2016.06.018.
49. Chang CL, Su LH, Lu CM, Tai FT, Huang YC, Chang KK. Outbreak of ertapenem-resistant *Enterobacter cloacae* urinary tract infections due to a contaminated ureteroscope. J Hosp Infect. 2013;85(2):118–24. https://doi.org/10.1016/j.jhin.2013.06.010.
50. Ofstead CL, Wetzler HP, Heymann OL, Johnson EA, Eiland JE, Shaw MJ. Longitudinal assessment of reprocessing effectiveness for colonoscopes and gastroscopes: results of visual inspections, biochemical markers, and microbial cultures. Am J Infect Control. 2017;45(2):e26–33. https://doi.org/10.1016/j.ajic.2016.10.017.
51. Carey RI, Gomez CS, Maurici G, Lynne CM, Leveillee RJ, Bird VG. Frequency of ureteroscope damage seen at a tertiary care center. J Urol. 2006;176(2):607–10. https://doi.org/10.1016/j.juro.2006.03.059.
52. Afane JS, Olweny EO, Bercowsky E, Sundaram CP, Dunn MD, Shalhav AL, Mcdougall EM, Clayman RV. Flexible ureteroscopes: a single center evaluation of the durability and function of the new endoscopes smaller than 9 Fr. J Urol. 2000;164(4):1164–8. https://doi.org/10.1016/S0022-5347(05)67133-9.
53. Jose Benito A, Abraham Corollos S, Abdelshehid Hak J, Lee Geoffrey N, Box Leslie A, Deane Todd, Le Forrest, Jellison James F, Borin Anthony, Manipon Elspeth M, McDougall Ralph V, Clayman. J Endourol. 2007;21(9):985–92. https://doi.org/10.1089/end.2007.0181.
54. Semins MJ, George S, Allaf ME, Matlaga BR. Ureteroscope cleaning and sterilization by the urology operating room team: the effect on repair costs. J Endourol. 2009;23(6):903–5. https://doi.org/10.1089/end.2008.0489.

Lasers in Flexible Ureteroscopy

Khurshid R. Ghani

Abstract

Laser technology has propelled ureteroscopy to become the most common surgical procedure for kidney stones in North America. This chapter begins with a history of lasers in endourology and the mechanistic aspects of fragmentation. The basics of laser settings and parameter selection, laser fiber selection, and the importance of laser fiber to stone distance for fragmentation are covered. Optimal settings for "dusting" and "fragmentation and retrieval" for laser lithotripsy are reviewed. The efficacy of advanced pulse-modulated holmium lasers and new systems such as the thulium fiber laser is covered, including aspects on laser settings and heat generation, to ensure safe use of lasers in patients.

Keywords

Ureteroscopy · Lasers · Lithotripsy

1 Introduction

In the United States (US), ureteroscopy is now the most common treatment modality for upper urinary tract stones. The increasing use and sophistication of flexible ureteroscopy to treat renal and ureteral calculi has been possible because of parallel advances in surgical laser technology. Since the advent of the pulsed dye laser in the 1980s to fragment stones, a variety of laser wavelengths have been tried and tested. The current standard is the holmium:yttrium–aluminum–garnet (Ho:YAG) laser. In the last decade, next-generation Ho:YAG systems have been developed that can provide the surgeon with a range of laser settings and parameters for stone fragmentation, tumor ablation, or stricture incision. Recently, the thulium fiber laser (TFL), which operates at a different wavelength to Ho:YAG, was launched and has renewed the enthusiasm for lasers.

In this chapter, I provide a brief history of lasers in endourology. Focusing on stones, I discuss the mechanism of fragmentation. The basics of laser settings, parameter and laser fiber selection, and other technical aspects such as fiber to stone distance and stone retropulsion are covered. Optimal settings for "dusting" and "fragmentation and retrieval" for laser lithotripsy are discussed, followed by an overview of the strategies of contact and non-contact phases of dusting. I conclude with the thulium fiber laser (TFL), which at the time of writing has been in clinical use in the United States for less than a year.

K. R. Ghani (✉)
Department of Urology, University of Michigan, Ann Arbor, MI, USA
e-mail: kghani@med.umich.edu

G. Zeng et al. (eds.), *Flexible Ureteroscopy*, https://doi.org/10.1007/978-981-19-2936-6_5

2 Background and Brief History

Laser stands for Light Amplification by Stimulated Emission of Radiation. Surgical lasers consist of a laser medium, which can be crystal, liquid, or gas, that is placed within an optical cavity. The medium is excited through an electrical current so that photons are emitted which has the wavelength of the chosen medium. Mirrors on either side of the cavity reflect the photons, and through this process, a repetitive amplification takes place, and eventually a small beam of light escapes through a hole in the cavity. This light is controlled to enter a flexible silica fiber which is then directed to the surgical target.

The first laser was developed in 1960 by Theodore Maiman using a ruby crystal as the medium. The journey for lasers in stone surgery has included the pulsed-dye (504 nm), FREDDY, and Alexandrite lasers [1]. Due to limited fragmentation for harder stones and lack of soft tissue action, along with stability and maintenance issues, these lasers were supplanted by the Ho:YAG laser when it was introduced in 1995. Over the years, this laser has undergone incremental changes in technology, with next-generation platforms released every few years. Like developments in the mobile phone industry, each generation provides the user with faster speed and versatility. We are currently on the fourth-generation Ho:YAG system which has pulse modulation with the Moses Technology™, launched by Lumenis in 2017. In 2020, the TFL was launched in the US and Europe by Olympus. Figure 1 demonstrates different lasers based on their wavelength spectrum.

3 Mechanistic Aspects of Laser Lithotripsy

Energy cannot be created nor destroyed. Figure 2 illustrates the light to tissue interactions occurring when the laser is fired on a stone during laser lithotripsy. A small amount of the energy through vapor bubble collapse is reflected back as light, called sonoluminescence. The majority of the light is absorbed, both by the stone and surrounding fluid. Kidney stones absorb the energy to undergo fragmentation. Greater absorption coefficients mean that light is more effectively absorbed. However, greater absorption coefficients also result in a smaller absorption length. Taken together, there is a maximum value for absorption coefficient where fragmentation depth is maximized. Exceeding that threshold will result in less fragmentation [2].

Importantly, the absorption characteristics are dependent on the wavelength of the laser. Because laser energy is so readily absorbed in fluid, which is an important safety feature, one must be mindful that fluid temperatures can increase to injurious levels when using high-power laser settings combined with low irrigation rates.

Three mechanistic processes are proposed for laser lithotripsy: photothermal, photoacoustic, and thermomechanical ablation.

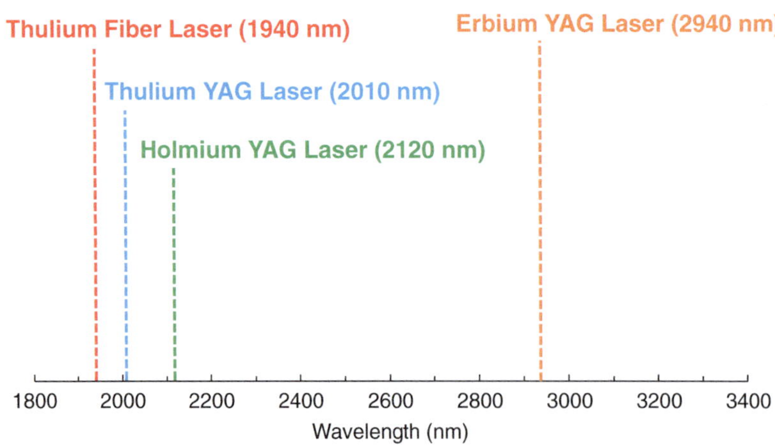

Fig. 1 Surgical lasers in endourology according to their wavelength

Photothermal ablation is the predominant mechanism, where the goal is to maximize energy transfer to the stone, through the process of contact laser lithotripsy. Photoacoustic ablation is thought to occur as a minor component depending on the pulse duration and energy. Recently, there has been interest in thermo-mechanical ablation, also known as explosive vaporization, where the goal is to maximize energy transfer to the water in the pores of the stone. It is hypothesized that this process is important for fragmentation with the TFL [3].

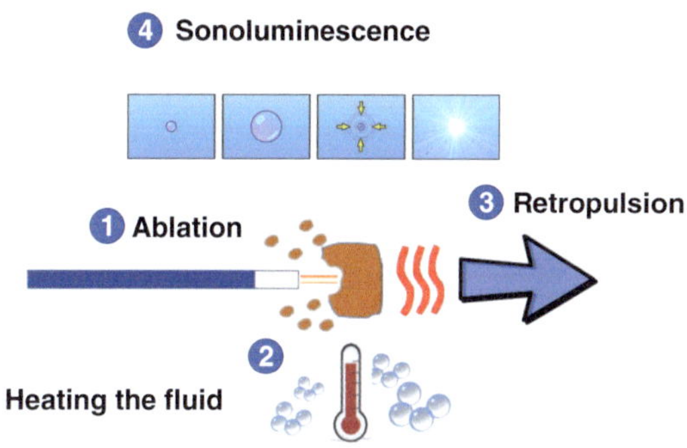

Fig. 2 Laser energy to tissue interactions occurring during laser lithotripsy

3.1 Fiber to Stone Distance

Fluid absorption and its relationship to the laser fiber tip to stone working distance is critical during laser lithotripsy. Ho:YAG and TFL perform the best when the laser is activated with the fiber tip on contact with the stone. If the fiber tip distance increases, it reduces fragmentation efficacy. This is because the energy reaching the stone diminishes as the distance between the laser fiber and stone increases. Figure 3 demonstrates that with holmium, the fragmentation volume is reduced by as much as 40% when 1 J is applied with the fiber tip just 1 mm away from the stone surface [4]. At 3 mm distance, there is no fragmentation. In comparison, the TFL operates at a different wavelength where the laser energy is four times more absorbed in fluid [3]. The consequence of this is that at greater than 1–2 mm fiber to stone distances, it may have no ablation effect on the stone, making it a truly contact laser.

Fig. 3 Mean crater volume following single pulse at 1.0 J at different laser fiber to stone distances utilizing short pulse mode. (Adapted from Aldoukhi et al. J Endo 2019)

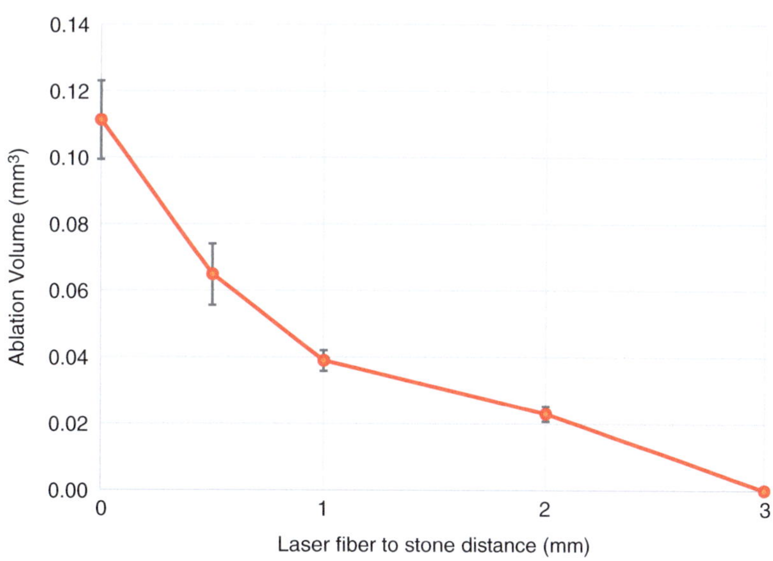

4 Holmium Laser

The Ho:YAG laser is a solid-state flashlamp-pumped laser that emits pulsed energy at 2120 nm wavelength. Holmium energy is highly absorbed by water with a low penetration depth that limits the amount of energy reaching surrounding tissue, which is an important safety feature. Laser activation causes the release of energy from the fiber tip creating a vapor channel allowing for direct absorbance of radiation by the stone. This direct irradiance leads to a photothermal reaction which causes chemical decomposition of the calculus [5]. Though collapse of the cavitation bubble has been noted to generate shockwaves, they are not strong enough to contribute significantly to total fragmentation [2]. The ability of the Ho:YAG laser to fragment stones of any composition, through the use of small flexible fibers that permit endoscope irrigation and flexibility, with its long track record of safety has made it the current standard for lithotripsy during ureteroscopy [6]. By incorporating multiple rods and flashlamps, it then became possible to increase the total power and expand the range of parameters.

4.1 Laser Settings and Parameters

Modern day systems allow the user to adjust pulse energy, frequency, pulse duration, and if available, pulse modulation—where the energy is delivered over two pulses. Some parameters such as peak power cannot be selected but are a product of the pulse energy and duration. The time-averaged power (Watts) is a function of the pulse energy and frequency and is displayed on the system (Fig. 4). Total power can have implications for safety. All of these parameters influence different aspects of lithotripsy performance including fragmentation, retropulsion, and fiber-tip degradation. Their appropriate selection helps optimize fragmentation efficiency.

4.1.1 Pulse Energy

Pulse energy (PE) is the optical energy emitted from the fiber-tip during one pulse and is measured in Joules (J). PE varies from 0.2 to 6.0 J, and its range is dependent on the power of the Ho:YAG system. Figure 5 shows the optical pulse profile of a holmium pulse, with its shark's fin appearance and high peak power. Peak power, which is the maximum optical power of a pulse, is an important consideration. Pulses with high peak power can increase fragmentation, but the drawback is greater stone retropulsion. Higher PE also increases laser fiber tip degradation, also known as burnback.

Factors that influence the selection of PE include stone composition, location, and desired fragment size, with commonly used settings during ureteroscopy ranging from 0.2 to 1.4 J. Low-power systems (e.g., 20 W) have a limited PE range, and often cannot go lower than 0.5 J. Low PE such as 0.2–0.4 J is employed when utilizing a dusting technique to create very small fragments that are left in situ for spontaneous passage. Using a low PE setting of 0.2 J leads to the smallest fragment size [7]. Increasing the PE leads to more fragmentation. Some hard stones like calcium oxalate monohydrate may require greater PE for fragmentation [8]. Higher PE settings such as 0.8–1.0 J are ideal for lithotripsy followed by active basket retrieval.

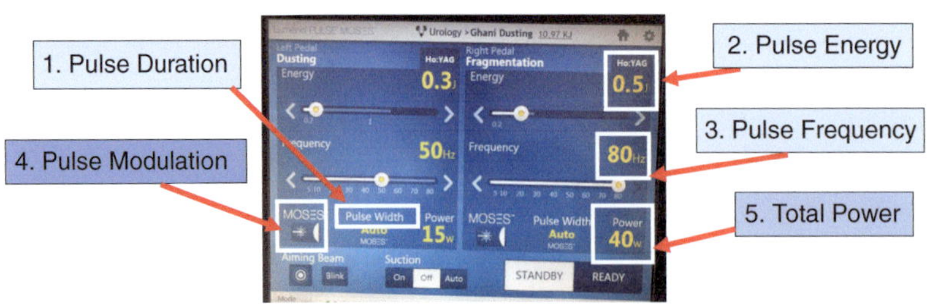

Fig. 4 Ho:YAG laser screen demonstrating multiple parameters that can be altered for laser lithotripsy (MosesP120, Lumenis)

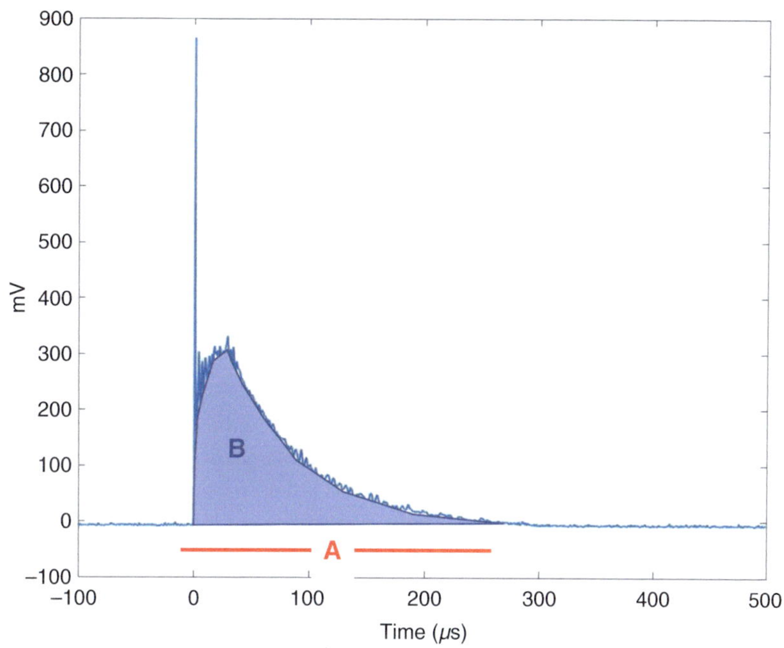

Fig. 5 Optical pulse profile of Ho:YAG pulse. (**a**) Pulse duration: duration of an optical pulse. (**b**) Peak power: maximum optical power of a pulse

4.1.2 Frequency

Frequency is the number of optical pulses emitted from the fiber-tip in 1 s and expressed in Hertz (Hz). The range available is dependent on the constraints of the holmium system, with low-power lasers limited to maximum frequencies of 15–20 Hz. High-power systems can achieve frequencies as high as 120 Hz, supporting techniques such as high-frequency dusting. Tweaking the frequency setting determines the clinical strategy of either fragmentation and retrieval, or dusting. Increasing the frequency while keeping PE constant can result in faster fragmentation especially when using low PE settings such as 0.2 J. High frequencies, especially if using higher PE settings will increase stone retropulsion. In my experience, the higher frequency high-power systems improve efficiency, especially for large kidney stones for rapid ablation at low PE. However, there is a threshold after which increasing the frequency brings minimal gain in fragmentation [9]. Furthermore, visibility must be considered when using higher frequencies as it can become too cloudy from the debris and fragments, to perform efficient lithotripsy if the irrigation parameters cannot safely maintain adequate vision.

4.1.3 Pulse Duration

Pulse duration is the time in which a single optical pulse is emitted, measured in microseconds (μs). Conventional Ho:YAG systems use fixed pulse duration settings of ~150–350 μs, commonly known as short pulse (SP). Next-generation systems allow for the selection of long pulse (LP) modes up to 1200 μs. LP delivers the same amount of total energy as SP, but over a longer period, and thus has a lower peak power. While SP and high peak powers may result in photoacoustic effects and large fragments, in the modern day the focus has been on optimizing photothermal ablation with LP duration to get fine fragments. The main advantage of using LP is to decrease stone retropulsion [10]. Laser fiber tip burnback is also reduced when using LP [11].

4.1.4 Pulse Modulation

When using traditional modes of SP or LP, all the energy is delivered in one pulse. The bubble that forms when laser energy is transmitted through fluid was described by Isner and associates as the Moses Effect; the energy causes a vapor tunnel that serves as a pathway permitting transmission of radiation between the “parted seas of water” [12]. During this process, most of the energy is lost in vapor channel formation. Pulse modulation is a novel parameter that reduces the energy lost to fluid absorption. This involves sequencing two pulses closely together. An initial pulse serves to create the vapor channel while the remaining energy is released in a second pulse which takes advantage of the first vapor bubble and transmits a greater portion of the pulse energy to the stone. This is in effect a multi-pulse mechanism, and the first system to do this was called the Moses Technology™ [13].

In the Moses Technology™, there are two settings to choose from: Moses Contact (MC), intended for operation at a close distance, and Moses Distance (MD) which is designed for lithotripsy at a distance of 1–2 mm. The major pulse profile difference between the two modes is that in MD, the first vapor bubble is big, and equal in size to the second bubble. In MC, the first bubble is smaller, and the second bubble much larger. This advance in pulse sequencing technology translates to more fragmentation. In vitro studies have shown that compared to SP and LP modes, using MD mode with the laser fiber tip in contact with the stone resulted in approximately 30% greater fragmentation [4]. MD mode also results in significantly more ablation when the fiber to stone distance is at 1 mm distance. In a clinical trial of patients with ureteral and renal calculi treated with ureteroscopy from Montreal, Canada, use of the Moses mode led to a 32% reduction in fragmentation time [14].

The "Virtual Basket" from Quanta Lasers (Italy) is a multi-pulse mode developed after Moses Technology™, where the sequencing of the two pulses is slightly different. The energy delivered is greater in the second pulse (similar to MD pulse). Instead, the second pulse is delivered just before the maximum bubble profile of the first pulse. Unlike Moses Technology™ which can go up to 120 Hz, it is limited to a maximum of 70 Hz. Figure 6 summarizes the different pulse modes currently available, as well as the concept of pulse trains which are in development.

4.1.5 Power and Heat Generation

As time-averaged power increases during laser lithotripsy, it is important to consider thermal effects. Temperatures can increase to concerning levels when using prolonged high-power settings and low irrigation rates. In vivo porcine studies demonstrate that laser activation utilizing high-power settings such as 40 W settings can increase temperatures to concerning levels if the irrigation rate is low [15]. The concern is thermal tissue injury.

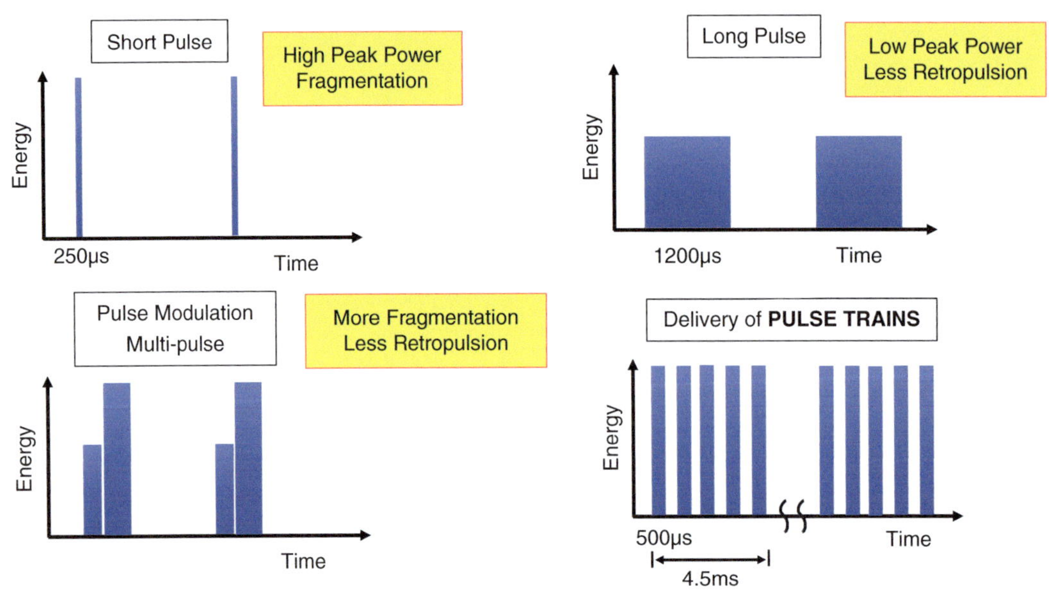

Fig. 6 Different pulse modes for Ho:YAG lasers and their overall effect on laser lithotripsy

As a principle, I do not use more than 10 W in the ureter for laser lithotripsy. In the kidney I will use high-power settings if there is mitigation. These measures include higher irrigation rates (30–40 mL/min), using room temperature or cooled irrigating fluid, and regulating the energy with intermittent laser firing. However, increasing the irrigation rate may increase intrarenal pressure which may lead to complications. To prevent injury associated with higher intrarenal temperatures, ureteral access sheaths can be used to increase outflow drainage and consequently increase the irrigation rate in a safe manner. Suction technology that removes irrigation fluid from the collecting system presents another potential solution to mitigating thermal injury and is under development.

5 Stone Retropulsion

Collapse of the laser vapor bubble leads to unwanted movement of stone debris, known as retropulsion. Higher PEs lead to a proportional increase in retropulsion; the larger vapor bubbles result in greater collapse and retropulsion. Retropulsion decreases lithotripsy efficiency by increasing the distance between the fiber tip and stone, resulting in less energy reaching the stone. Consequences of retropulsion are migration of stone (such as from ureter to renal pelvis), thereby increasing procedural time. Both LP and pulse modulated modes reduce stone retropulsion and are helpful for controlled fragmentation [10, 13].

6 Laser Fibers

Specially designed fibers consisting of different layers of material deliver energy from the laser to the surgical target during laser lithotripsy. The fiber consists of an inner core which is made of pure fused-silica that transmits the light energy. The middle "cladding" layer is made with fluorine-doped silica to provide a lower refractive index and keeps the energy within the core. An outer layer made of colored plastic limits the strain resulting from bending the fibers. Because the fiber is made of glass, its tip can be damaged during laser lithotripsy which can result in reduced energy output.

Fiber size can affect the efficiency of laser lithotripsy. The go-to fiber size for flexible ureteroscopy is the smaller 200–270 μm core diameter fiber, as it provides superior irrigation through the working channel and is flexible enough to allow lower pole lithotripsy. Vision is especially important for efficiency if a dusting technique is utilized as one needs to see through the small fragments and debris. The fiber size also determines the size of fragments produced during lithotripsy, with smaller fragments obtained with the smaller core fibers, especially if using a low PE setting. Furthermore, smaller core fibers are associated with less retropulsion compared to larger fibers. This is due to the small recoil momentum for the small fibers. Fragmentation is similar among the fiber sizes when using low pulse energies ($\leq$1.0 J) but greater for larger fibers when using higher pulse energies. Larger fibers (i.e., 365 μm) have been traditionally used for semirigid ureteroscopy where fragmentation and basketing are common. However, I prefer to use the smaller core fibers regardless of scope used, primarily for vision purposes. The performance of modern-day single-use small core fibers is excellent. Some centers may prefer to use reusable fibers because of the cost.

6.1 Laser Fiber Tip Configuration

The power output from the laser fiber depends on the lasing time and cleaving method. Power output is highest when the fiber is new and has a smooth surface at the tip. It diminishes with time due to tip damage. For fiber cleaving, cleaving tools are superior to scalpel and Mayo suture scissors by providing a higher power output initially. However, the power output from the fiber is equivalent after a few minutes of laser firing regardless of the cleaving method or laser setting. Some surgeons prefer to strip or cut the fiber tip prior to lithotripsy, making it flush with the colored coated sheath (called the coated tip) [16]. This can help with easier identification of the tip during laser lithotripsy. However, in vitro studies have shown that using a new or cleaved and stripped laser fiber tip results in better fragmentation compared to coated tips that are created by cutting with scissors [17, 18].

Fibers with a rounded ball-tip design have been developed to reduce friction within the working channel during its insertion, thereby reducing the likelihood of reusable flexible ureteroscope damage. They have comparable comminution, tip degradation, and ureteroscope deflection to standard flat-tip fibers. These fibers are helpful when treating stones in the lower pole, as the fiber can be inserted through the working channel while the scope is deflected [19]. Sometimes with a fiber already out of the working channel, it can be hard to deflect into an acute angled lower pole calyx. It is important to know the ball-tip can erode during the case as energy is applied, which means it loses its cardinal benefit for lower pole lithotripsy. For these reasons, I always treat the lower pole stone first when using this fiber. However, they are more expensive and should be considered on a selective basis.

6.2 Laser Fiber-Tip Degradation

Energy delivery through the fiber tip causes chemical and mechanical breakdown of the silica, leading to distal end damage and shortening. This tip degradation, known as "burnback," reduces energy transmission and reduces the efficiency of fragmentation. Degradation of the tip can lead to increased operative time by needing to replace the fiber with a new one, or the time needed to undertake fiber cleaving. In general, higher PE leads to more burnback. Degradation of the fiber decreases its length and damages the tip, reducing the amount of energy reaching the stone. Contact with the stone can be impaired if the fiber degrades beyond the colored sheath which reduces fragmentation efficiency further.

Laser fiber-tip burnback is affected by both pulse duration and PE. Using LP instead of SP will decrease the amount of tip degradation. Frequency on its own has little impact on burnback, which is more influenced by the total power, especially if using high PE settings. For example, when using a 35 W setting of 0.5 J × 70 Hz on SP mode, there is significantly less burnback than using a 40 W setting of 1 J × 40 Hz on SP mode [11]. Careful selection of PE, frequency, and pulse mode can optimize operative efficiency (Table 1).

Table 1 Relationship between pulse energy, frequency, pulse duration and pulse modulation on laser lithotripsy performance

	Pulse energy (J)		Frequency (Hz)		Pulse duration		Pulse modulation
	Hi	Lo	Hi	Lo	Short	Long	Moses Technology™
Fragmentation	↑	↓	↑	↓	No effect	No effect	↑
Retropulsion	↑	↓	=/↑	No effect	↑	↓	↓
Burnback	↑	↓	↑*	No effect	↑	↓	↓

Adapted from Black KM, Aldoukhi AH, Ghani KR. A Users Guide to Holmium Laser Lithotripsy Settings in the Modern Era. Front Surg. 2019 Aug 14;6:48. doi: 10.3389/fsurg.2019.00048

↑*=Increase in burnback only if total power increases

7 Surgical Strategies for Laser Lithotripsy: Dusting vs. Fragmentation

The surgical strategy for treating upper urinary tract stones with flexible ureteroscopy consists of either fragmentation and active basket retrieval or fragmentation, resulting in fine fragments that are left in situ for spontaneous passage, also known as dusting technique [20]. Some surgeons may use a hybrid approach, dust the stone initially, and retrieve larger fragments at the end. "Dust" is not a new term and was described by John Blandy and Manmeet Singh in 1976 when describing outcomes for open renal stone surgery [21], by Stevan Streem in 1996 when reporting results from shockwave lithotripsy [22, 23], and importantly by Michael Grasso in 1996 [6] when detailing his experience with the holmium laser for ureteroscopy.

First-generation holmium lasers were only capable of ≤15–20 Hz pulse frequency. High PE such as 0.8–1.0 J and low frequency such as 8–12 Hz were typically used to allow a "fragmentation" strategy where the laser is placed in direct contact with the stone, pinning it against the urothelium to sequentially fracture and divide the stone into extractable fragments. To avoid excessive retropulsion, fragmentation and retrieval are performed using lower frequency settings. Because of the limited low frequency on low power systems, the use of dusting was not initially widespread, as it would take too long. High-power (100–120 W) holmium laser systems, capable of 50–120 Hz pulse frequency, and low PEs such as 0.2–0.3 J, have expanded the available settings for laser lithotripsy and made dusting more popular (Table 2). In contrast, higher frequencies when using low PE do not have as much impact on retropulsion.

Dusting is particularly attractive for treating renal stones. A multi-center prospective study from the United States, comparing outcomes after dusting to those done with pure fragmentation and retrieval, demonstrated no significant differences in stone-free rates or complications [24]. However, dusting was significantly faster, taking half the operative time of retrieval. When performing a dusting technique to treat a renal stone, there are two phases to consider.

7.1 Dusting: Contact Laser Lithotripsy

This is the initial phase to debulk the stone, where the laser fiber tip touches the stone surface on contact as much as possible. The goal is to carefully fragment the stone using low-PE and high-frequency settings to get the smallest size fragment (<0.5, <1 mm) breaking off the surface. By using techniques of dancing, chipping, and painting (Fig. 7), especially for large stones [24], the surgeon constantly interrogates the stone surface, making sure not to stay in one area too long, otherwise fissures appear with larger chunks breaking off. In contrast to fragmentation, the goal is not to get large fragments. In the ureter, if a dusting technique is used, I work centrally on the stone to avoid touching the ureteral wall (<10 W settings).

In the kidney, the principle is to work peripherally on the stone, and intermittently shave off the center areas of the stone. Because of the constant movement, the laser pedal is always on, and a good proportion of the laser pulses are fired at distance. For these reasons, I prefer using relatively

Table 2 Laser lithotripsy modes and typical settings for Ho:YAG laser lithotripsy

Mode	Pulse energy/frequency	Laser settings	Power (W)
Fragmentation	High/low	0.8 J × 8 Hz 1 J × 8 Hz	6.4–8
Dusting	Low/high	0.2–0.4 J × 50–80 Hz	10–32
Pop-corning	High/moderate	1 J × 15–20 Hz	15–20
Pop-dusting	Moderate/high	0.5 J × 50–80 Hz	25–40

The pulse energy and frequency range will be dependent on the machine. The latest systems have extended frequency ranges of 100–120 Hz

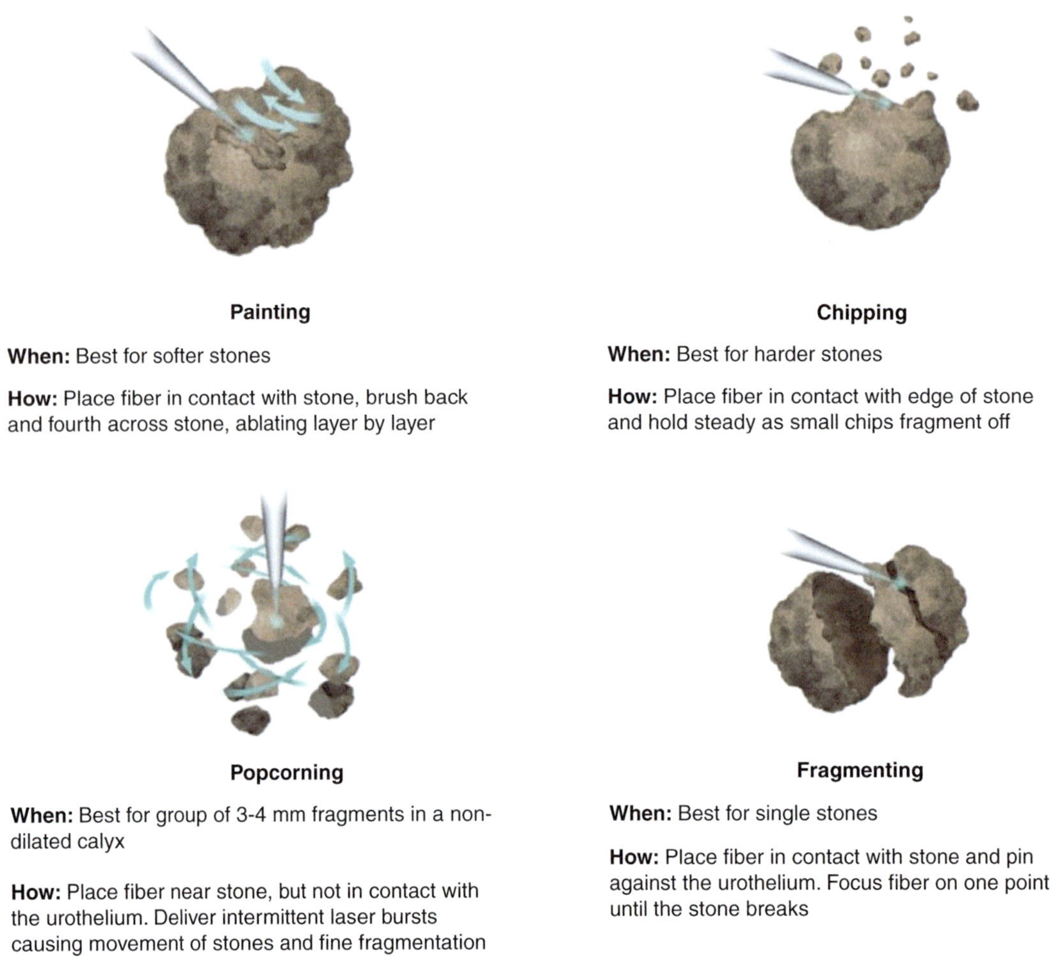

Fig. 7 Fragmentation and dusting techniques for laser lithotripsy of renal stones. (Adapted from Ghani KR, Roberts WW. Dusting vs Extraction Strategies during Ureteroscopy for Renal Calculi. AUA Lesson 5. Update Series 2020 Volume 39)

mid-range power settings (e.g., 20–30 W), along with pulse modulation as this mode is optimized for both contact and at distance from the stone. Work from the University of Michigan Endourology laboratory shows that during dusting technique approximately 50% of pulses are fired when the fiber to stone distance is >1 mm [9].

I also prefer to nudge the stone into a calyx or infundibulum at the very beginning where it is much easier to manage, and in the correct spot for the second phase of dusting. While the stone bulk reduces, the stone may wobble which is an indication that lower power settings need to be used for less retropulsion and effective dusting. With hard stones, higher PE settings may be needed to obtain smaller fragments. Yet, no matter how skillful the technique or settings, the stone will eventually break into smaller chunks. These larger fragments are then pulverized with non-contact laser lithotripsy.

7.2 Dusting: Non-Contact Laser Lithotripsy

In this technique, stone fragments are pulverized in a calyx with the laser fiber activated in bursts, placed a few millimeters away from the fragments in a non-contact manner. This results in a whirlpool-like effect that causes the fragments to move around and come in direct contact with the laser tip and undergo fragmentation. First described by Demetrius Bagley in 2008, it is also commonly known as the "popcorn" effect due to the chaotic and noisy movement of fragments [25]. The technique allows the surgeon to not spend time repositioning the laser on the stone between pulses.

Multiple studies have tried to determine what are the best settings and technique. Bagley found that a laser setting of 1.5 J and 40 Hz was the most efficient for stone fragmentation, resulting in 63% loss of stone mass after 2 min of continuous laser firing [25]. However, this type of setting with a high PE of 1.5 J will lead to significant fiber burnback. Emiliani and Traxer found that high pulse energy (1.5 J) and high pulse frequency (40 Hz) resulted in more efficient popcorning [26]. They also found longer lithotripsy time (4 vs. 2 min) and smaller laser fiber (273 vs. 365 μm) led to higher fragmentation success, which was defined as 50% reduction of stone volume. Our research team studied this where we treated stones in glass bulbs to simulate a calyx and varied the pulse energy (0.5 J, 1.0 J), frequency settings (20, 40, 80 Hz), size of the bulb (small and large), and fiber tip to stone distance (0 and 2 mm) [27]. Higher pulse frequencies and power settings, performing it in a smaller bulb, and keeping the fiber positioned closer to the stone surface significantly improved sub-millimeter fragmentation outcomes. The best setting was 0.5 J × 80 Hz. At the University of Michigan, we coined the term "Pop-dusting," to differentiate it from 1 J × 15–20 Hz setting typically used for popcorn technique [28]. Regardless of the setting used, if the calyx is too dilated for effective popcorning, it may be more appropriate to retrieve the fragments.

8 Thulium Fiber Laser

In the thulium fiber laser (TFL), energy is generated in a chemically doped small laser fiber that is tightly coiled within a system that has a much smaller footprint compared to Ho:YAG (Fig. 8) [29]. The energy is then routed to a smaller silica fiber that is then delivered to the target tissue. TFL can operate at either 1908 or 1940 nm. This wavelength has a higher absorption peak in water compared to Ho:YAG. PE settings with TFL can go as low as 0.025 J and frequency as high as 2400 Hz. The pulse duration is also much longer than that of HoYAG, up to 50 ms. It has a low peak power (<500 W) compared to Ho:YAG which is in the range of 1500–3000 W. Low peak power means less retropulsion, which is an advantage for the dusting technique. In contrast, the low peak power may hinder an effective fragmentation technique which requires greater energy to fracture hard stones.

A major advantage of THL is that it can be coupled to laser fibers with core diameters as small as 100–150 μm. These smaller fibers open

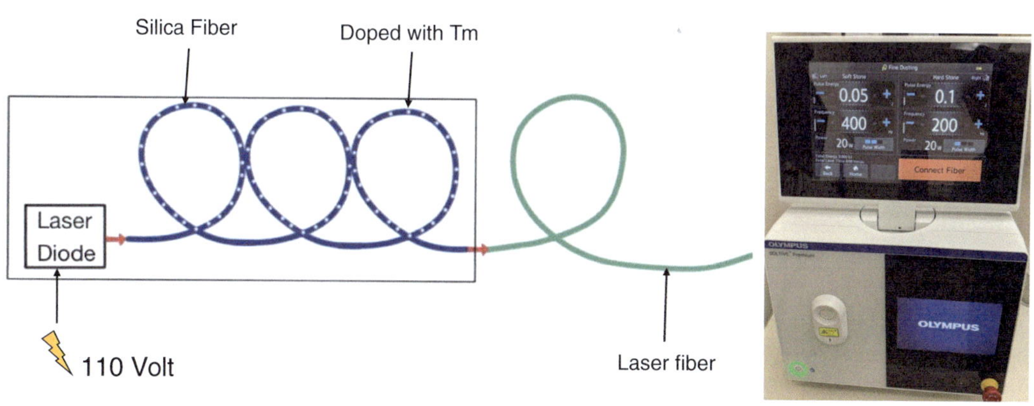

Fig. 8 Schematic of thulium fiber laser (left). Soltive system (Olympus) demonstrated (right)

the door for higher irrigation rates and better ureteroscope maneuverability, as well as smaller scopes in the future. Because its architecture does not rely on flashlamp plugs and a sophisticated cooling system, it is quieter and more stable. Unlike the high-power HoYAG system, it does not require a specialized electrical circuit, and can be plugged to a normal electrical outlet. This means it can be used in any operating room.

In vitro studies comparing HoYAG with TFL demonstrated that TFL resulted in greater fragmentation for uric acid and calcium oxalate monohydrate stones [29]. While the TFL is a promising technology, more clinical studies are needed to better understand the use of TFL for lithotripsy in comparison with the holmium laser. For example, hot flashes and sparks are possible when using this system. Long pulse duration lasers are known to be associated with collateral and thermal tissue damage [2]. While such durations are not seen with Ho:YAG, they can be with the TFL depending on the settings. The optimal settings for TFL are not fully understood at this time and require refinement.

9 Conclusion

The emergence of the thulium fiber laser (TFL) has provided a competitor to the advanced holmium laser. Time will tell which laser system will become the dominant machine in clinical practice. One thing is clear, we have entered a new era of laser systems that are more powerful and versatile and offer a range of settings that provide greater precision for the task at hand. However, with this array of gadgetry and sophistication comes the possibility to do harm. An understanding of the principles of laser technology and their safe use during ureteroscopy is essential for the modern day endourologist.

Acknowledgements I want to thank all the Endourology laboratory research fellows who have worked with me at the University of Michigan: Ali Aldoukhi MD, Kristian Black MD, Sami Majdalny MD, Brandon Levin, and Nikta Khajeh; and my partners Dr. Tim Hall and Dr. William Roberts.

Conflict of Interest/Disclosures Dr. Ghani receives grant funding from Boston Scientific to study optimal laser settings in the laboratory. He serves as a consultant for Lumenis, Boston Scientific, Olympus, Coloplast, and Karl Storz.

References

1. Zarrabi A, Gross AJ. The evolution of lasers in urology. Ther Adv Urol. 2011;3(2):81–9.
2. Chan KF, Pfefer TJ, Teichman JMH, Welch AJ. A perspective on laser lithotripsy: the fragmentation processes. J Endourol. 2001;15:257–73.
3. Fried NM, Irby PB. Advances in laser technology and fibre-optic delivery systems in lithotripsy. Nat Rev Urol. 2018;15:563–73.
4. Aldoukhi AH, Roberts WW, Hall TL, Ghani KR. Watch your distance: the role of laser fiber working distance on fragmentation when altering pulse width or modulation. J Endourol. 2019;33(2):120–6. https://doi.org/10.1089/end.2018.0572.
5. Chan KF, Vassar GJ, Pfefer TJ, et al. Holmium:YAG laser lithotripsy: a dominant photothermal ablative mechanism with chemical decomposition of urinary calculi. Lasers Surg Med. 1999;25:22–37.
6. Grasso M. Experience with the holmium laser as an endoscopic lithotrite. Urology. 1996;48:199–206.
7. Sea J, Jonat LM, Chew BH, et al. Optimal power settings for holmium:YAG lithotripsy. J Urol. 2012;187:914–9.
8. Spore SS, Teichman JM, Corbin NS, Champion PC, Williamson EA, Glickman RD. Holmium: YAG lithotripsy: optimal power settings. J Endourol. 1999;13:559–66.
9. Aldoukhi AH, Hall TL, Ghani KR, Roberts WW. Strike rate: analysis of laser fiber to stone distance during different modes of laser lithotripsy. J Endourol. 2021;35:355–9.
10. Bader MJ, Pongratz T, Khoder W, Stief CG, Herrmann T, Nagele U, Sroka R. Impact of pulse duration on Ho: YAG laser lithotripsy: fragmentation and dusting performance. World J Urol. 2015;33:471–7.
11. Levin BA, Aldoukhi AH, Black KM, Hall TL, Roberts WW, Ghani KR. Burnback: the role of pulse duration and energy on fiber-tip degradation during high-power laser lithotripsy. Lasers Med Sci. 2021;36(9):1817–22. https://doi.org/10.1007/s10103-020-03199-5.
12. Isner JM, DeJesus SR, Clarke RH, Gal D, Rongione AJ, Donaldson RF. Mechanism of laser ablation in an absorbing fluid field. Lasers Surg Med. 1988;8:543–54.
13. Elhilali MM, Badaan S, Ibrahim A, Andonian S. Use of the Moses Technology to improve holmium laser lithotripsy outcomes: a preclinical study. J Endourol. 2017;31(6):598–604.

14. Ibrahim A, Elhilali MM, Fahmy N, Carrier S, Andonian S. Double-blinded prospective randomized clinical trial comparing regular and Moses modes of holmium laser lithotripsy. J Endourol. 2020;34:624–8.
15. Aldoukhi AH, Hall TL, Ghani KR, Maxwell AD, MacConaghy B, Roberts WW. Caliceal fluid temperature during high-power holmium laser lithotripsy in an in vivo porcine model. J Endourol. 2018;32:724–9.
16. Kronenberg P, Traxer O. Are we all doing it wrong? Influence of stripping and cleaving methods of laser fibers on laser lithotripsy performance. J Urol. 2015;193:1030–5.
17. Aldoukhi AH, Knudsen BE, Black KM, Hall TL, Roberts WW, Ghani KR. Are we cutting ourselves short? Laser lithotripsy performance based on differences in fiber-tip preparation. Urology. 2019;134:79–83.
18. Vassantachart JM, Lightfoot M, Yeo A, et al. Laser fiber cleaving techniques: effects on tip morphology and power output. J Endourol. 2015;29:84–9.
19. Shin RH, Lautz JM, Cabrera FJ, Shami CJ, Goldsmith ZG, Kuntz NJ, Kaplan AG, Neisius A, Simmons WN, Preminger GM, Lipkin ME. Evaluation of novel ball-tip holmium laser fiber: impact on ureteroscope performance and fragmentation efficiency. J Endourol. 2016;30:189–94.
20. Aldoukhi AH, Roberts WW, Hall TL, Ghani KR. Holmium laser lithotripsy in the new stone age: dust or bust? Front Surg. 2017;29(4):57. https://doi.org/10.3389/fsurg.2017.00057.
21. Blandy JP, Singh M. The case for a more aggressive approach to staghorn stones. J Urol. 1976;115(5):505–6.
22. Streem SB, Yost A, Mascha E. Clinical implications of clinically insignificant store fragments after extracorporeal shock wave lithotripsy. J Urol. 1996;155(4):1186–90.
23. Humphreys MR, Shah OD, Monga M, et al. Dusting versus basketing during ureteroscopy—which technique is more efficacious? A prospective multicenter trial from the EDGE research consortium. J Urol. 2018;199:1272–6.
24. Hecht SL, Wolf JS Jr. Techniques for holmium laser lithotripsy of intrarenal calculi. Urology. 2013;81:442–5.
25. Chawla SN, Chang MF, Chang A, Lenoir J, Bagley DH. Effectiveness of high-frequency holmium:YAG laser stone fragmentation: the "popcorn effect". J Endourol. 2008;22:645–50.
26. Emiliani E, Talso M, Cho SY, et al. Optimal settings for the noncontact holmium:YAG stone fragmentation popcorn technique. J Urol. 2017;198:702–6.
27. Aldoukhi AH, Roberts WW, Hall TL, Teichman JMH, Ghani KR. Understanding the popcorn effect during holmium laser lithotripsy for dusting. Urology. 2018;122:52–7.
28. Tracey J, Gagin G, Morhardt D, Hollingsworth J, Ghani KR. Ureteroscopic high-frequency dusting utilizing a 120-W holmium laser. J Endourol. 2018;32:290–5.
29. Blackmon RL, Irby PB, Fried NM. Holmium:YAG (lambda = 2120 nm) versus thulium fiber (lambda = 1908 nm) laser lithotripsy. Lasers Surg Med. 2010;42:232–6.

Preoperative Assessment, Patient Preparation and Anaesthesia for Flexible Ureteroscopy

Simon K. S. Choong and Simeon West

Abstract

Ureteroscopy is a moderate risk operation, but risk factors for stone formation in certain high-risk patient groups require careful management in the perioperative period.

Preoperative assessment is an important strategy to identify and mitigate risks.

Knowledge of underlying patient comorbidities, such as obesity, diabetes, chronic kidney disease, and spinal cord injury, can help improve postoperative outcome. UTIs must be treated preoperatively, and appropriate antibiotics given at induction of anaesthesia. Anticoagulants and powerful antiplatelet medication must be managed or stopped perioperatively and a bridging plan put in place. High-risk patients should be identified and electively managed after their surgery in a high dependency unit.

Keywords

Ureteroscopy · Kidney stones · Preoperative assessment · UTI · Sepsis · Raised BMI · Spina bifida · Anticoagulation · Multidisciplinary planning

S. K. S. Choong (✉) · S. West
Institute of Urology, University College London Hospitals, London, UK
e-mail: simon.choong1@nhs.net

1 Preoperative Assessment

Preoperative assessment is key to ensuring that the patient presenting for surgery is as well prepared as possible. This ensures that complications from surgery are kept to a minimum, and on the day, cancellations are reduced.

Preoperative assessment largely comprises of the following steps:

- A face to face or telephone interview and medical case notes review to establish current problems, contemporary prescriptions and past medical and anaesthetic history. Traditionally, this was performed by the anaesthetist on the day of surgery, but it is now usual to do this within a preoperative assessment clinic. It is usually done by specialist nurses using scripted questionnaires/proformas.
- Examination, including airway assessment.
- Review of results of relevant investigations (see below).
- (MRSA) screening and risk of venous thromboembolism.
- Where risks are flagged up, nurses have access to a consultant anaesthetist for review of history/test results, or the option to have a face to face review.
- The need for further tests to give the patient more information about their individual risk. This might include risk scoring systems such as the ASA classification, P-POSSUM, SORT

G. Zeng et al. (eds.), *Flexible Ureteroscopy*, https://doi.org/10.1007/978-981-19-2936-6_6

score, and frailty assessments such as the Edmonton Scale.

A number of comorbidities are seen in association with nephrolithiasis, and these are considered here specifically:

Raised BMI—patients with an increased bodyweight are at increased risk of stones formation. Body habitus may preclude the use of Extra Corporeal Shock Wave Lithotripsy and PCNL, and so they may reflect a disproportionate number of patients presenting for retrograde stones surgeries. Obesity increases postoperative morbidity for a number of reasons. The main concerns are an increased prevalence of sleep apnoea, difficult intubation and cannulation, and postoperative hypoxaemia.

Chronic kidney disease (CKD)—the presence of kidney stones increases the risk of CKD, especially where obstruction has occurred. All patients presenting with kidney stones should be screened for CKD. Where CKD is found, anaesthetic management should be tailored using drugs to reduce the risk of worsening renal function, e.g. avoidance of non-steroidal anti-inflammatory drugs, and the use of drugs where renal clearance is important, e.g. morphine.

Diabetes—diabetic patients have an increased risk of stone formation. The principles of preoperative management of diabetes are to ensure adequate longer-term blood sugar control, e.g. HBA1C of <69 mmol/mol (or <8.5%). Achievement of this should be prioritised through consultation with the patients' endocrinologist. Where the risk of stone growth or obstruction is high, then an MDT approach should be used to balance risks of unstable diabetes and of waiting for surgery.

Other groups with contraindications to Extracorporeal Shock Wave Therapy (ECST)—a number of conditions may preclude the use of ECST in those otherwise suitable, leading to these patients presenting in increased numbers for retrograde endoscopic surgical techniques. These include those with coagulation disorders, pregnancy, and patients with implantable cardioverter defibrillators. The continued use of perioperative anticoagulants should be considered only in patients where there is a high risk of perioperative thrombotic event. A discussion with the speciality commencing the anticoagulant should be undertaken, and a risk benefit decision taken in tandem.

Spina bifida and spinal cord injuries (SCI)—the incidence of spina bifida (SB) is ~1:1000, and risk of stone disease is substantially raised in SB due to a neurogenic bladder. Similarly, SCI raises the risk of stone recurrence and urosepsis. Patients with spina bifida and SCI can present multiple concerns for anaesthesia and surgery, including reduced respiratory function, muscle spasms and contractures and (in SCI) autonomic dysreflexia (see below).

The following investigations are routinely performed on patients during their preoperative assessment for ureteroscopy.

- Full blood count and differential
- Renal profile
- Calcium and urate
- MRSA culture screen
- Urine—microscopy and culture (MSU)
- COVID-19 Swab

Timing for COVID-19 swabs should adhere to local guidelines, and advice from virology should be sought for those testing unexpectedly positive.

Additionally, as per national guidelines, the following tests are sometimes carried out:

ECG—should be done where ASA is 2 or greater, especially in patients with pre-existing hypertension or ischaemic heart disease. Consider in all patients over 65 years of age.

Lung function tests—should be done in all patients with lung disease with substantive functional limitation, i.e. ASA 3 or greater.

Echocardiogram—consider resting echocardiography if the person has a new heart murmur or signs or symptoms of heart failure, e.g. dyspnoea not of a respiratory cause, syncope, peripheral oedema, etc.

2 MSU and Management of UTI Preoperatively

Preventing infections is paramount in this surgery because this complication is the most life threatening. A urine culture must be performed before any treatment. In patients with negative urine culture, single-dose antibiotic prophylaxis most appropriate for the local resistance profile must be offered perioperatively. At induction, a cephalosporin or gentamicin or an antibiotic chosen for documented sensitivity should be given intravenously.

Infected urine in a symptomatic patient should be treated and urine rechecked to ensure the infection has been eradicated before surgery. In an asymptomatic patient with a positive urine culture, antibiotics are started 3 days before and continue into surgery, following which, a further 3–5 days of antibiotics may be given.

Stone fragments should be sent for culture and sensitivity testing in infected cases. The incidence of infectious complications after ureteroscopy is around 8–10%. Pyuria, operative duration, raised intrarenal pressures and infectious stones are risk factors for infectious complications following ureteroscopy.

Antibiotics treat bacteria in the urine but usually cannot treat bacteria inside an infected stone or penetrate the bacterial biofilms on a stent. Bacteria is released from an infected stone or a stent during an operation and a longer course of antibiotics postoperatively should be considered.

3 Patient Preparation

Prior to surgery, the following should be considered and managed

- Discussion of the type of surgery being undertaken, understanding of the consent and ensuring that shared-decision principles are followed. A discussion of major risks of the anaesthetic and surgery.
- A discussion of the options for anaesthesia (see below), an opportunity to ask questions and agreement to the anaesthetic technique proposed. Outlining plans for postoperative pain relief.
- A plan for preoperative fasting, including use of carbohydrate loading if appropriate.
- A discussion around benefits for smoking/alcohol cessation in the perioperative period.
- A plan for the perioperative management of anticoagulant drugs, diabetic drugs and other current medications.
- A process of medicine reconciliation by a pharmacist or pharmacy technician should be in place preoperatively.
- The documentation of details of any discussion in the anaesthetic record.

4 Anaesthetic Management

Anaesthetic strategies for ureteroscopy fall into three main groups: local anaesthesia alone +/− sedation, neuraxial techniques and general anaesthesia.

4.1 Local Anaesthetics

Ureteroscopy can be performed safely and with minimal discomfort under local anaesthetics alone (usually Lidocaine gel +/− penile block in males), or in combination with conscious sedation. Patients must be counselled effectively about what to expect, and plans must be made for what to do if the patient experiences undue discomfort, i.e. conversion to general anaesthesia or abandoning the procedure. This technique is often reserved for patients who would be otherwise unfit for alternative methods of anaesthesia.

4.2 Spinal Anaesthesia

This is a well-described technique using the injection of local anaesthetics +/− opioids into the intrathecal space so that dense loss of sensation is produced in the lower half of the body. Usually, hyperbaric solutions of local anaesthetics are used, e.g. 0.5% "heavy" Bupivacaine or 2% "heavy" Prilocaine. These allow the anaesthetist to use the spinal curvature to increase the block height in a controlled fashion. Block height should be appropriate to the position of the stone, T10 is sufficient for the lower tract, whilst T6 is necessary for the upper tract. Local anaesthetic choice is influenced by surgical time. Prilocaine will provide around 90 min of surgical anaesthesia, with block regression in full by around 4 h. Bupivacaine can provide surgical anaesthesia for up to 3 h, but its regression is much slower, typically up to 6 h, with a higher risk of postoperative urinary retention. For this reason, prilocaine is a better choice if same day discharge surgery is planned. Spinal anaesthesia can be combined with conscious sedation for patient comfort. Spinal anaesthesia is commonly employed in SCI to prevent/mitigate autonomic dysreflexia.

4.3 General Anaesthesia

General anaesthesia is probably the most commonly employed technique. Ureteroscopy lends itself to a wide variety of anaesthetic types. Most cases can be managed using a spontaneously breathing technique employing a laryngeal mask airway. Muscle relaxation may be required occasionally if kidney movement during respiration is excessive. Where a significant aspiration risk exists, then the airway should be secured with endotracheal intubation.

4.4 Patient Positioning

Cases are done in the lithotomy position. Special care needs to be taken to avoid nerve damage, particularly the femoral and common peroneal nerve. Do not flex hips or knees beyond 90°, hip abduction should be less than 45° and there should be neutral hip rotation. This can be challenging in patients with contractures or fixed deformities.

The lithotomy position causes major physiological alterations. Functional residual capacity decreases leading to atelectasis and hypoxia. Initial elevation of the legs drains blood into the central circulation. Mean blood pressure increases, usually without change in cardiac output. Rapid lowering of the legs from the lithotomy or Trendelenburg position acutely decreases venous return and can result in hypotension. Blood pressure measurements should be taken immediately and sequentially after the legs are lowered.

Compartment syndrome is a significant but rare risk with this position in prolonged surgeries. In the lithotomy position, ischaemia occurs from compression via the external leg supports coupled with reduced blood flow from leg elevation and compression of the popliteal artery, leading to ischaemia/reperfusion injury with subsequent compartment syndrome. Other compounding risks are the concomitant use of the Trendelenburg position, ankle dorsiflexion and hypotension/hypovolaemia.

4.5 Laser Precautions

These are taken during use of the surgical laser, e.g. use of Laser Protective Eyewear (LPE), Laser in Use signs, a closed theatre and readiness for laser fire.

4.6 Autonomic Dysreflexia

This is a potentially fatal condition of patients with SCI above T6, where a massively disordered sympathetic response occurs to stimuli below the level of the injury. Common precipitants include bladder dilation and constipation. In the surgical patient, distension of the bladder during urological procedures is a well-recognised risk factor. It consists of an increase in blood pressure of at least 20%, headache, flushing, sweating, chills, nasal congestion, piloerection and pallor. Severe hypertension leads to raised intracranial pressure (ICP), resulting in seizures and haemorrhage. Cardiac complications include myocardial ischaemia, arrhythmias and pulmonary oedema. Often patients with SCI for ureteroscopy are managed without anaesthesia, but the anaesthetist must be on standby for managing dysreflexia (this is usually by the administration of GTN/sublingual Nifedipine). Patients with a previous history are usually given a spinal anaesthetic, or occasionally a general anaesthetic.

4.7 Postoperative Management

Mild to moderate pain in the flank or groin is expected after surgery. This is usually controlled with short-acting intravenous opioids such as fentanyl initially, followed by oral opioid and paracetamol analgesics in the following days. Care must be taken not to use non-steroidal anti-inflammatory drugs if there is a risk of acute kidney injury, due to their potential for nephrotoxicity, though these can be safely used in simple cases.

Patients often experience significant discomfort related to catheters and/or ureteral stents. Treatment of this pain often requires alpha-blockers or anticholinergics.

Sepsis is the most significant postoperative complication, and it should be vigilantly watched for in patients with risk factors e.g. prolonged insertion of previous stent, significant encrustation, current urosepsis and infected stones. Consider management on high dependency for patients at significant risk, or with significant comorbidities.

5 Planning and Safety Meeting

A weekly multidisciplinary meeting involving urologists, radiologists, microbiologists, nephrologists, specialist nurses and the team is useful to assess upcoming ureteroscopy cases, especially the complex patients. The patients' cases and circumstances, blood and urine results are checked. Complex patients are optimised, and a decision is made regarding elective admission to a high-dependency unit postoperatively. These meetings help to familiarise the team with patients, ensure a smooth hospital journey and avoid unnecessary last-minute surprises and cancellations.

6 Summary

- Principle is delivery of safe and appropriate surgery and anaesthesia.
- Preoperative assessment is used to optimise patients in order to improve outcomes and reduce perioperative risk.
- MSU results must be checked and a UTI treated prior to a ureteroscopy.
- High-risk patients must be assessed by a consultant anaesthetist and considered for elective admission to a high-dependency unit postoperatively.
- Multidisciplinary planning meetings are useful to optimise safety and ensure a smooth hospital journey for the patient.

Indications and Contraindications of Flexible Ureteroscopy

Norberto Bernardo and Maximiliano López Silva

Abstract

Flexible ureteroscopy is today the most versatile dispositive for the treatment of stones located in proximal ureter and kidneys. Spectrum of recommendations for active treatment of urolithiasis with flexible ureteroscopy is wide and includes symptomatic stones and asymptomatic ones in selected patients. Flexible ureteroscopy has become the first-line therapy in most cases of stones up to 20 mm and every day more often in stones larger than 20 mm. Contraindications for flexible ureteroscopy are few, but the most important is the presence of active urinary tract infection. In this chapter, indications and contraindications will be analyzed in detail.

Keywords

Flexible ureteroscopy · Urinary stones Indications · Contraindications

N. Bernardo (✉)
Hospital de Clínicas "José de San Martín", Buenos Aires, Argentina

Universidad de Buenos Aires, Buenos Aires, Argentina

Clínica San Camilo, Buenos Aires, Argentina
e-mail: urologia@hospitaldeclinicas.uba.ar

M. L. Silva
Hospital de Clínicas "José de San Martín", Buenos Aires, Argentina

Clínica San Camilo, Buenos Aires, Argentina

1 Introduction

Flexible ureteroscopy constitutes, at present, the most versatile tool used for treating upper urinary tract kidney stones. Together with the technology developments of the last years, it has been able to evolve to solve larger stones and in more complex locations. This is a very useful tool also in the treatment of upper urinary tract tumors, which will not be addressed in this chapter.

The beginnings of the flexible ureteroscopy date back to 1987, when Demetrius Bagley introduced the modern flexible ureteroscope concept [1]. Rudimentary first steps were made with equipment full of weaknesses in comparison to the current ones, such as a difficult ureteral catheterization due to its thickness, low flow level, limited angle of deflection and low visual resolution [2]. With the technology development achieved by the end of the 1980s and beginning of the 1990s, the progress on flexible ureteroscopy was notable: reduction of the equipment diameter, use of fiber optic to capture image and lightning, expansion of the working channels, improvement of flexion, and deflection active mechanisms. In parallel, supplementary elements for the endoscopic work were also evolving: a larger variety of baskets and of lower diameter, upgraded guides, and improvements on the laser intracorporeal lithotripsy systems [3].

But it was not until the beginning of the twenty-first century that flexible ureteroscopes became the tool they are today, and this was hand

G. Zeng et al. (eds.), *Flexible Ureteroscopy*, https://doi.org/10.1007/978-981-19-2936-6_7

in hand with digital technology that allowed an optimum visualization of the urinary tract and the adoption of ureteroscopes to treat stones of greater complexity [4].

Prevalence of lithiasis in western countries is increasing, with reports estimating a minimum amount of surgeries throughout the life of a patient that suffers from urinary lithiasis of at least two procedures [5]. These data dare to minimize impassivity in the treatment, and flexible ureteroscopy is the path as a single treatment or as a complement of the percutaneous nephrolithotripsy (PCNL) to achieve it.

2 Anatomy

2.1 Ureter

Ureters are paired tubular structures in the retroperitoneum whose function is to propel urine from the renal pelvis up to the bladder. Its normal length is between 22 and 30 cm, and the inner diameter between 1.5 and 3 mm (4–9 Fr) [6]. The classic anatomical description is divided into three sections [7, 8]:

1. Proximal ureter, it is the portion from its origin in the renal pelvis, up to the top border of the sacrum.
2. Medium ureter, it is the portion from the top border of the sacrum, up to the distal border of the same bone structure.
3. Distal ureter, it is the portion from the distal border of the sacrum up to entering the bladder.

Three natural narrowed areas are described inside the path of the ureter, which are important from the endoscopic point of view: at the pyeloureteral junction level, in its beginning; in the anterior crossing of the iliac vessels; and at the vesical orifice, being this last the ureter's narrowest area [8].

From the radiological point of view, when a contrast agent is injected, we can observe the ureters descend straight from the renal pelvis, up to the high of L5 vertebra, where they get close to medial. In a lateral sight, ureters are behind the anterior border of the vertebral bodies up to the L5 height, when they become anterior [8]. It is extremely important not to confuse some variations that might appear during the radiological observation of the ureter with pathological processes (ureteral peristaltism, gonadal vessels crossing) [9].

Finally, a fundamental aspect for the management of the ureteroscopy is to understand the endoscopic ureteral anatomy.

The first point is the access to the ureter through the ureteral orifice. The ureteral orifice is located in the lateral border of the intermetal bar. The configuration of the ureteral orifice is classified into four categories according to visual appearance: grade 0 (cone shaped), grade 1 (stadium orifice), grade 2 (horseshoe orifice) and grade 3 (golf hole orifice) [10]. Normally, clear urine outflow from the orifices is visible every 20–30 s [8]. The bladder emptying may collaborate in the possibility of finding the orifices and facilitate their access.

At the ureter entry, the ureteral mucosa presents a clear pink aspect, with superficial vessels passing by its wall. At the same time, ureteral rhythmic contractions may be observed as we move forward endoscopically inside the ureter until we get to the renal pelvis [11].

2.1.1 Are Blockers Useful to Prepare the Ureter?

Alpha-blockers have been investigated in their role to reduce ureteral muscle tone and peristalsis, due to the abundance of alpha 1 receptors in distal ureter muscle [12]. A recent meta-analysis that included 1352 individuals has shown that among patients scheduled for ureteroscopy because of ureteral stones, use of preoperative a-blockers is associated with a significant reduction in the need for ureteral dilation at the time of ureteroscopy, increase in patient stone-free status at follow-up, and a higher rate of ureteroscopic access to stones, although reducing operative time. These findings offer clinicians and patients moderate quality evidence of the benefit of preoperative a-blockers for ureteroscopic removal of ureteral stones [13].

Furthermore, it is still not confirmed the possibility that a-blockers improve the chance of placing a ureteral access sheath (UAS). Porcine models have shown a better ureteral relaxation by using sedatives such as isoproterenol, [14] making easier the ascent of ureteral sheath of different diameters, although this is not proved on human yet [15].

2.2 Renal Pelvis

Knowing the intrarenal collecting system is essential for a right upper urinary tract endoscopic handling. One of the most accurate and currently used classifications is the one created by Sampaio [16]. Minor calyces might drain in an infundibulum to the major calyces, or join directly various minor calyces to form a major calyx, while major calyces flow into an infundibulum to the renal pelvis [8].

Thus, two groups of pyelocaliceal systems are evidenced:

Group A: It has two major systems (upper and lower), the medium area dependent on one of these groups. It is the mostly found configuration.

A1. The medium area is drained by minor calyces that flow into the upper and/or lower systems.

A2. The medium area is drained by crossing calyces that flow simultaneously into the upper and/or lower groups.

Group B: The medium area has a drainage independent from the upper and lower groups.

B1. A major calix drains the medium area.

B2. Multiple minor calyces drain the medium area directly into the renal pelvis [16].

Based on the previous knowledge of the anatomy supplied by the pre-surgical studies, and with the help of a radioscopic guide during the procedure, better results are achieved in relation to stone-free rate (SFR) on flexible ureteroscopy.

3 Indications

It is important to understand, in the first place, the recommendations for active treatment in urolithiasis. Nowadays, guides for the management of urolithiasis from the American Urological Association (AUA) and the European Association of Urology (EAU) summarize the main recommendations [17–19].

Recommendations of active treatment: according to the AUA guidelines, surgical treatment is indicated for patients with symptomatic stones and/or obstruction; treatment for asymptomatic stones is reserved for those cases of stone growth, associated infection, and profession or traveling reasons [18]. EAU guidelines recommend active treatment in the presence of symptoms or in case of stones bigger than 15 mm. If the stones are smaller than 15 mm and asymptomatic, treatment is indicated in case of obstruction caused by stones, stone growth, stones in high-risk patients for stone formation, infection, patient preference, comorbidity, social situation of the patient (e.g., profession or traveling), and choice of treatment [17].

Regarding the choice of treatment

In all the cases of patients with bleeding diathesis, anticoagulation, and/or antiaggregation, flexible ureteroscopy (FU) should be considered as first-line method.

On lower pole stones smaller than 10 mm, Retrograde Intra Renal Surgery (RIRS) as well as Extracorporeal Shockwave Lithotripsy (ESWL) share the first-line option, taking into account that those patients with unfavorable factors for ESWL [stones >1000 UH or distance of the skin >10 cm, steep infundibular-pelvic angle, long lower pole calyx (>10 mm), and narrow infundibulum (<5 mm)], are cases where ureteroscopy may be the first indication.

Lower pole stones between 10 and 20 mm are first-line treatment with FU or percutaneous nephrolithotomy (PCNL).

Stones of up to 20 mm in other locations are first-line treatment with FU or ESWL.

In stones >20 mm, the classic indication is PCNL, but, in selected cases, FU is a very useful alternative, considering the possibility that various procedures might be performed to achieve the stone-free stage [17, 18].

Below, each particular location will be described.

3.1 Distal and Mid Ureteral Stones

Usually stones in distal and mid ureter are treated with semirigid ureteroscopy, but in some cases, FU is needed with SFR higher than 95% [17].

3.2 Proximal Ureteral Stones

Both FU and ESWL are accepted as first-line treatment options by international guidelines [17–19]. ESWL is a less-invasive procedure, but it is associated with a lower success rate and higher retreatment rate [20]; also, Pace et al. showed a significant decrease in ESWL success after a failed initial attempt [21].

FU has showed in many publications high rate of success in the treatment of proximal ureteral stones with stone-free rates (SFR) higher than 95% [21–24].

The high success rate of fURS in the treatment of proximal ureteral stones was recently redemonstrated in a prospective, multi-institutional study that included 71 patients with solitary proximal ureteral stones with an overall SFR of 95% and SFR of 100% for stones less than 1 cm [24]. No patient had double-J previously placed, and stone-free status was determined on 4- to 6-week postoperative imaging with ultrasound or urinary X-rays.

Kijvikai et al. [25] evaluated the outcomes of ESWL and FU in the management of proximal ureteral stones less than or equal to 20 mm. They found a significantly better outcome after FU for stones over 10 mm. However, the review included heterogeneous data from studies of both semirigid ureteroscopy and FU.

3.3 Intrarenal Stones Less Than 20 mm

Both FU and ESWL are recommended as first-line management options especially for stones measuring between 11 and 20 mm in international guidelines [17–19].

Efficacy of RIRS has been reported between 80 and 95% [22, 26–28]. When it is compared with ESWL, stone-free rates (SFR) are similar in stones less than 10 mm; Pearle et al. [29] compared in a randomized controlled trial RIRS with ESWL for the management of small size (<10 mm) lower pole stones. They found no statistically significant difference of SFRs between RIRS (50%) and ESWL group (35%); ESWL showed better acceptance and higher satisfaction among patients, probably because of faster recovery to regular activities and the minimal use of anesthesia during ESWL.

When stone size increases, there is a decline in the use of ESWL with a parallel rising application of RIRS, because of better results regarding SFR [30, 31]. El-Nahas et al. [27] performed a study with lower pole stones 10–20 mm; RIRS evidenced higher SFR compared with ESWL (86.5% vs. 67.7%, respectively). In the same way, the study by Sener et al. [32] evidenced better SFR and low complication rate in favor of RIRS group of patients, but this study may have flawed results because of different stone sizes and considerations regarding lower pole infundibulopelvic angle in the different groups.

Bozkurt et al. [33] compared RIRS with Percutaneous Nephrolithotomy (PCNL) or MiniPerc in midsize stones (15–20 mm) with similar results regarding SFRs in RIRS and PCNL (89.2% vs. 92.8%, respectively) for lower pole stones 15–20 mm. They found no differences regarding complication comparing both the groups. They finally concluded an acceptable efficacy for RIRS in medium-sized stones located in the lower pole and achieved with lower morbidity. Of course PCNL is a more invasive procedure than RIRS; this generates more frequently the necessity of blood transfusions in this group of patients. Zhang et al. [30] meta-analysis evidenced the use of blood transfusion exclusively in percutaneous procedures.

3.4 Lower Pole Stones

It is well known that position of lower calyces limits spontaneous passage of stone fragments after ESWL treatment, and FU evidences higher SFR in this stones locations [34]. Kumar et al. [35] showed that both the treatment groups (FU and ESWL) had similar SFR after 3 months of procedures, but with differences in the retreatment rate. ESWL group of patients had a higher rate of retreatment compared with those treated with FU (61.1% vs. 11.1%, respectively). Additional retreatment impacts also the associated cost of the procedures.

Different strategies are used to approach lower pole stones. Differences between digital and optical scopes in the possibility to access to lower calyx are described. Dragos et al. found less effectiveness to access in the sharp angled inferior calyx and limited end-tip deflection angle for digital ureteroscopes compared with fiber optic ones (Fig. 1), because of this, when a difficult inferior calyx is going to be approached, it may be better to use a fiber optic ureteroscope [36]. The rate of failure to access in the lower calyx with FU reach up 7% [26]. Different anatomical factors play a role in this difficult accesses to inferior calyx, as infundibulopelvic angle minor than 30° and infundibular length longer than 30 mm [37]; also infundibular width may play a role when low calyx stones may not be reached, but this situation may be solved by laser incision [37].

If it is possible, an attempt to relocate the stone with a nitinol basket to a more favorable position (upper pole preferentially or renal pelvis) has to be performed [38] (Fig. 2). This maneuver helps to reduce the possibility of rupture of the scope during the procedure and facilitates stone target. At the same time, stones and their fragments located in upper pole makes easier re-entries with the scope to grasp and extract fragments (basketing technique) or improves the possibility of spontaneous pass of fragments (dusting technique) [1].

In those stones of maximum diameter larger than 10 mm, usually it is not possible to relocate it in upper pole by the use of grasps. These cases require performing laser lithotripsy in situ, some-

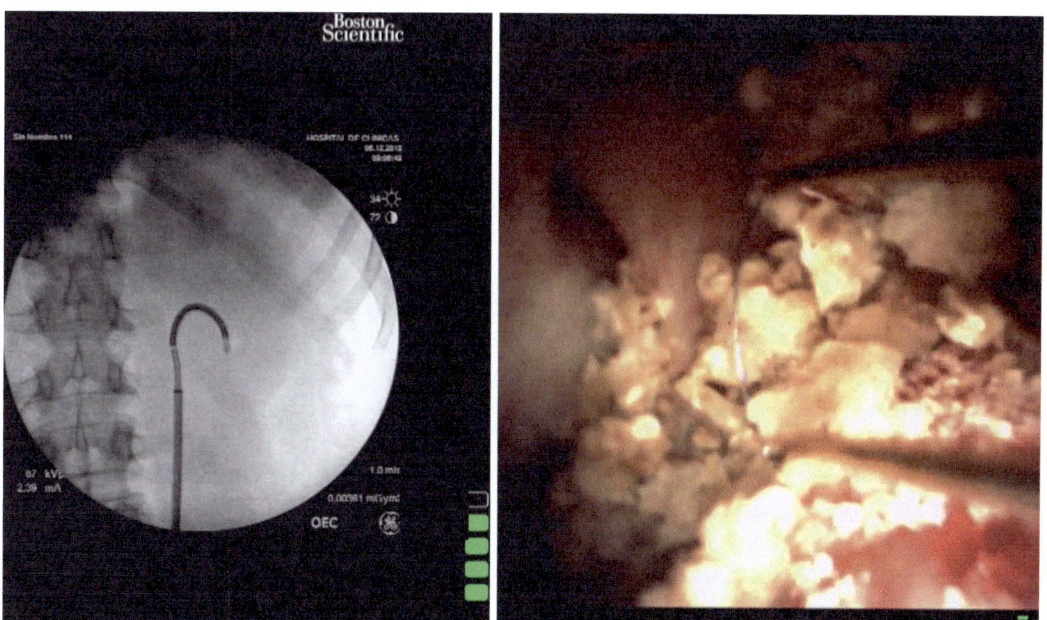

Fig. 1 Laser lithotripsy in lower calyx

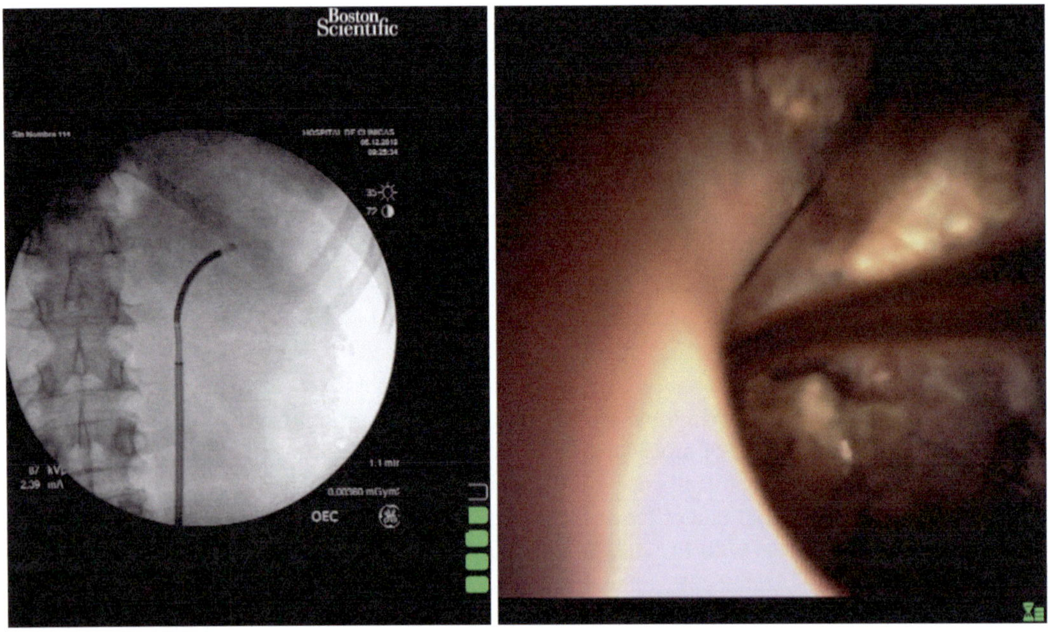

Fig. 2 Stone relocation in an upper calyx to perform laser lithotripsy

times with the scope in maximum deflection, increasing the risk of laser fiber failure and also the risk of ureteroscope damage [39]. A recommendation for this kind of cases is to insert the laser fiber with the minimal deflection and after the fiber reaches the top of the scope perform the required deflection; this reduces the risk of damage of the working channel. It is important to consider that with the fiber in place, ureteroscope cannot reach its maximum deflection, and the access to lower poles with acute angles may be challenging [40]. To solve this problem, in the present, we have new laser fibers with ball-tip shape. The objective of this kind of shape is to reduce the friction between the laser fiber and working channel when the scope is deflected [41]. The issue with this new fiber is durability; special tip of this fiber is lost after the first minute of use because of fiber degradation, especially if high pulse energy is being used [42]; therefore, this fiber is able to be inserted only once with the scope in maximum deflection.

Haddad et al. showed that laser fiber diameter, curve, and settings to treat stones are important with regard to fiber durability. The use of dusting parameters in laser devices may break 272-µm fibers when the fiber curve reaches 9 mm or below, while the use of fragmentation parameters may break these fibers when the curve reaches 12 mm. In 365-µm fibers, the curves to generate rupture are 9 mm in dusting mode and 15 mm in fragmentation mode. Due to previous descirption regarding fiber fragility, to prevent fiber rupture, it is better to use the thinner fiber as possible and in dusting parameters [43].

Bozkurt et al. [44] performed a retrospective study comparing FU and PCNL (including MiniPerc) for the treatment of lower pole stones less than 20 mm. They showed a similar SFR in both the groups without differences regarding complications rate. Surgical time was shorter in PCNL and MiniPerc group, but higher fluoroscopy time and longer stay were found in this group [45].

3.5 Intrarenal Stones Larger Than 20 mm

Usually standard treatment of stones larger than 20 mm is PCNL over RIRS, but, in the last years, technology and technique advancements have dramatically increased the therapeutic potential of RIRS. Recent studies have reported that RIRS can offer an acceptable efficacy with low morbidity in selected patients with large intrarenal stones [30, 46, 47], especially in high-risk patients.

One of the first data about this issue is by Grasso et al. [23]. They treated 45 large intrarenal stones using FU and Holmium:YAG laser lithotripsy. The SFR of residual fragments less than 2 mm was achieved in 76% of FU patients after first procedure and 91% after second FU with low post surgical complications rate.

Aboumarzouk et al. [47] published a meta-analysis with a total of 445 patients treated with FU and with stones larger than 20 mm. The mean stone-free rate was 93.7% (77–96.7%), with an average of 1.6 procedures per patient. The mean stone size was 25 mm. This is comparable with PCNL success rate. It is expected that the treatment of larger stones may be associated with a greater FU complication rate. In their meta-analysis, Aboumarzouk et al. evidenced 10.1% of complication rate with major complications (including sub-capsular hematoma, obstructive pyelonephritis, steinstrasse) reported in 5.3% of the cases, while minor complications (specially self-limited hematuria and post-procedure fever) were reported in 4.8% of the cases. In the subgroup of patients with stones between 20 and 30 mm, no major complications were revealed [45].

In a paired matched analysis, performed by Akman et al. [46], 34 patients with stones between 20 and 40 mm were studied comparing FU with PCNL. Focusing the analysis on the first procedure, there is a SFR in favor of PCNL (73.5% for FU vs. 91.2% for PCNL), but this difference decrease when is taken into account the second FU procedure, achieving a final SFR of 88.2%. Surgical time is shorter in PCNL with longer hospital stay as is expected and without differences regarding complication rate.

The use of UAS in some publication was reported as a factor to improve success [45]. This is because UAS could facilitate re-entries to the kidney and improve visibility in some cases, but is not fully demonstrated.

However, FU was found to be significantly inferior in treating intrarenal stones greater than 20 mm compared to MiniPerc (18 Fr tract) in another matched-pair analysis [20]. The success rate was only 43.4% after the first FU procedure.

In conclusion, for kidney stones bigger than 20 mm, RIRS cannot be recommended as first-line treatment because SFR is lower than that for PCNL and many times staged procedures are needed. But, for those patients with contraindications in percutaneous procedures, RIRS is a first-line option [17].

3.6 Endoscopic Combined Intrarenal Surgery

In order to reduce the number of tracts utilized and its associated complications, FU is also described together to PCNL. Both the procedures used in a combined fashion are really useful to treat staghorn stones [45].

Hamamoto et al. [48] reported 42 patients with staghorn stones treated with ECIRS with an SFR of 83.3%, using only one percutaneous access and FU after the procedure.

3.7 Flexible Ureteroscopy in Special Situations

3.7.1 Anticoagulated Patients

PCNL and ESWL are contraindicated in anticoagulated patients, because of significant bleeding risk; meanwhile FU has been proven to be safe and effective in this group of patients [45].

Watterson et al. [49] performed a retrospective study with patients treated with FU and with known and uncorrected bleeding diathesis. They analyzed 25 patients with urinary stones who were treated with ureteroscopy and endoscopic lithotripsy with holmium laser. Seventeen of the patients were receiving warfarin as medication, three patients suffered of liver disfunction, and one patient suffered of von Willebran's disease. Overall, the stone-free rate was 96% (27 of 28 cases) and were completed successfully without significant complication in Holmium:YAG patients.

Similar findings were report by Turna et al. [50]. In their publication, this group examined the safety of FU and Holmium:YAG laser lithotripsy for the treatment of kidney stones in patients under anticoagulant treatment. They found no difference in intra and post surgical complications with control group with similar SFR rates.

Studies concluded that upper tract urinary calculi in patients with uncorrected bleeding diathesis can be safely managed with holmium laser, and lithotripsy with holmium laser without correcting hemostatic parameters preoperatively reduces thromboembolic complications and costs associated with hospital stay.

The rest of special situations such as obesity, pregnancy, urolithiasis in children, and lithiasis anatomic anomalies will be developed in detail in Chaps. 14 and 15.

4 Contraindications

There are a few contraindications to perform flexible ureteroscopy (FU).

General or spinal anesthesia are required to perform FU; therefore, in patients with anesthetics contraindications, FU cannot be performed.

A relative contraindication is the presence of bleeding diatheses or ongoing anticoagulant or antiplatelet therapy. This must be assessed on each patient indication, but usually FU can be performed safely in this group of patients [51] as previously described in Sect. 3.7.

Urinary tract anatomic difficulties may constitute a contraindication, as impassable anatomy involving the ureteral orifice, prostate, trigone, or distal ureter due to cancer or other disorders, or ureteral narrowing [52].

But, the most important contraindication of FU is the presence of active urinary tract infection, because performing FU in this condition may result in urinary sepsis and even patients' death in severe sepsis events. In the presence of these clinical scenarios, the first step is to perform adequate resolution before FU. This may include the placement of double-J stent or nephrostomy tube to drain urinary tract and the use of specific antibiotics [53].

There is a lack of evidence in endoscopic surgery about the use of prophylactic antibiotics in patients with presurgical negative urine culture [17], but actual recommendations are to use prior to surgery in a one-dose scheme of first-generation cephalosporin or a fluoroquinolone [54, 55].

The use of ureteral access sheath (UAS) during FU is another topic without definitive guideline recommendations about placing and the suggested diameter; some publications have demonstrated that its use may prevent pressure increasing during FU with reduction for the risk of lymphatic and venous bacterial backflow [17, 56, 57]. This reduces the possibility of bacterial dissemination and endotoxin resorption during stone fragmentation [53, 58].

Infectious complications in many opportunities occur because of high-pressure irrigation in the urinary tract. It is fundamental to check during the procedures the continuous saline drainage form the UAS (in the case of this is being used); the use of endoluminal isoproterenol irrigation could be useful in cases where high pressure is needed [59].

An important topic to highlight the way to reduce septic complications is surgical time; this may not be longer than 2 h, with staged procedures, if necessary [60]. During postoperative period, the majority of cases of septic complication occur within 6 h after surgery, because of this a careful observation during the first 6 postoperative hours is needed [53]. It is important to keep safety rules to avoid the increase of risks [53].

Finally, in the last years, some interesting tools, as procalcitonin serum levels, have been developed to identify early the septic patient and to choose a fast antimicrobial treatment to obtain a better and faster resolution of this clinical scenarios [61, 62].

5 Conclusions

Flexible ureteroscopy has been proven to be an effective and safe treatment for urolithiasis. Together with technological advances, indications have increased (and probably may increase even more in the next years). Contraindications for FU are really few, highlighting the importance of treating urinary infectious disease prior to performing the procedure.

References

1. Doizi S, Traxer O. Flexible ureteroscopy: technique, tips and tricks. Urolithiasis. 2018;46(1):47–58.
2. Takayasu H, Aso Y. Recent development for pyeloureteroscopy: guide tube method for its introduction into the ureter. J Urol. 1974;112(2):176–8.
3. Geavlete P, Multescu R, Geavlete B. Pushing the boundaries of ureteroscopy: current status and future perspectives. Nat Rev Urol. 2014;11(7):373–82.
4. Andonian S, Okeke Z, Smith AD. Digital ureteroscopy: the next step. J Endourol. 2008;22:603–6.
5. Johnson B, Best S, Nakada S, Tracy C, Steinberg R, Thomas L, Marien T, Miller N, Kolitz E, Cohen A, Pearle M, Lotan Y, Antonelli J. Initial Results from the M-STONE Group: a multi-center collaboration to study treatment outcomes in nephrolithiasis evaluation. J Endourol. 2020;34(9):919–23.
6. Zelenko N, Coll D, Rosenfeld AT, Smith RC. Normal ureter size on unenhanced helical CT. AJR Am J Roentgenol. 2004;182(4):1039–41.
7. Frober R. Surgical anatomy of the ureter. BJU Int. 2007;100(4):949–65.
8. Testut L, Latarjet A. Human anatomy. Tomo IV. Barcelona: Salvat Editors; 1968.
9. Bergman H. The ureter. 2nd ed. New York: Springer; 1981.
10. Lyon RP, Marshall S, Tanagho EA. The ureteral orifice: its configuration and competency. J Urol. 1969;102(4):504–9.
11. Hamamoto S, Okada S, Inoue T, Sugino T, Unno R, Taguchi R, Ando R, Okada A, Miura H, Matsuda T, Yasui T. Prospective evaluation and classification of endoscopic findings for ureteral calculi. Sci Rep. 2020;10(1):12292.
12. Johnson LJ, Davenport D, Venkatesh R. Effects of alphablockade on ureteral peristalsis and intrapelvic pressure in an in vivo stented porcine model. J Endourol. 2016;30:417–21.
13. Alsaikhan B, Koziarz A, Lee J, Pace K. Preoperative alpha-blockers for ureteroscopy for ureteral stones: a systematic review and meta-analysis of randomized controlled trials. J Endourol. 2020;34(1):33–41.
14. Lildal S, Andreassen K, Christiansen F, Jung H, Pedersen M, Osther P. Pharmacological relaxation of the ureter when using ureteral access sheaths during ureterorenoscopy. Ther Adv Urol. 2016;2016:8064648.
15. De Coninck V, Keller E, Rodrıguez-Monsalve M, Audouin M, Doizi S, Traxer O. Systematic review of ureteral access sheaths: facts and myths. BJU Int. 2018;122:959–69.
16. Sampaio FJB. Anatomic classification of the pelviocaliceal system. Urologic and radiologic implications. In: Sampaio FJB, Uflacker R, editors. Renal anatomy applied to urology, endourology, and interventional radiology. New York: Thieme Medical Publishers; 1993. p. 1–5.
17. Türk C, Neisius A, Petřík A, Seitz C, Skolarikos A, Somani B, Thomas K, Gambaro G. EAU guidelines on urolithiasis. In Presented at the EAU Annual Congress Milan 2021. 2021.
18. Assimos D, Krambeck A, Miller N, Monga M, Murad M, Nelson C, Pace K, Pais V Jr, Pearle M, Preminger G, Razvi H, Shah O, Matlaga B. Surgical management of stones: American Urological Association/Endourological Society Guideline, Part I. J Urol. 2016;196(4):1153–60.
19. Assimos D, Krambeck A, Miller N, Monga M, Murad M, Nelson C, Pace K, Pais V Jr, Pearle M, Preminger G, Razvi H, Shah O, Matlaga B. Surgical management of stones: American Urological Association/Endourological Society Guideline, Part II. J Urol. 2016;196(4):1161–9.
20. Aboumarzouk OM, Kata SG, Keeley FX, McClinton S, Nabi G. Extracorporeal shock wave lithotripsy (ESWL) versus ureteroscopic management for ureteric calculi (review). Cochrane Database Syst Rev. 2012;5:1–44.
21. Pace KT, Weir MJ, Tariq N, Honey RJ. Low success rate of repeat shock wave lithotripsy for ureteral stones after failed initial treatment. J Urol. 2000;164:1905–7.
22. Sofer M, Watterson JD, Wollin TA, Nott L, Razvi H, Denstedt JD. Holmium:YAG laser lithotripsy for upper urinary tract calculi in 598 patients. J Urol. 2002;167:31–4.
23. Grasso M, Conlin M, Bagley D. Retrograde ureteropyeloscopic treatment of 2 cm or greater upper urinary tract and minor staghorn calculi. J Urol. 1998;160:346–51.
24. Hyams ES, Monga M, Pearle MS, Antonelli JA, Semins MJ, Assimos DG, et al. A prospective, multi-institutional study of flexible ureteroscopy for proximal ureteral stones <2 cm. J Urol. 2014;193:165–9.
25. Kijvikai K, Haleblian GE, Preminger GM, de la Rosette J. Shock wave lithotripsy or ureteroscopy for the management of proximal ureteral calculi: an old discussion revisited. J Urol. 2007;178:1157–63.
26. Grasso M, Ficazzola M. Retrograde ureteropyeloscopy for lower pole caliceal calculi. J Urol. 1999;162:1904–8.

27. El-Nahas AR, Ibrahim HM, Youssef RF, Sheir K. Flexible ureterorenoscopy versus extracorporeal shock wave lithotripsy for treatment of lower pole stones of 10–20 mm. BJU Int. 2012;110:898–902.
28. Cohen J, Cohen S, Grasso M. Ureteropyeloscopic treatment of large, complex intrarenal and proximal ureteral calculi. BJU Int. 2014;111:E127–31.
29. Pearle MS, Lingeman JE, Leveillee R, et al. Prospective, randomized trial comparing shock wave lithotripsy and ureteroscopy for lower pole caliceal calculi 1 cm or less. J Urol. 2005;173:2005–9.
30. Zhang W, Zhou T, Wu T, Gao X, Peng Y, Xu C, Chen Q, Song R, Sun Y. Retrograde intrarenal surgery versus percutaneous nephrolithotomy versus extracorporeal shockwave lithotripsy for treatment of lower pole renal stones: a meta-analysis and systematic review. J Endourol. 2015;29(7):745–59.
31. Chung BI, Aron M, Hegarty NJ, Desai MM. Ureteroscopic versus percutaneous treatment for medium-size (1–2-cm) renal calculi. J Endourol. 2008;22:343–6.
32. Sener NC, Imamoglu MA, Bas O, et al. Prospective randomized trial comparing shock wave lithotripsy and flexible ureterorenoscopy for lower pole stones smaller than 1 cm. Urolithiasis. 2014;42:127–31.
33. Bozkurt OF, Resorlu B, Yildiz Y, et al. Retrograde intrarenal surgery versus percutaneous nephrolithotomy in the management of lower-pole renal stones with a diameter of 15–20 mm. J Endourol. 2011;25:1131–5.
34. Elbahnasy AM, Shalhav AL, Hoenig DM, Elashry OM, Smith DS, Mcdougall EM, et al. Lower caliceal stone clearance after shock wave lithotripsy or ureteroscopy: the impact of lower pole radiographic anatomy. J Urol. 1998;159:676–82.
35. Kumar A, Vasudeva P, Nanda B, Kumar N, Das MK, Jha SK. A prospective randomized comparison between shock wave lithotripsy and flexible ureterorenoscopy for lower caliceal stones 2 cm: a single-center experience. J Endourol. 2015;29:575–9.
36. Dragos LB, Somani BK, Sener ET, Buttice S, Proietti S, Ploumidis A, Iacoboaie CT, Doizi S, Traxer O. Which flexible ureteroscopes (digital vs. fiber-optic) can easily reach the difficult lower pole calices and have better end-tip deflection: in vitro study on K-box. A PETRA evaluation. J Endourol. 2017;31(7):630–7.
37. Jessen JP, Honeck P, Knoll T, Wendt-Nordahl G. Flexible ureterorenoscopy for lower pole stones: influence of the collecting system's anatomy. J Endourol. 2014;28:146–51.
38. Auge BK, Dahm P, Wu NZ, Preminger GM. Ureteroscopic management of lower-pole renal calculi: technique of calculus displacement. J Endourol. 2001;15(8):835–8.
39. Seto C, Ishiura Y, Egawa M, Komatsu K, Namiki M. Durability of working channel in flexible ureteroscopes when inserting ureteroscopic devices. J Endourol. 2006;20(3):223–6.
40. Baghdadi M, Emiliani E, Talso M, Servián P, Barreiro A, Orosa A, Proietti S, Traxer O. Comparison of laser fiber passage in ureteroscopic maximum deflection and their influence on deflection and irrigation: do we really need the ball tip concept? World J Urol. 2017;35(2):313–8.
41. Shin RH, Lautz JM, Cabrera FJ, Shami CJ, Goldsmith ZG, Kuntz NJ, Kaplan AG, Neisius A, Simmons WN, Preminger GM, Lipkin ME. Evaluation of novel ball-tip holmium laser fiber: impact on ureteroscope performance and fragmentation efficiency. J Endourol. 2016;30(2):189–94.
42. Kronenberg P, Traxer O. Lithotripsy performance of specially designed laser fiber tips. J Urol. 2016;195(5):1606–12.
43. Haddad M, Emiliani E, Rouchausse Y, Coste F, Doizi S, Berthe L, Butticè S, Somani B, Traxer O. Impact of the curve diameter and laser settings on laser fiber fracture. J Endourol. 2017;31(9):918–21.
44. Bozkurt OF, Resorlu B, Yildiz Y, Can CE, Unsal A. Retrograde intrarenal surgery versus percutaneous nephrolithotomy in the management of lower-pole renal stones with a diameter of 15–20 mm. J Endourol. 2011;25:1131–5.
45. Alenezi D. Flexible ureteroscopy: technological advancements, current indications and outcomes in the treatment of urolithiasis. Asian J Urol. 2015;2(3):133–41.
46. Akman T, Binbay M, Ozgor F, et al. Comparison of percutaneous nephrolithotomy and retrograde flexible nephrolithotripsy for the management of 2–4 cm stones: a matched-pair analysis. BJU Int. 2012;109:1384–9.
47. Aboumarzouk OM, Monga M, Kata SG, Traxer O, Somani B. Flexible ureteroscopy and laser lithotripsy for stones >2 cm: a systematic review and meta-analysis. J Endourol. 2012;26:1257–63.
48. Hamamoto S, Yasui T, Okada A, Koiwa S, Taguchi K, Itoh Y, et al. Efficacy of endoscopic combined intrarenal surgery in the prone split-leg position for staghorn calculi. J Endourol. 2015;29:19–24.
49. Watterson JD, Girvan AR, Cook AJ, Beiko DT, Nott L, Auge BK, et al. Safety and efficacy of holmium: YAG laser lithotripsy in patients with bleeding diatheses. J Urol. 2002;168:442–5.
50. Turna B, Stein RJ, Smaldone MC, Santos BR, Kefer JC, Jackman SV, et al. Safety and efficacy of flexible ureterorenoscopy and holmium:YAG lithotripsy for intrarenal stones in anticoagulated cases. J Urol. 2008;179:1415–9.
51. Sharaf A, Amer T, Somani BK, Aboumarzouk OM. Ureteroscopy in patients with bleeding diatheses, anticoagulated, and on anti-platelet agents: a systematic review and meta-analysis of the literature. J Endourol. 2017;31(12):1217–25.
52. Wason S, Monfared S, Ionson A, Leslie S. Ureteroscopy. Orlando: Stat Pearls Publishing LLC; 2021.

53. Cindolo L, Castellan P, Scoffone C, Cracco C, Celia A, Paccaduscio A, Schips L, Proietti S, Breda A, Giusti G. Mortality and flexible ureteroscopy: analysis of six cases. World J Urol. 2016;34(3):305–10.
54. Gravas S, et al. Postoperative infection rates in low risk patients undergoing percutaneous nephrolithotomy with and without antibiotic prophylaxis: a matched case control study. J Urol. 2012;188:843.
55. Chew BH, et al. A single dose of intraoperative antibiotics is sufficient to prevent urinary tract infection during ureteroscopy. J Endourol. 2016;30:63.
56. Jung H, Nørby B, Frimodt-Møller PC, Osther PJ. Endoluminal isoproterenol irrigation decreases renal pelvic pressure during flexible ureterorenoscopy: a clinical randomized, controlled study. Eur Urol. 2018;54(6):1404–13.
57. Mc Aleer IM, Kaplan GW, Bradley JS, Carroll SF, Griffith DP. Endotoxin content in renal calculi. J Urol. 2003;169(5):1813–4.
58. Stern JM, Yiee J, Park S. Safety and efficacy of ureteral access sheaths. J Endourol. 2007;21:119–23.
59. Jung H, Nørby B, Frimodt-Møller PC, Osther PJ. Endoluminal isoproterenol irrigation decreases renal pelvic pressure during flexible ureterorenoscopy: a clinical randomized, controlled study. Eur Urol. 2008;54(6):1404–13.
60. Giusti G, Proietti S, Peschechera R, et al. Sky is no limit for ureteroscopy: extending the indications and special circumstances. World J Urol. 2015;33(2):257–73.
61. Salluh JI, Nobre V, Povoa P. Using procalcitonin to guide antimicrobial duration in sepsis: asking the same questions will not bring different answers. Crit Care. 2014;18(3):142–4.
62. Zheng J, Li Q, Fu W, et al. Procalcitonin as an early diagnostic and monitoring tool in urosepsis following percutaneous nephrolithotomy. Urolithiasis. 2015;43(1):41–7.

Clinical and Operating Room Setup for Flexible Ureteroscopy

Abdulmalik Addar, Ahmed Aljuhayman, and Saeed Bin Hamri

Abstract

Optimizing the setting inside the operating room is a vital element in all surgical procedures including flexible ureteroscopy. In this chapter, we address how to optimize and achieve a safe and efficient environment for flexible ureteroscopy. It is crucial for all personnel in the urology operating team to familiarize themselves with all equipment, consumables, and the organization inside the operating room. This may be tailored to individual surgeon preference; however, we present here our style of setting up the operating room which is a combination of the most established setups among urologists.

Keywords

Flexible ureteroscopy · OR setup · Patient positioning · Clinical setup · Cystoscopy table · Operating table

Flexible ureteroscopy is a procedure that utilizes expensive and highly intensive instruments. The setup is space limited, and any misplaced piece or poor organization will cause major disturbance and frustration that will cause inconvenience to the surgeon and staff and place the patient at risk of potential harms and injuries. This will also prolong operative time and may cause financial losses by wasting and damaging instruments or improper use of consumables.

Safety is critical inside the operating room. In order to achieve a safe environment, certain knowledge must be obtained. Being familiar with potential hazards and how to prevent and recognize them will lead to successful outcomes. Hypothermia in the setting of flexible ureteroscopy can be catastrophic and affect patient overall morbidity. The two main causes of hypothermia are anesthetic agents (by vasodilatation) and conductive heat loss. This may be hindered by using warmed air blankets, and warm irrigation and intravenous fluids. Another important element is patient positioning [1, 2]. Patient positioning is the responsibility of all members of the team including anesthetist and anesthetist assistant,

A. Addar
Division of Urology, College of Medicine, King Abdulaziz Medical City, King Abdullah International Medical Research Center, King Saud bin Abdulaziz University for Health Sciences, Riyadh, Saudi Arabia

A. Aljuhayman
Department of Urology, College of Medicine, Majmaah University, Al-Majmaah, Saudi Arabia

S. Bin Hamri (✉)
Division of Urology, Department of Surgery, Ministry of National Guard Health Affairs, King Abdullah International Medical Research Center. College of Medicine, King Saud bin Abdulaziz University for Health Sciences, Riyadh, Saudi Arabia

G. Zeng et al. (eds.), *Flexible Ureteroscopy*, https://doi.org/10.1007/978-981-19-2936-6_8

nursing team, and surgeons. In flexible ureteroscopy, patients are positioned when anatomically feasible in a lithotomy position. Many injuries, especially neuropathic and thrombotic, may arise from improper positioning as a result of excessive stretching and prolonged compression [3, 4]. The hamstring muscles should be relaxed and padding applied on pressure points in order prevent nerve injury [3, 4]. A crucial element is to position both lower limbs concurrently and flexion of the hip joint to 80°–100° and abduction at 30°–40°. The leg may be slightly extended, and the hip abducted; this will help in decreasing the angulation of the ureter. Particular attention should also be made to the upper limb safety during positioning and to securing the patient to the operating table via a safety belt [4, 5].

Prepping the skin is done using antiseptic agents usually iodine as it is less irritative than alcohol agents on genitalia. The area extending from the mons pubis superiorly down to the perineum inferiorly and laterally to the groin is prepped, then a drape is applied ideally only exposing the penis in male and the vagina in female.

The basic equipment needed during flexible ureteroscopy on the instruments table are simple and include a prep tray, cystoscope and its adjuncts, drapes for cystoscope, ureteroscope and C-arm, irrigation tubing, light cables, guidewires, wet basin with wet sponges and syringe, dry sponges in a dry area and contrast and a contrast syringe (Fig. 1). The table should be well organized so that all the urologists have all instruments within their grasp. Our style is to divide the instruments table into four quadrants: (1) a dirty corner where all dirty and used instruments are placed within reach of the circulating nurse, (2) a wet corner where a wet basin with wet sponges, syringes, instruments, contrast basin, and lubricating gel, (3) a dry corner with dry gauze and dry equipment, (4) a working corner where working instruments are placed (Fig. 2). Supplementary equipment such as forceps including grasping and biopsy, baskets, ureteric and urethral catheters, lithotripsy instruments, ureteral access sheaths, dilators, and special guidewires among others should not be opened initially. They should be close by on a supplementary instruments table in the operating room and only opened when asked for in order to minimize wastage. Before opening these supplementary instruments, the circulating nurse should double check with the surgeon, assistant, or scrub nurse that it is the one required in this step.

X-ray use via a C-arm fluoroscopy is part of a standard flexible ureteroscopy procedure. The C-arm is ideally placed on the right side of the patient adjacent to the endoscopic tower; this is usually at surgeon's preference [6]. Being acquainted with radiation safety is a fundamental part of being

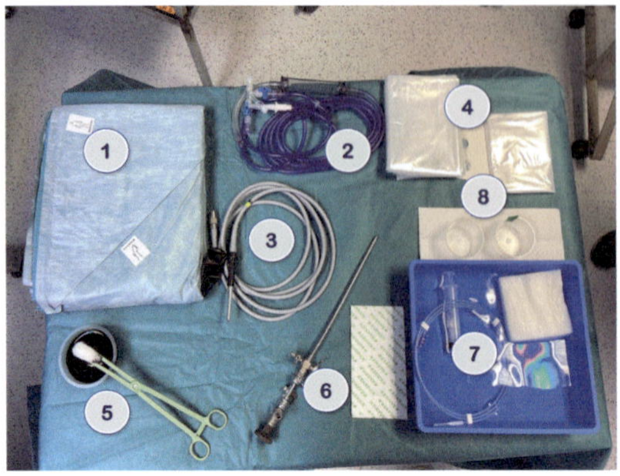

Fig. 1 Initial table preparation; 1: sterile drape, 2: irrigation pump, 3: light cable, 4: camera head and C-arm drapes, 5: prep set, 6: cystoscope, 7: wet basin with wet sponges and syringe, 8: containers for lubricating gel and contrast

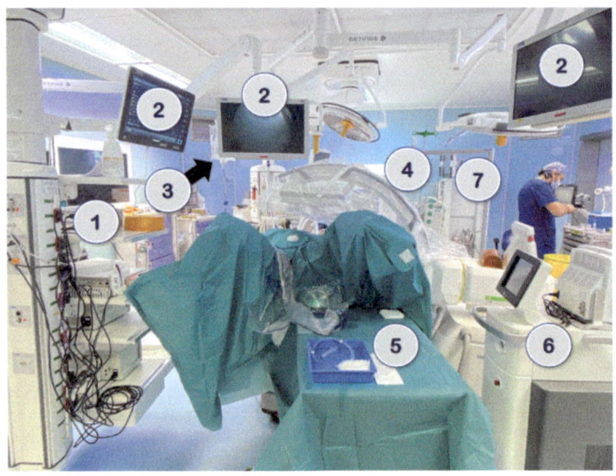

Fig. 2 Room layout, 1: endoscopic tower, 2: screens for endoscopy and fluoroscopy, 3: irrigation fluids, 4: C-arm, 5: instruments table, 6: laser machine, 7: X-ray shield for anesthetist

inside an operating room where flexible ureteroscopy is being conducted. All staff should wear all-around X-ray gowns including a thyroid collar or an X-ray shield for non-circulating team members. The person operating the C-arm should alert all personnel inside the operating room before using the machine to ensure that accidental exposure is prevented. The C-arm should be placed contralateral to the endoscopic tower and laser machine.

A crucial player in the setup of the operating room is the scrub nurse. Her/his role is to make sure that all the equipment is present, assembled, and ready for use. She/he is also responsible for overseeing the general setup and prepared in anticipation for all what might arise during the procedure. She/he also ensures the integrity of the sterile field by overseeing proper handling of instruments and the sterility of the surgical environment and breaches that may arise.

By dividing the operating theater into the mentioned setting, flexible ureteroscopy would be a more efficient, safe, and dynamic procedure. Having the positions of endoscopic tower, laser machine, instruments table, and C-arm as mentioned will provide more space in the operating theatre allowing for easier access of instruments. This ergonomic organization allows clear eye-to-eye contact between the surgeon and anesthetist and keeps communication easy at emergencies or for surgeon request, for example, asking for apnea during lithotripsy (Fig. 3). This setup prevents crossing of cables which minimizes danger in the operating room as well as helps in a smooth flowing procedure as crossing of instruments and guidewires is avoided. When it comes to organizing the instrument table into the mentioned areas, we found that flexible ureteroscopy became more efficient in terms of operative time and reproducibility of the procedure.

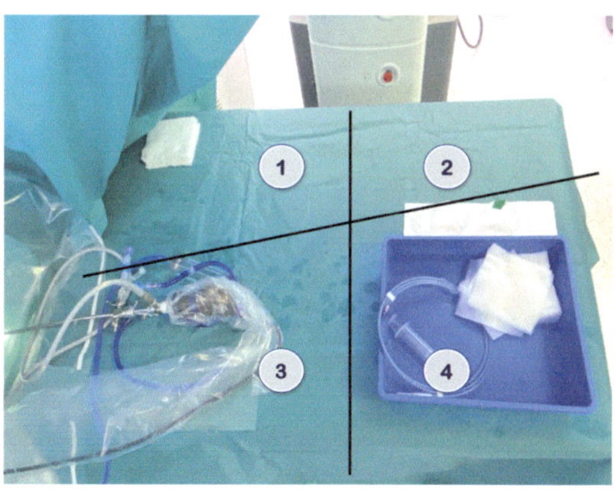

Fig. 3 Working table organization during procedure 1: dry corner, 2: dirty corner, 3: working corner, 4: wet corner

This helps the surgeon's assistant or resident to quickly access needed instruments and avoid wasting of disposables where they might fall into the ground or lose sterility by touching surfaces. Furthermore, we found it more of a dynamic process where the assistant can simultaneously hand on instruments to the surgeon and put back any disposable handed by the surgeon into its designated area. The surgeon's assistant or resident also plays a major role in helping with introducing disposables, holding baskets, and pumping fluid which all accumulate into a quick, safe, and efficient procedure. By doing so, the assistant holds the role of assistant and scrub nurse at the same time, which makes the environment less crowded.

It is the authors' experience that applying the mentioned organization and setting would facilitate flexible ureteroscopy and help provide a safe and efficient structure to the procedure. Furthermore, it helps as well in the teaching process where a well-formed structure of setting, steps, and roles that can be reproduced in each flexible ureteroscopy. The proposed design provides a safe environment with less operative time and cost effectiveness to flexible ureteroscopy.

References

1. Madrid E, Urrútia G, Roqué i Figuls M, Pardo-Hernandez H, Campos JM, Paniagua P, Maestre L, Alonso-Coello P. Active body surface warming systems for preventing complications caused by inadvertent perioperative hypothermia in adults. Cochrane Database Syst Rev. 2016;4:CD009016. https://doi.org/10.1002/14651858.CD009016.pub2.
2. Basillote J, Lee D, Eichel L, Clayman R. Ureteroscopes: flexible, rigid, and semirigid. Urol Clin N Am. 2004;31:21–32. https://doi.org/10.1016/S0094-0143(03)00094-6.

3. Graversen JA, et al. Ureteroscopy: patient positioning and room setup. In: Monga M, editor. Ureteroscopy. Current clinical urology. Totowa: Humana Press; 2013. https://doi.org/10.1007/978-1-62703-206-3_19.
4. American Society of Anesthesiologists. Advisory for the prevention of perioperative peripheral neuropathies 2018: an updated report by the American Society of Anesthesiologists Task Force on Prevention of Perioperative Peripheral Neuropathies. Anesthesiology. 2018;128(1):11–26.
5. Smith A. Smith's textbook of endourology. 2nd ed. Hamilton: BC Decker; 2007. p. 67–75.
6. Giusti G, Proietti S, Villa L, Cloutier J, Rosso M, Gadda G, Doizi S, Suardi N, Montorsi F, Gaboardi F, Traxer O. Current standard technique for modern flexible ureteroscopy: tips and tricks. Eur Urol. 2016;70(1):188–94.

How to Perform Flexible Ureteroscopy for Renal Stones

Kandarp Parikh, Ravi Jain, Rahul Soni, and Aditya Parikh

Keywords

Renal stone · Flexible ureteroscopy · RIRS · Ergonomics · Procedure

Abbreviations

AUA	American Urology Association
CT IVU	Computed tomography intravenous urography
EAU	European Association of Urology
ESWL	Extracorporeal shock wave lithotripsy
Fr	French
FURS	Flexible ureteroscopy
Ho:YAG	Holmium:YAG
HPGP	Hydrogen peroxide gas plasma
IRP	Intrarenal pressure
IVU	Intravenous urography
KUB	Kidney ureter bladder
NCCT KUB	Non-contrast computed tomography kidney ureter bladder
PCNL	Percutaneous nephrolithotomy
PCS	Pelvi-calyceal system
PTFE	Polytetrafluoroethylene
RGP	Retrograde pyelography
RIRS	Retrograde intrarenal surgery
SAP	Single action pump
TCC	Transitional cell carcinoma
UAS	Ureteric access sheath
UO	Ureteric orifice
UPJ	Uretero-pelvic junction

Urolithiasis is a common health problem worldwide causing a lot of human suffering and morbidity with grave socio-economic concerns [1]. Recent EAU guidelines clearly mention Retrograde Intra Renal Surgery (RIRS) as the treatment modality of choice for renal calculi less than 2 cm [2]. Ureteroscopy evolved way back in 1964 when Marshall first reported ureteroscopy with fiberoscope, whereas flexible ureteroscopy (fURS) was introduced by Bagley in 1987 [3, 4].

Since its inception, the technology and technique of RIRS have evolved manyfold. The art and craft of a successful surgery depend on the proper technique, good instrumentation, and reasonable experience of the surgeon. Every surgeon has his or her way of doing things; hence, there is no single technique that can be called ideal. Our technique is an amalgamation of our own experi-

K. Parikh (✉) · R. Soni
Shyam Urosurgical Hospital, Ahmedabad, Gujarat, India
e-mail: drkandarp@shyamurosurgical.com

R. Jain
Department of Urology, Institute of Kidney Disease and Research Center, Ahmedabad, Gujarat, India

A. Parikh
MPUH, Nadiad, Gujarat, India

G. Zeng et al. (eds.), *Flexible Ureteroscopy*, https://doi.org/10.1007/978-981-19-2936-6_9

ences of performing more than 1000 RIRS over more than 13 years. However, it is prudent to learn and master the technique of performing successful RIRS as well as to take care of the delicate and costly endoscopes and accessories involved.

1 Preoperative Planning

To begin with, an appropriate preoperative workup of the patient is essential. Proper history, physical examination, routine laboratory investigations (hemogram, renal function tests, urine analysis, and culture) with appropriate radiological investigations (ultrasound KUB, X-ray KUB, NCCT KUB, IVU, or CT IVU as required) should be done. Preoperative fitness by the physician or anesthetist is essential. It is imperative to have sterile urine culture preoperatively. However, in the case of positive urine culture with signs of uro-sepsis, it may be necessary to pre-stent and/or give antibiotics for few days. Routinely, pre-stenting is not required in our experience, except in selected cases [5].

RIRS has very low risk of bleeding and is preferred over percutaneous nephrolithotomy (PCNL) and extracorporeal shock wave lithotripsy (ESWL) among patients on anti-coagulants and with cardiac issues. It is advisable to discontinue aspirin and clopidogrel for 3–5 days prior to surgery if feasible. If not, clopidogrel is advised to be discontinued, whereas aspirin can be continued peri-operatively [6]. A cardiologist opinion and fitness are essential.

2 Informed Written Consent

Informed written consent, explaining the pros and cons of the procedure, need for additional procedures such as Re RIRS, ESWL, etc. should be obtained. We have a special and separate consent form for RIRS in English and the local language of the patient in which, the technique, expected outcome after RIRS, and the possible complications such as urinary tract infection, bleeding, failure to perform the procedure followed by pre-stenting, residual stones, etc. are explained in detail. A preoperative single dose of injectable third-generation cephalosporin antibiotic is preferred at our center. In the case of positive urine culture, we prefer to give culture-specific antibiotics for few days followed by a repeat urine culture to ensure it is sterile.

3 Anesthesia

General anesthesia is usually preferred since it provides better control of the patient's respiratory movement by modulating the tidal volume, and short periods of apnea can be utilized to minimize the respiratory movement during precise laser lithotripsy [7].

The procedure can also be performed under spinal anesthesia if general anesthesia is contraindicated [8]. It is more relevant in the era of the COVID-19 pandemic in order to decrease the risk of virus transmission due to aerosol-generating procedures.

4 Preoperative Checklist

Before the start of the procedure, it is prudent to check the endoscopes, accessories and laser machine, and laser fiber by a dedicated OT personnel to avoid any intra-op crisis. The following checklist can be useful before the start of the procedure along with routine surgical instruments:

1. Cystoscope with sheath and bridge (17 or 20 Fr).
2. Semi-rigid ureteroscope (4.5 or 6/7.5 Fr).

3. Flexible ureteroscope and/or digital ureteroscope (Fig. 1).
4. The guidewire of choice (Terumo rigid shaft/Sensor/Bi-wire).
5. Stent removal forceps (in cases of pre-stenting).
6. The ureteric dilator of choice (ureteric balloon dilator/single-step Nottingham dilator/ureteric serial dilators).
7. Ureteric access sheath (UAS) of choice (select appropriate length and size as per the case).
8. Double lumen ureteric catheter (selected cases).
9. Radio-contrast (for retrograde pyelography).
10. Dormia Baskets (Zero tip N-Circle/Engage, etc.)
11. Laser machine (Ho:YAG or thulium fiber laser).
12. Laser fiber of choice (200/272/365 μm).
13. Irrigation mechanism of choice (100 cm extension tube with 20 ccs syringe/Traxer Flo/Automated Irrigation flow, etc.)
14. Radiation protection equipment.

All endoscopes and accessories should ideally be sterilized with plasma sterilization or ethylene oxide (as per the availability). We use Plasma Sterilization Sterrad NX based on hydrogen peroxide gas plasma (HPGP) technology and we have found extremely low rates of uro-sepsis postoperatively [9].

It is important to achieve adequate room cooling of the operation theater before the start of the procedure to avoid laser malfunction in many laser machines. Wide trolleys for keeping the flexible endoscope and accessories like guidewires, baskets, laser fiber, and other surgical instruments help prevent accidental damage to the endoscopes and other armamentarium. The laser machine should always be on standby mode when not in use.

5 Ergonomics

Ergonomics is a Greek word, where "Ergon" means work and "nomos" means law. So it means "laws of work" or "science of work." Ergonomics is very important in any surgery especially RIRS to achieve optimal results without much fatigue. RIRS demands good coordination of the surgeon's eyes, hands, legs, and mind. A few technical points are suggested to improve the ergonomics (Fig. 2).

While the patient is in the supine lithotomy position and the surgeon is at the foot end of the patient, the surgeon should be positioned like an archer with his neck and body in the same line and both the arms by the side of the body. The right hand should be flexed at the elbow by 60°–70°, while the left hand should be flexed at the elbow by 110°–120°. The right leg should be slightly in a forward position to press the laser foot-paddle. All the light cables, camera cables, and irrigation systems should be free enough for movement without undue dangling or twisting. We have suggested a simple way to keep fixed guidewire and laser fiber

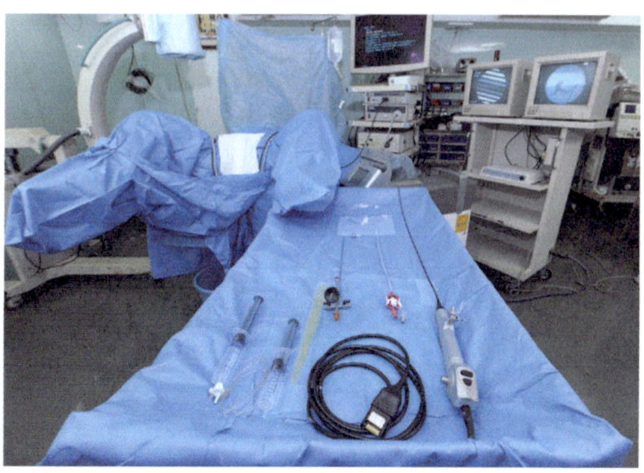

Fig. 1 Operation theater setup

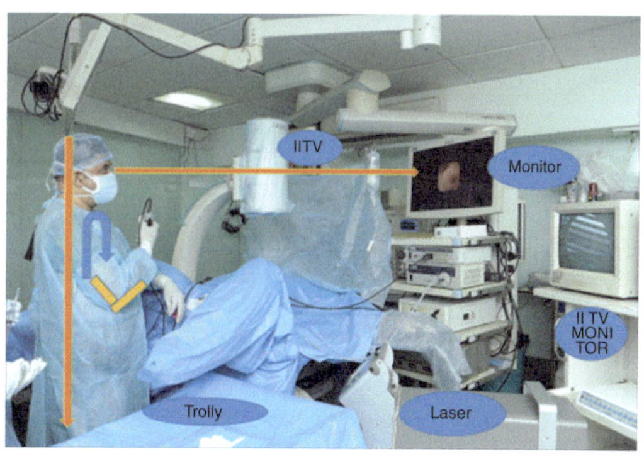

Fig. 2 Viewing monitor on the right side of the surgeon and IITV on the left side

during the procedure so that there are minimum chances of accidental slippage of guidewire or damage to laser fiber. Guidewire is parked in its jacket over the patient's thigh to prevent its accidental slippage and also laser fiber should be covered with a wet mop and not with any towel clip or artery forceps to avoid undue breakage (Fig. 3). All the movements of the flexible scope handle should occur at the wrist joint. Finger grip with partial palm grip to hold the flexible scope is suggested (Fig. 4). We prefer to perform to stand while performing surgery, but the surgeon can comfortably sit especially for larger stones when longer operative time is expected, when the stone is in the straight line of flexible scope (pelvic or upper calyceal stone), or when more number of cases are lined up. Sitting posture is also adopted in robotic ureteroscopy.

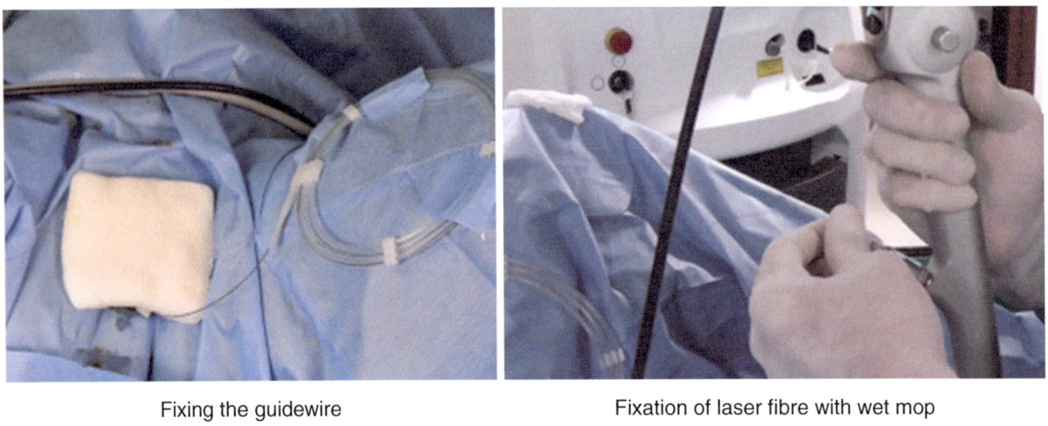

Fig. 3 Fixation of guidewire and laser fiber

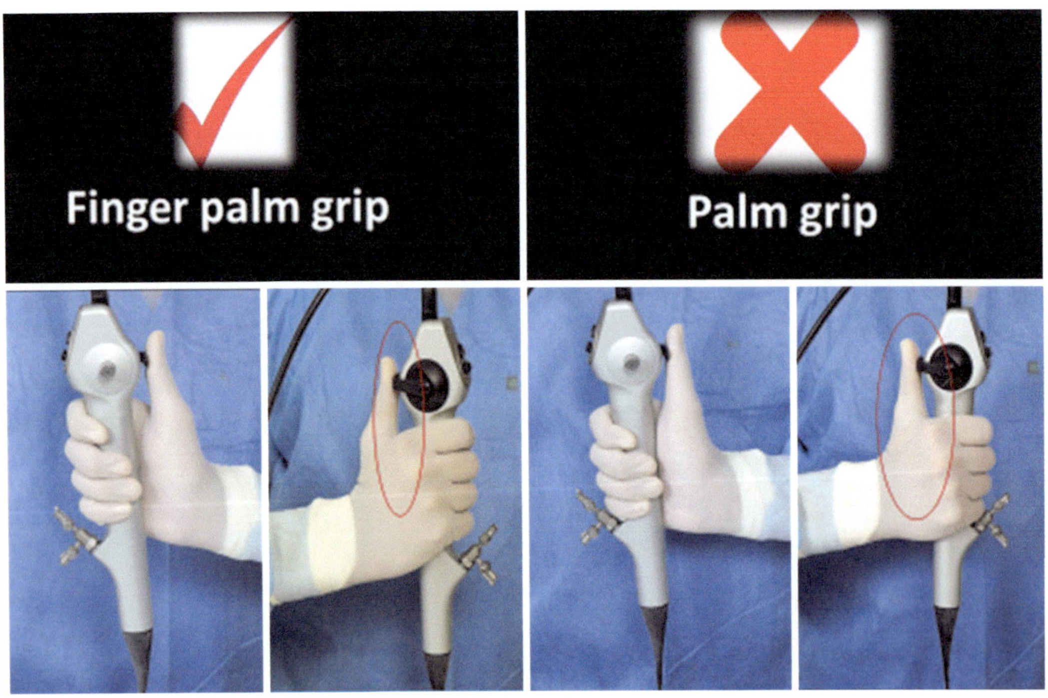

Fig. 4 Finger palm grip is preferred than palm grip

5.1 Cysto-Urethroscopy

To start with the procedure, first of all cysto-urethroscopy was done with cystoscope to delineate the anatomy of the urethra, any bladder calculus or pathology, size and shape of the ureteric orifice (UO) and to put guidewire in the respective pelvic-calyceal system (PCS). As per our experience, the ureteric orifice can be identified as small, medium, and large size (Table 1; Fig. 5).

To avoid injury due to a large size cystoscope sheath in the urethra, we prefer to do cysto-urethroscopy with 4.5 Fr ureteroscope to assess the urethra, urinary bladder, and ureteric orifice.

5.2 Semirigid Ureteroscopy

Semirigid ureteroscopy is preferred by the same 4.5 Fr ureteroscope. Ureteroscopy may also be performed with a 6/7.5 Fr semirigid ureteroscope. This serves the following purposes:

Table 1 Different caliber of ureteric orifice

Small UO	Medium UO	Large UO
Usually requires ureteric dilatation for UAS insertion	Usually allows 9.5/11.5 Fr or 10/12 Fr UAS without ureteric dilatation	Usually allows 11/13 or 12/14 Fr UAS. Common in pre-stented patients

- To study the course of the ureter.
- To identify any surprise findings (stone/tumor).
- Retrograde pyelographic contrast study (RGP) to evaluate upper tract (in abnormal ureteric anatomy, not routinely done).
- Passive dilatation of the ureteric orifice and lower ureter.
- Under vision insertion of a guidewire through it. (This can reduce the use of radiation for insertion of the guidewire).

5.3 Ureteric Dilatation

Ureteric dilatation is required in cases of a narrow ureteric orifice. Balloon dilatation is usually preferred, but serial Teflon ureteric dilatation or single-step Nottingham dilator can be used. We normally inflate the balloon with saline; however, contrast is ideally preferred. In cases of tight ureters, dilation of the ureter can be achieved with Double Lumen Ureteric Catheter. Double Lumen Ureteric Catheter is usually of 10 Fr diameter with a floppy tip. It can serve several purposes like passing a safety guidewire, RGP, and dilation of the ureter. The guidewire insertion in the PCS is an important step because it will facilitate the successful deployment of UAS and/or fURS. In our experience, hybrid wires such as sensor guidewire (Boston Scientific) with a hydrophilic tip and rigid shaft of PTFE guidewire or rigid

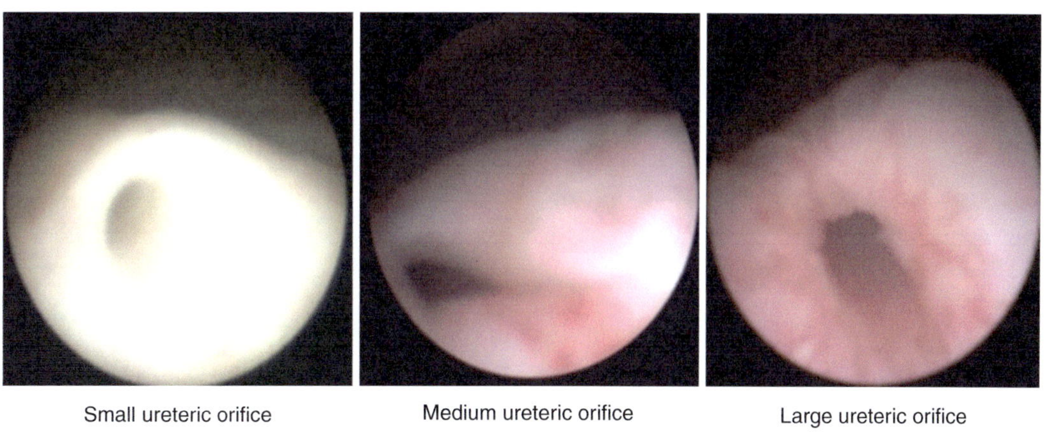

Fig. 5 Small, medium, and large ureteric orifice

shaft Terumo guidewire are useful as they do not slip out easily and also have the least chances of mucosal perforation. Guidewire negotiation in difficult anatomy cases such as ureteric kink can be technically challenging. In such cases, a semi-rigid or flexible ureteroscope can be useful in guidewire placement [10]. Though suggested by many experts, few practitioners question the routine use of safety guidewire during ureteroscopy [11]. In our practice, we usually do not place a safety guidewire because ureters in the Indian population are narrow and do not accommodate UAS and safety guidewire together in most of the cases, but according to EAU and AUA guidelines, it is suggested to place safety guidewire.

5.4 Ureteral Access Sheath (UAS) Placement

This is followed by the placement of UAS of appropriate size. Whether to place UAS or not is itself a matter of debate, and there are several advantages and disadvantages to both [12, 13]. This chapter focuses on the technique of performing RIRS; hence, we shall not discuss it. Our choice of UAS is 9.5/11.5 or 10/12 Fr UAS as this will accommodate flexible ureteroscopes of most companies, can be successfully placed in most of the un-stented patients, and also ensure low intrarenal pressure (IRP). Routinely, UAS is placed under fluoroscopic guidance. The tip is not to push the UAS if undue resistance is encountered. In cases of tight ureters, sheathless fURS (described later) or staging the procedure by ureteric stenting can minimize the chances of ureteric trauma. The upper end of UAS should ideally be parked at the upper ureter level, to allow complete deflection of fURS in the PCS, especially lower calyx, and to avoid injury to uretero-pelvic junction (UPJ). In cases when the UAS is not used, the flexible ureteroscope should be back-loaded over a guidewire to allow easy introduction across the UPJ. At all steps, the tip and the shaft of the fURS should be kept straight to avoid scope damage.

5.5 Stone Disintegration

Once the scope is placed in PCS, we gently irrigate the system, we preferred gravity-dependent irrigation with intermittent manual irrigation with a 20-cc syringe. The aim is to avoid high intra renal pressures (IRP) as it is the most important factor to prevent infection-related complications following RIRS. One may use Traxer flow, path finder, single action pump (SAP) device, automated pump device, or Peditro foot control device for irrigation (Fig. 6). We do not perform a contrast study at the beginning of the procedure as different densities of contrast and saline hamper the vision. This will also reduce the use of radiation during the procedure. In case if the contrast is used, one must wait for at least 2 min to clear up the contrast and vision to improve. The entire PCS is inspected and the plan of surgery is made according to the stone burden, number, and location as well as the anatomy of PCS. In the case of small- to medium-sized lower calyx stones with wide and broad infundibulum, the calculi are picked up with a Dormia basket and are put in the straight line of the endoscope in the suitable upper or middle calyx. If the stone burden is large and infundibular anatomy is not friendly, the stones in lower calyx are fragmented, and then small fragments are basketed in the upper or middle calyx, and subsequently, laser lithotripsy is done. This helps to avoid too much torque on the fURS and decreases the wear and tear. In the case of multiple upper or middle calyx stones, the smaller ones are fragmented first before going for the larger stone.

Stone burden (>2 cm), stone density (>1000 Hounsfield units), infundibular length (>2.5 cm), and lower calyx calculi with acute infundibulo-pelvic angle (<30°) are the adverse factors for stone clearance in the lower calyx [14]. Laser fiber should cover 1/4th of the screen diameter to improve safety during laser lithotripsy (Fig. 7) [15]. Most of the time, lower calyx stones can be addressed by producing maximum deflection of ureteroscope which is called the active deflection. But in cases where lower calyx is still unapproachable, one can produce exaggerated

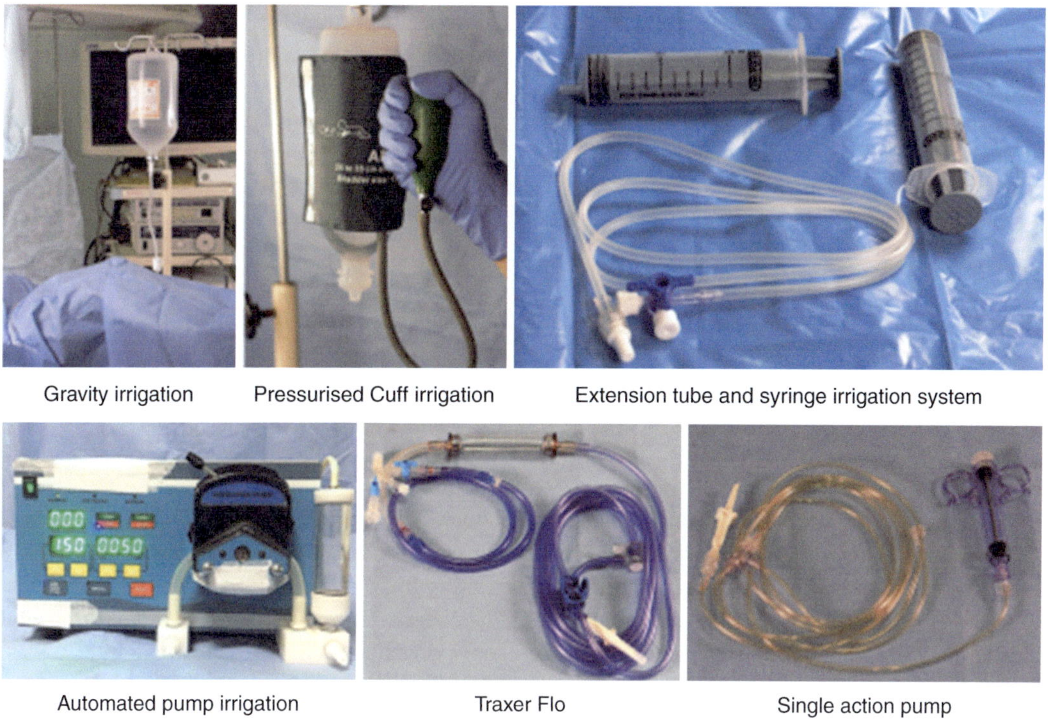

Fig. 6 Irrigation devices

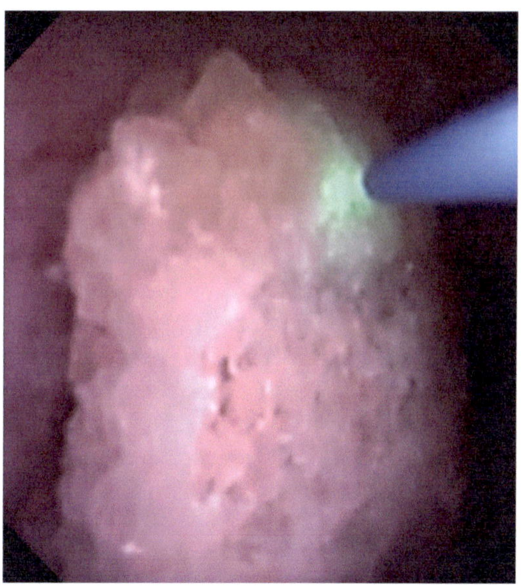

Fig. 7 Laser fiber occupying ¼th of the screen

deflection by pressing the ureteroscope against the wall of the pelvis which is known as passive deflection. The shaft of the flexible ureteroscope can be twisted with the fingers of the nondominant hand to achieve minor degrees of added movement of the tip to reach into the desired calyx, especially the lower anterior calyx. Ball tip laser fiber may also be used to insert the laser fiber with the tip of the scope deflected in lower calyx [16]. It is important to note that the ball tip is destroyed after its first use. Then the laser fiber can be used as a regular laser fiber but cannot be inserted with the scope tip deflected.

In cases where the stone fragments get clogged into the lower calyx and are difficult to clear on their own, the use of autologous blood around 5–8 mL can be done. Here, the autologous blood is instilled through a syringe and filled up in lower calyx. After waiting for 5 min, a coagulum is formed which can fill the entire lower calyx to prevent the entry of calculi fragments during lithotripsy [17]. To confirm the formation of the coagulum, RGP is done which shows non-opacification of lower calyx due to the coagulum. One can also use this autologous blood to form a coagulum to retrieve the very small calculi fragments which get stuck down in the coagulum and it becomes easy to remove the fragments with a blood clot.

Stone lithotripsy is mainly performed using two different techniques:

- Dusting—including painting or chipping technique.
- Fragmentation.

Our policy during the lithotripsy depends on the stone burden and location

- *Small* (<7–8 mm) *stone*—Fragmentation and removal with basket.
- *Stone* (>8 mm)—Dusting off the stone from periphery to center reduces a large stone to the small one with the formation of fine dust of around 200 μm which gets cleared on its own, and once the stone is reduced to a small size, fragmentation and removal with basket are done [18].

5.5.1 Popcorning

When the stone is large and fragmented in many pieces, popcorning is performed. The settings preferred for popcorning are adequate energy (around 0.8–1 J) and high frequency (15–20 Hz) for a 30–35 W Ho:YAG laser machine, which can vary among different laser machines. It is important to have a stone in a shallow cavity (calyx) to produce an effective whirlpool effect during popcorning (Table 2) [19].

At the conclusion of the procedure, we do a systematic inspection of the entire PCS to check for residual stone fragments. RGP is done to delineate PCS for any injury or contrast extravasation. This helps in identifying patients prone to develop complications post-RIRS especially urosepsis. It will also help to place the DJ stent. Under vision, removal of UAS is done to rule out any ureteric injury or residual stone fragment in the ureter.

5.6 Exit Strategy

DJ stent is placed at the end of the procedure. Retrograde ureteric catheter can be placed in selected cases where operative time was not too long, with complete stone clearance and when UAS was not used. Foley's catheter is placed at the end of the procedure.

Note: We restrict our operating time to 90 min

6 Postoperative Monitoring

Postoperatively, the patient is monitored for vital signs, any flank tenderness, and signs of sepsis. Oral diet is resumed usually within 4–6 h along with ambulation. In the absence of any complication, usually, the catheter is removed the next postoperative day and discharged. The patient has to report for follow-up after 4 weeks with NCCT KUB to check for any residual fragments and DJ removal.

7 Special Situations

Wireless or sheathless ureteroscopy, also known as the "No-Touch Ureteroscopy" was introduced by Bagley and popularized by M. Grasso. This technique aims to minimize the ureteric mucosal trauma by avoiding the use of guidewire (wireless) and ureteric access sheath (sheathless). This technique can be used for both diagnostic and therapeutic purposes. This technique was devised for the follow-up of patients with upper tract

Table 2 Different laser settings for stone surgery

Mode of stone lithotripsy	Energy	Frequency	Pulse duration
Dusting	Low	High	Long
Fragmentation	High	Low	Short
Popcorning	High	High	Long

There are no perfect settings for stone lithotripsy. Usually one should start with low energy and low frequency and then gradually increase as required transitional cell carcinoma (TCC) who were managed endoscopically. To avoid missing any lesion in the ureter and avoiding confusion between mucosal lesion vs. mucosal injury by guidewire or UAS, wireless fURS was developed [20]. Newer generation flexible ureteroscopes have made this feasible due to smaller caliber and better deflection mechanisms.

Robotic flexible ureteroscopy is the new horse in the market of fURS. The first reported use of robotic fURS was in interventional cardiology in 2008 using the Sensei-Magellan system. This system consisted of a catheter sheath and an inner catheter guide combined with a custom-built passive fiber-optic flexible ureteroscope. Desai et al. in 2008 first described a flexible robotic device for RIRS in porcine model [21, 22]. Roboflex Avicenna™ (Elmed Medical Systems, Ankara, Turkey) is a specially designed system for robotic fURS by Remzi Saglam in 2013 [23]. It is a classic master–slave model of robots which consists of a surgeon's console and manipulator of a flexible ureteroscope. The console provides an adjustable seat with armrests and two manipulators of the endoscope: the right wheel enables deflection and the left horizontal joystick allows rotation as well as advancing and retracting the instrument. Initial two multicentric studies demonstrated the safety and efficacy of Roboflex as well as significantly improved ergonomics. It however requires further randomized control trials in the future to establish this technique. The limitations with the robotic system are the availability and cost-effectiveness at the present date (Fig. 8).

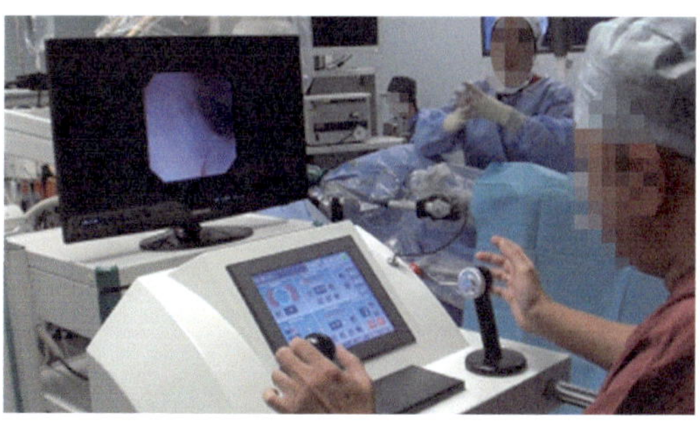

Fig. 8 Robotic flexi ureteroscopy

8 Summary

To conclude, developing a proper technique, protocol, and team are essential to improve the results of fURS. Proper understanding of the flexible ureteroscope mechanism and dedicated care by designated persons is vital to the longevity of the ureteroscope. Gentle care, liberal but judicious use of radiation, irrigation, ureteric access sheath, and other accessories can help in improving the learning curve of RIRS in a short time. The case selection of upper calyx and middle calyx stones and the initial phase can help improve surgeon confidence. Many technological innovations are happening in the field of flexible ureteroscopes and lasers. In the future, disposable flexible ureteroscopes with pressure sensors and smaller diameters with the possibility to aspirate stone dust, and advancements in laser technology will lead to further evolution of RIRS and expand the indications and scope of flexible ureteroscopy.

References

1. Romero V, Akpinar H, Assimos DG. Kidney stones: a global picture of prevalence, incidence, and associated risk factors. Rev Urol. 2010;12(e86):96.
2. Turk C, Knoll T, Petrik A, Sarica K, Skolarikos A, Straub M, et al. EAU guidelines on urolithiasis. European Association of Urology. 2020. https://uroweb.org/wp-content/uploads/EAU-Guidelines-on-Urolithiasis-2020.pdf.
3. Marshall VF. Fiber optics in urology. J Urol. 1964;91:110–4.
4. Bagley DH. Ureteral endoscopy with passively deflectable, irrigating flexible ureteroscopes. Urology. 1987;29:170–3.
5. Parikh KP, Jain RJ, Kandarp AP. Is retrograde intrarenal surgery the game changer in the management of upper tract calculi? A single-center single-surgeon experience of 131 cases. Urol Ann. 2018;10:29–34.
6. Bourdoumis A, Stasinou T, Kachrilas S, et al. Thromboprophylaxis and bleeding diathesis in minimally invasive stone surgery. Nat Rev Urol. 2014;11:51–8.
7. Emiliani E, Talso M, Baghdadi M, Ghanem S, Golmard J, Pinheiro H, Gkentzis A, Butticè S, Traxer O. The use of apnea during ureteroscopy. Urology. 2016;97:266.
8. Tran K, Cimon K, Severn M, Pessoa-Silva CL, Conly J. Aerosol generating procedures and risk

of transmission of acute respiratory infections to healthcare workers: a systematic review. PLoS One. 2012;7(4):e35797.

9. Parikh KP, Jain RJ, Parikh AK. Is plasma sterilization the modality of choice of sterilization today for endourological procedures such as ureterorenoscopy and retrograde intrarenal surgery? A single-center retrospective evaluation of 198 patients. Urol Ann. 2020;12:122–7.
10. Parikh KP, Jain RJ. Is upper ureteric kink a real nightmare for the urologists while performing flexible ureteroscopy (fURS)? A single-center experience of 15 cases of retrograde intra renal surgery (RIRS) in unstented patients with an upper ureteric kink. Gujarat Med J (Index Copernicus). 2019.
11. Dutta R, Vyas A, Landman J, Clayman RV. Death of the safety guidewire. J Endourol. 2016;30(9):941–4.
12. Auge BK, et al. Ureteral access sheath protects against elevated renal pressures during routine flexible ureteroscopic stone manipulation. J Endourol. 2004;18(1):33–6.
13. Traxer O, Thomas A. Prospective evaluation and classification of ureteral wall injuries resulting from insertion of a ureteral access sheath during retrograde intrarenal surgery. J Urol. 2013;189(2):580–4.
14. Xiao Y, Li D, Chen L, et al. The R.I.R.S. scoring system: an innovative scoring system for predicting stone-free rate following retrograde intrarenal surgery. BMC Urol. 2017;17(1):105. https://doi.org/10.1186/s12894-017-0297-0.
15. Giusti G, Proietti S, Villa L, Cloutier J, Rosso M, Gadda GM, Doizi S, Suardi N, Montorsi F, Gaboardi F, Traxer O. Current standard technique for modern flexible ureteroscopy: tips and tricks. Eur Urol. 2016;70(1):188–94.
16. Shin RH, Lautz JM, Cabrera FJ, Shami CJ, Goldsmith ZG, Kuntz NJ, Kaplan AG, Neisius A, Simmons WN, Preminger GM, Lipkin ME. Evaluation of novel ball-tip holmium laser fiber: impact on ureteroscope performance and fragmentation efficiency. J Endourol. 2016;30(2):189–94.
17. Cloutier J, Cordeiro ER, Kamphuis GM, Villa L, Letendre J, de la Rosette JJ, Traxer O. The glue-clot technique: a new technique description for small calyceal stone fragments removal. Urolithiasis. 2014;42(5):441–4.
18. Doizi S, Keller EX, De Coninck V, Traxer O. Dusting technique for lithotripsy: what does it mean? Nat Rev Urol. 2018;15(11):653–4. https://doi.org/10.1038/s41585-018-0042-9.
19. Chawla SN, Chang MF, Chang A, Lenoir J, Bagley DH. Effectiveness of high-frequency holmium:YAG laser stone fragmentation: the "popcorn effect". J Endourol. 2008;22(4):645–50. https://doi.org/10.1089/end.2007.9843.
20. Johnson G, Portela D, Grasso M. Advanced ureteroscopy: wireless and sheathless. J Endourol Endourol Soc. 2006;20:552–5. https://doi.org/10.1089/end.2006.20.552.
21. Desai MM, Aron M, Gill IS, Pascal-Haber G, Ukimura O, Kaouk JH, et al. Flexible robotic retrograde renoscopy: description of novel robotic device and preliminary laboratory experience. Urology. 2008;72:42–6.
22. Müller PF, Schlager D, Hein S, Bach C, Miernik A, Schoeb DS. Robotic stone surgery—current state and future prospects: a systematic review. Arab J Urol. 2017;16(3):357–64. https://doi.org/10.1016/j.aju.2017.09.004.
23. Rassweiler J, Fiedler M, Charalampogiannis N, Kabakci AS, Saglam R, Klein JT. Robot-assisted flexible ureteroscopy: an update. Urolithiasis. 2018;46(1):69–77.

Irrigation Mechanisms and Intrarenal Pressure in Flexible Ureteroscopy

Søren Kissow Lildal, Palle Osther, and Helene Jung

Abstract

Saline irrigation during flexible ureterorenoscopy (fURS) is necessary to maintain a clear vision during diagnostic and therapeutic procedures. Technological development has brought us different irrigation mechanisms, ranging from gravity irrigation to a variety of hand- and foot-controlled devices as well as automated pumps, the performance of which will be discussed in the clinical perspective.

As a result of scope manipulation and fluid irrigation, intrarenal pressure (IRP) unequivocally will increase during fURS. Data on IRP during experimental and clinical fURS is presented and discussed, including the role of ureteral access sheaths. Increases in IRP will often exceed thresholds for tubular (20–30 mmHg) and venous (30–50 mmHg) backflow, potentially resulting in septic complications. When IRP increases even further, forniceal rupture may occur, emerging into hemorrhagic complications. Additionally, IRP increments will produce strain in the pelvic/calyceal wall, thereby activating pacemaker cells that will initiate peristalsis, which may result in access-related problems. In this way, IRP variations represent the main determinant for adverse events in fURS. Preventive measures will be discussed, including potential role of pharmacological modulation of upper urinary tract dynamics.

Keywords

Ureteroscopy · Irrigation · Intrarenal pressure Pathophysiology · Complications · Prevention

S. K. Lildal
Department of Urology, Aarhus University Hospital, Aarhus, Denmark

Department of Clinical Medicine, Aarhus University, Aarhus, Denmark

P. Osther (✉) · H. Jung
Department of Urology, Vejle Hospital—A Part of Lillebaelt Hospital, University Hospital of Southern Denmark, Vejle, Denmark

Urological Research Center, Department of Regional Health Research, University of Southern Denmark, Odense, Denmark
e-mail: posther@health.sdu.dk; palle.joern.osther@slb.regiosyddanmark.dk

Abbreviations

fURS	Flexible ureteroscopy
IRP	Intrarenal pressure
PCNL	Percutaneous nephrolithotomy
sURS	Semirigid ureteroscopy
UAS	Ureteral access sheath

G. Zeng et al. (eds.), *Flexible Ureteroscopy*, https://doi.org/10.1007/978-981-19-2936-6_10

1 Introduction

Today, open surgery in the treatment of kidney stones is almost obsolete. The transition to endoscopic procedures, including the invention and ongoing technological development of endoscopic armamentarium, proved the obvious benefits of minimally invasive surgery. Lower morbidity and mortality justified the endoscopic techniques also in patients requiring urological treatment [1]. Despite its many advantages, endoscopic management also turned out to comprise potential risks and hazards. The need for continuous fluid irrigation to secure optimal visibility results in non-physiological high intrarenal pressures [2, 3]. Increased intrarenal pressure (IRP) may be followed by severe clinical complications such as sepsis and renal damage due to pyelorenal backflow and fluid absorption [4–6]. Stretching of the renal tubular cells followed by tubular atrophy, nephron loss, and accumulation of fibrotic interstitial tissue has been documented [7]. While attention initially—only to a very limited extent—was focused on this type of complications, the potential deteriorating effects of intrarenal backflow have been subject to several clinical and experimental studies during recent years [8]. Thomsen et al. discovered the pathoanatomic changes caused by elevated pressure levels in the kidney in 1983 [9], and since then the connection between extensive irrigation and complications to ureteroscopic procedures has been documented [10–13]. Of particular concern is the development of infectious complications, which are observed in up to 18% of patients undergoing retrograde intrarenal stone surgery [14]. Technical improvements and refinements, but also patients' requirements and expectations, have allowed for surgeries on patients with severe comorbidity and increasing complex conditions. This calls for an intensified awareness of pre-, peri-, and postoperative factors that may give rise to complications. Therefore, it seems of great relevance to continue investigating the clinical implications of elevated IRP during endourological procedures.

In this chapter, we will focus on irrigation methods and mechanisms, the resulting intrarenal pressures during ureteroscopic procedures and the potential pathophysiological consequences.

2 Irrigation Methods and Mechanisms in Flexible Ureteroscopy

Flexible ureteroscopy (fURS) necessitates the use of irrigation in order to clear the field of view from dust, debris, and blood and thus maintain a clear vision. As with other areas of fURS, irrigation has for the past years been subject to many technical developments in order to advance the ability to operate easier, safer, and more efficiently. However, when developing new methods to advance in one direction, there is always a risk that negative downsides will follow.

Higher fluid pressure deployed through endoscopes will yield better flow and thus aid in visibility and evacuation of stone dust and debris, and ultimately shorten duration of surgery [15]. On the other hand, increasing the irrigation flow rates, among other factors, may result in the development of increased IRP, which by now has been observed in several studies [3, 8, 6, 16]. Increased IRP may result in postoperative sepsis or other complications due to a well-established mechanism of intra renal backflow of irrigation fluid.

Guzelburc et al. [17] performed a clinical study on cases operated for renal stones larger than 2 cm. With irrigation fluid pressure set at 60 cmH_2O by gravity and limited use of hand pump irrigation, utilizing ureteral access sheath (UAS) 9.5/11.5 Fr., fluid absorption was observed in all patients (20–573 mL). Examining the effect of high pressure endoscopic irrigation on renal histology. Loftus et al. [18] performed an experiment on ex vivo pig kidneys. The mean percentages of kidney tissue penetration by irrigation fluid with pressure settings of 50, 100, and 200 mmHg were found to be 33.1, 21.0, and 99.3% without a UAS, respectively, and 0, 0, and 18.8% with a UAS. These studies show that pressurized irrigation unequivocally leads to fluid extravasation.

3 Methods of Irrigation

Several irrigation systems have been developed and used for ureteroscopy. Gravity irrigation is the simplest and least equipment requiring method. Using this, the irrigation pressure can be raised simply by elevating the fluid bag to a higher level above the patient. In this way, it is assured that the IRP will never exceed the pressure of the water column between the kidney level and the pressure bag (Fig. 1). Another simple way of applying more pressure to obtain better flow is to use a pressurized irrigation bag system where the fluid bag is placed in an air inflated pressure bag device, which can be inflated to a desired pressure, which is then transferred to the fluid bag to yield higher irrigation pressure. Using this does however require an assistant to monitor and regulate the pressure bag inflation as the fluid bag empties. Using this method, it has to be remembered that the pressure noted on the manometer of the inflated bag does not directly correspond to the IRP, and it may be difficult to control irrigation pressure with the risk of applying very high pressures at the kidney level. Other systems for pressurized irrigation include manual pump systems that can be controlled by the surgeon or by an assistant. Devices exist for hand or foot action and control and consist of either a syringe or balloon/reservoir device connected to irrigation systems via valves and tubes (Fig. 2). Thus, they can be used either alone with irrigation only when activated or in combination with gravity irrigation to have the option of enhancing the flow when needed. In recent years, automated systems have been introduced allowing for steady controlled application of irrigation pressure and lately even systems with pressure feedback and regulation have evolved. Concomitantly to this evolution, several studies have been published on the advantages and disadvantages of the different methods.

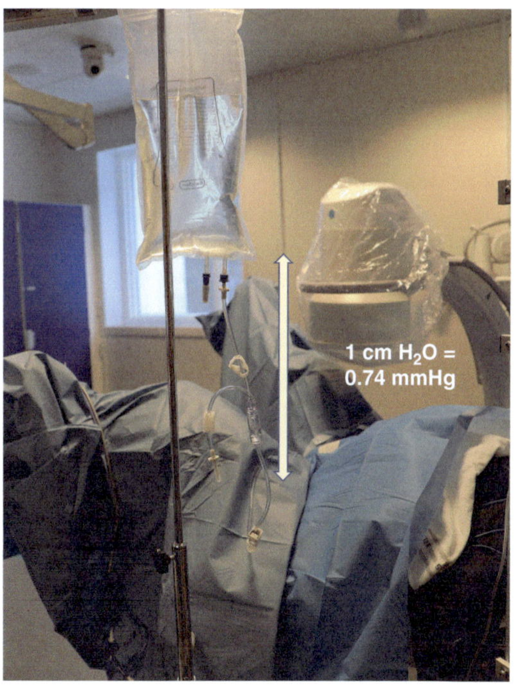

Fig. 1 Gravity irrigation

In 2005, Blew et al. [19] compared the Peditrol® hands-free irrigation device (foot pump) (Fig. 2) to 100 cmH_2O gravity irrigation (GI), and 300 cmH_2O pressure bag irrigation (PI) and to irrigation using a 60-cc syringe, in fURS of a cadaveric pig kidney. They concluded that with or without instruments in the working channel, the foot pump resulted in superior flow rates over GI and PI and comparable to syringe irrigation. At the same time, IRP was observed to be 30, 58, 92, and 97 cmH_2O without a UAS and 5, 13, 31, and 34 with a UAS, respectively, for the four irrigation methods. Appreciating the fact that handheld irrigation pumps may give rise to high IRP, MacCraith et al. [20] conducted an experiment on different combinations of endoscopes, UASs, and irrigation systems on harvested pig urinary tracts. Principally and in thread with other studies, they found that IRP was reduced by the combination of a larger UAS and smaller diameter ureteroscopes. More specifically, they found that of the three hand pumps examined, the Pathfinder Plus™ delivered the lowest IRP profile; however, this may be somewhat questionable as the pressure from any handheld device is highly dependent on the pressure delivered from the individual user. Accordingly, Proietti et al. [21] evaluated maximum pressure generation in an in vitro artificial kidney model, comparing three groups of people divided after

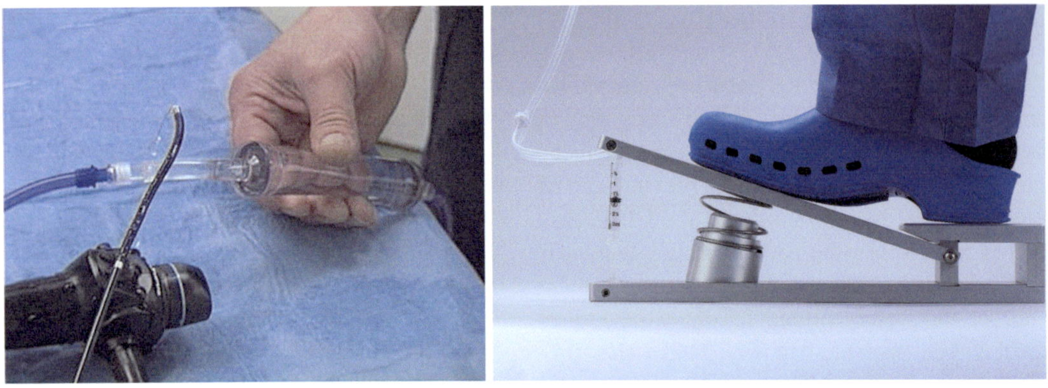

Fig. 2 On-demand flushing. Two examples of on-demand flushing during ureterorenoscopy. Left: hand-assisted irrigation with the T-flow™ (Roccamed). Right: foot-assisted irrigation with the Peditrol® device (Wismed)

physical strength using six different on-demand irrigation systems. The stratification between the groups showed that the most powerful group could produce the highest pressure in the kidney model with all the irrigation devices in almost any situation. The exception to this was the T-Flow system (Fig. 2), in which no statistical differences were detected between groups.

High IRP, to unsafe levels, using manual HI was seen in the in vivo pig study by Noureldin et al. using a Flex-x2 ureteroscope [22]. Using only GI, the IRP was 23 cmH_2O or lower with or without a UAS, but during manual pumping, the IRP rose to 45 without a UAS and 46 with a 9.5/11.5 UAS. They did however see very low IRP levels of 18 and 1 cmH_2O using larger 12/14 and 14/16 Fr. UASs, demonstrating that the UAS/ureteroscope diameter relationship greatly affects the release of intraluminal fluid and affects the IRP accordingly. This relationship was also examined and quantified by Fang et al. in an in vitro study using fresh cadaveric porcine kidney-ureter-bladder specimens. Several combinations of four different fURS and six UAS sizes 11/13 Fr. to 13/15 Fr. were combined to conclude that to maintain a low IRP and acceptable flow rate, the ratio of endoscope-sheath diameter should be kept below 0.75.

Inoue et al. [23] tested two automated irrigation pumps (ENDOFLOW® II and UROMAT® Endoscopic Automatic System for Irrigation (EASI)) against each other and against gravity-based irrigation regarding efficiency of flow measured at the tip of the ureteroscope. When the irrigation pressure in automated pumps increases, and when the bags are elevated in gravity irrigation, flow rate will increase. The two automated systems performed equally well, but the irrigation efficiency of a gravity-based system under the same pressure was significantly lower. The UROMAT® EASI was compared to a pressure infusion bag system (Ethox Infu-Surg®) by Lama et al. [24] under pressure settings of 150 and 200 mmHg with and without instruments in the working channel of a flexible ureteroscope. Conclusively, they found that the flow rates were similar during the first 5 min of irrigation, whereafter the PI needed to be re-inflated and moreover that the irrigant pressure at inflow to the ureteroscope was significantly variable regarding the PI system, making this type of irrigation subject to a need for regular attention from the OR staff.

Doersch et al. [25] compared AIP to HI in regard to clinical patient outcomes in a retrospective study of URS procedures without use of UAS. The AIP maximum pressure was set for 150 mmHg and the HI was used as little as possible to obtain visibility. The recorded complication rates were 11.2% for AIP and 8.3% for HI; 14.1% and 25%, respectively, had emergency department returns and 11.2% and 16.7% had post-procedural pain. Thus, there was no significant difference between these two groups. But unfortunately, no comparison was done with a GI alone group. A comparison was however done between GI and HI by Farag et al. [13] in a retrospective analysis of 234 fURS procedures. GI procedures were done using fixed pressures in the range 60–204 cmH_2O, and HI was done with a pump delivering 1–10 mL per flush. In the group of patients operated using HI, significantly higher rates of SIRS, emergency room consultations, and postoperative fever were observed. There was no significant difference in SFR or auxiliary procedures. Due to the retrospective nature of the study, these data might be flawed by selection and confirmation bias.

Looking at comfort of use, Jefferson et al. [26] performed a prospective randomized comparison of HI vs AIP with the findings that AIP usage resulted in significantly reduced total pump time and number of irrigation-related concerns of the surgeon, and a significantly higher nurse satisfaction during fURS.

4 Irrigation Flow: Endoscopes, Baskets, and Laser Fibers

The flow rate of fluids through a tube is dependent on the diameter of the tube in an exponential way, meaning that the irrigation flow during fURS is greatly affected by how much of the cross-sectional area of the working channel is available or occupied. Bedke et al. [27] tested flow rates of irrigation in semirigid URS (sURS) and fURS, 5 Fr. and 3.6 Fr. working channels, respectively, with different sizes of baskets inserted. With empty working channels, the flow rate was 197 mL/min for sURS and 44 for fURS, showing that a 39% increase in working channel diameter results in a 450% increase in irrigation flow provided that the same method of irrigation was used. Insertion of baskets sized 1.2–2.2 Fr in the straight fURS significantly lowered the flow rate from 20.4 to 1.5 mL/min, correspondingly (13.6-fold). Similarly, Inoue et al. [23] showed in an in vitro study that in order to maintain an equal flow rate with instruments in the working channel, the applied irrigation pressure has to be raised significantly. A range of instruments were tested, which showed that the diameter of an instrument decides how much the resulting flow declines and thus how much the irrigant pressure needs to be increased. An example of this is that when using a 200-μm laser fiber, the influx pressure needs to be approximately doubled to maintain a constant flow at the tip of the endoscope. Kruck et al. [28] tested five flexible ureteroscopes—all with 3.6 Fr. working channels—regarding resulting flow when applying a pressure of 100 cmH_2O. Expectedly, the flow rates were quite uniform for all the scopes ranging from 44 to 50 mL/min with an empty working channel and decreasing to 9–12 mL/min with a 1.9 Fr. basket inserted. Flexion of the scopes had no significant effect on the flow rate.

Aside from that, concerning the need for sufficient irrigation during usage of high-power laser treatment of kidney stones, Noureldin et al. [29] found in an animal study that gravity irrigation was not enough to maintain safe intrarenal temperatures (IRT). Applying 20 W of energy for 20 s IRT was considered hazardous without the use of UAS. With a UAS used, IRT was borderline, but with increasing laser energy levels, the effect of a UAS was not sufficient with IRT measured up to 60 °C. Oppositely, it was found that under pump irrigation with laser at highest power setting of 60 W for 60 s, the IRT remained at safe levels below 45 °C at all times even without a UAS. Similarly, Hein et al. [30] described in a test tube experiment that no and low irrigation during high-energy laser application results in rapid increases in temperatures to very high levels, but when using high irrigation rates of 100 mL/min, the temperature rise was only 5 °C at the highest laser power setting of 100 W.

5 Irrigation, Pressure Monitoring and Control

In 2016 Deng et al. [31] developed a system for controlling the IRP during fURS, consisting of a UAS with a pressure-sensitive tip, allowing intelligent computerized real-time regulation of irrigation/suction via the UAS. They evaluated it in a retrospective analysis of 93 cases for renal/ureteral lithiasis with a set perfusion flow of 100 mL/min and reported controlled IRP lower than 20 mmHg and clear visibility, with an SFR of 95.6% and no major complications. Again, the retrospective design calls for caution, and presently no firm conclusions can be drawn with this system.

In a recent study on characterization of intracalyceal pressures during fURS by Patel et al. [32], a secondary observation was that in some of the calyces the mean pressure was significantly higher when using a manual hand pump compared to an automated system (Thermedx® FluidSmart™), likely due to higher peak pressures and flow rates. The intended irrigation pressure applied was 150 mmHg, which for the hand pump infusion system was checked every 5 min. As described in this publication, the two methods were routinely used at the facility, and thus the observation in the study shows that automated systems of irrigation may have a positive effect on the ability to control the resulting intraluminal flow rate, and thus avoiding high-pressure peaks during surgery. When utilizing an automated system, the user may be inclined to trust the settings of the system. However, Fedrigon et al. [33] tested the Thermedx FluidSmart® and the Cogentix RocaFlow® (ENDOFLOW® II) AIPs in an in vitro setting and found that the output pressure of both the systems exceeded the chosen settings over the entire tested range (30–300 mmHg) with 15.7 and 5.2 mmHg, respectively. Testing of the fluid heating capabilities found that they had similar maximum temperatures of 34.0 °C, but that it took 8–18 min to reach this temperature, respectively. Even though it was concluded that these systems were safe to use, not least because of their ability to provide steady and safe pressures of irrigation, this shows that it is always important that the surgeon and staff gains detailed knowledge of new automated appliances before taking them into use. Another in vitro study from De et al. [34] evaluated a Thermedx Fluid Management System AIP and found similarly that the system underestimated the resulting pressure at the tip of the endoscope by 8–17%, while at the same time, and probably of less importance, overestimating flow rates and temperatures by 2–8% and 4–6 °C.

Using a pressure sensor wire, Doizi et al. [35] successfully monitored the IRP during five fURS for stone treatment in a pilot study. An Endoflow II® with a set pressure of 80 cmH_2O was used, and in addition to this, a T-Flow handheld pump (Fig. 2) was used for on-demand forced irrigation. Recorded baseline pressure was 6 cmH_2O, and mean IRP during ureteroscopy alone was 63 cmH_2O. During laser lithotripsy with on-demand forced irrigation, the mean IRP was 115.3 cmH_2O with recorded maximum pressure peaks of 289–437 cmH_2O. Thus, this study confirms previously recorded high intraoperative IRPs, but at the same time, it opens for future possibilities of monitoring the resulting pressures and thereby take measures to try avoiding them.

In conclusion, different situations call for different needs for irrigation during URS. High pressure/flow irrigation has many positive effects, but at the same time, it can be a double-edged sword. Pressurized irrigation results in higher flow rates, yielding immediate and very clear payoffs such as better visibility, lower temperatures, and better evacuation of stone dust, but these winnings may come at the price of higher intrarenal pressure and thus the risk of pre- and postoperative complications.

6 Intrarenals Pressure Values (IRP) During Ureterorenoscopy

6.1 Intrarenal Pressure

The intraluminal or the intrarenal pressure (IRP) is the pressure that can be recorded inside the lumen of the renal pelvis. Initial recordings were achieved by Kiil and coworkers in 1953 utilizing pressure transducers connected to ureteral plastic catheters and an oscillator–amplifier [36]. Due to many anatomical and physiological similarities with humans, pigs are commonly used to study the IRP in experimental settings. For that purpose, a nephrostomy tube is often inserted for pressure measurements. However, due to ethical considerations, deployment of a nephrostomy tube is unlikely to be accommodated in human studies. As a result, retrogradely inserted ureteral catheters are more frequently used in clinical settings. The presence of a foreign body in the ureter might alter ureteral peristalsis and give rise to small pressure variations [37]. However, the pelvic pressures observed using a retrograde ureteral catheter were fully comparable with the pressure measurements obtained in a study utilizing an antegradely inserted device [38, 39]. Recently, Doizi et al. evaluated the feasibility of measuring the IRP during flexible ureteroscopy with a 0.014″ wire attached to a pressure sensor. The pressure wire, which is normally used for interventional cardiology procedures, could easily be deployed in the renal pelvis through a double lumen ureteral catheter and pressure recordings similar to those found in studies using nephrostomy tubes or ureteral catheters for pressure measurements were obtained [35]. The potential of using a small-diameter wire for pressure measurement in the renal pelvis implies great advantages, as the placement of a nephrostomy tube without a medical indication is not justifiable in human clinical studies. A ureteral catheter also comprises certain challenges as it takes up a considerable amount of space in ureter which may affect the pelvic pressure and complicate the endoscopic procedure.

Intrarenal pelvic pressure depends on several factors including the compliance and the tension of the pelvic and ureteral walls, the actual urine flow, the system capacity, and external pressures exerted by surrounding structures. The physiological intraluminal pressure in the un-obstructed kidney is found to be 0–10 mmHg [36, 37, 40]. In hydronephrotic kidneys, higher levels of intrarenal pressure in the range of 10–20 mmHg have been documented. It is worth noticing that increased bladder pressure is reflected in the renal pressure, which emphasizes the importance of sufficient bladder drainage during endourological procedures to avoid further IRP increments.

Intrarenal backflow, which can be defined as the accumulation of renal pelvic contents beyond the limits of the calyces either to the collecting ducts or to the renal interstitium, is demonstrated to occur at 30–35 mmHg [41–43]. However, unfavorable conditions such as low urine flow, previous ischemic damage of the renal parenchyma, and vesico-ureteral reflux lower the limit for both pyelotubular and pyelointerstitial backflow. Also, anatomic alterations such as dilated ducts of Bellini in Medullary Sponge Kidney may result in lower thresholds of intrarenal backflow [44, 45]. Pyelovenous backflow characterized as pelvic urine entering the main renal vein may be observed at pressures as low as 15–20 mmHg [46]. According to both experimental and human clinical studies, intrarenal backflow is frequently occurring during ureteroscopic procedures and is considered to be an important contributing factor to several unwanted effects such as excessive fluid absorption, intraparenchymal renal damage, infection, and sepsis [4, 9, 12, 47]. For example, Loftus and coworkers found that pressurized endoscopic irrigation in porcine kidneys led to significant extravasation of fluid into the renal tissue [18]. These findings were confirmed by Guzelburc et al., who demonstrated up to 573 mL of fluid absorption during retrograde intrarenal stone surgery in patients with kidney stones larger than 2 cm [17]. These findings may represent part of the explanation for the sepsis occurring after upper urinary tract endoscopy.

7 Intrarenal Pressure During Ureterorenoscopy

The increased focus on the potential harmful effects of raised IRPs has resulted in both experimental and human studies on pressure variations during upper urinary tract endoscopy. In this context, ureterorenoscopic procedures represent a certain challenge as they are executed in the small, closed space of the renal pelvis, which allows for limited drainage through the narrow ureter.

Clinical studies evaluating the IRP during ureteroscopy differ with respect to pressure measurement methods, irrigation devices, and endoscopic equipment. Both antegrade and retrograde approaches as well as flexible and semi-rigid ureteroscopes form the basis of the investigations, and pressure pumps, gravity, and handheld devices are used for irrigation. The pelvic pressures recorded vary accordingly, but all studies have in common that extremely high pressures, far exceeding the level for intrarenal backflow, have been documented. It is worth mentioning that the irrigation pressure strongly correlates with, but does not uniformly represent, the measured intrarenal pressure. For example, Shao et al. found a mean IRP of 122 ± 24 mmHg during an inflow irrigant pressure of 200 mmHg and a mean IRP of 73 ± 11 mmHg at irrigant pressures of 100 mmHg [48]. Patel and coworkers concluded that the IRP varies depending on the exact anatomic localization in the calyx system being significantly higher in the upper pole and lowest in the lower pole [32]. This may explain why renal forniceal rupture and urine leakage as a result of ureteric obstruction are often observed at the upper pole calices.

Wilson and Preminger were among the first to report IRP levels during upper urinary tract endoscopy, and the dramatically increased high pressures of up to 440 mmHg when using forceful manual irrigation with a 60-mL syringe formed the base for further studies [49]. Pressure increments up to mean 142 mmHg but peaking at revolting 362 mmHg when using a 10-mL syringe were shown during fURS in kidney stone patients [50]. Moreover, the mean IRP of 35 mmHg increased to a mean of 47 mmHg when using a laser fiber for stone fragmentation, indicating that pelvic pressure increases with movements of the endoscope and when employing different devices for stone treatment, possibly by inducing contractions [50]. In experimental studies, the occupancy of the working channel with laser fibers or baskets elicited lower pressure increments due to decreased irrigation flow through the endoscope [51]. However, in a clinical setting, the movements of the scope and the manipulation with stones may "overrule" the pressure decline caused by reduced inflow.

In Table 1, IRPs during ureterorenoscopy in human studies are listed [32, 48–50, 52, 53].

In experimental settings, IRP is most often studied in anesthetized or cadaveric pigs (Table 2). Intrarenal pressure recordings in pigs are in general comparable to those found in humans. Interestingly, McCraith et al. found a significant difference in IRPs when using a 9.5 F ureteroscope compared to a 8.7 F ureteroscope [20]. They concluded that the larger the ureteral access sheath and the smaller the ureteroscope, the lower IRP to be expected. Moreover, they showed significant variations in IRPs depending on the irrigation system used, ranging from 30

Table 1 Intrarenal pressures in ureterorenoscopy in humans

Study	No. of patients	Endoscope	Pressure measurement	Irrigation	Mean IRP, mmHg	Maximum IRP, mmHg	Irrigation pressure, mmHg
Auge et al. [53]	5	fURS	Nephrostomy tube	Gravity + manual	94.4	N.A.	N.A.
Jung et al. [38]	7	fURS	Retrograde ureteral catheter	Irrigation pump 8 mL/min + hand-held	35–47	361	N.A.
Jung et al. [52]	12	fURS	Retrograde ureteral catheter	Irrigation pump 8 mL/min + hand-held	33 ± 12	328	N.A.
Patel et al. [32]	8	fURS	Verrata® pressure guidewire	Hand-held pump	41.3 ± 31.2	N.A.	150 mmHg
Shao et al. [48]	15	fURS	Nephrostomy tube	Irrigation pump	34 73 122	149	50 100 200
Wilson and Preminger [4]	6	sURS + fURS	Nephrostomy tube	Gravity + manual syringe	30 45	410 440	N.A.

Table 2 Intrarenal pressures (IRP) in experimental studies

Study	Experimental setup	Endoscope	Pressure measurement	Irrigation	Mean IRP, mmHg	Maximum IRP, mmHg	Irrigation pressure
Doizi et al. [35]	In vitro silicon model	fURS	Pressure wire guidewire retrogradely	Irrigation pump	31.2 34	N.A.	30 mmHg 142 mmHg
Jakobsen (2009)	In vivo anesthetized pigs	sURS	Nephrostomy tube	Irrigation pump 4–33 mL/min	28	75	N.A.
Jung et al. [52]	In vivo anesthetized pigs	fURS	Retrograde ureteral catheter	Irrigation pump 8 mL/min	38	46	N.A.
MacCraith et al. [20]	Cadaveric pig kidneys	fURS 9.5 F	5 F pressure transducer in renal pelvis	SAPS single action pumping system	60 ± 22	74 ± 12	100 cmH_2O
Noureldin et al. [22]	In vivo anesthetized pigs	fURS sURS	Nephrostomy tube	Gravity	17 22	33 77	100 cmH_2O
Schwalb et al. [2]	In vitro pigs	sURS	Nephostomy tube	N.A.	N.A.	439	90–150 mmHg

(bag squeeze) to 74 mmHg (single-action pumping system, SAPS™, Boston Scientific). Schwalb et al. described the "scope effect" characterized by a 20–25 mmHg additional pressure increase produced by moving the endoscope in the ureter without flow [2]. Conclusively, porcine experiments confirm extensive pressure increments during irrigation and instrumentation of the collecting system but also indicate that the IRP level is under the influence of different parameters such as the irrigation method and the size of the ureteroscope. Moreover, occupancy of the working channels and active therapeutical use of the endoscope inside the collecting system, for example, laser treatment of stones, usage of baskets, may contribute to further pressure elevation due to induction of pelvic contractions.

Figure 3 (left) A typical pressure profile during fURS [3]

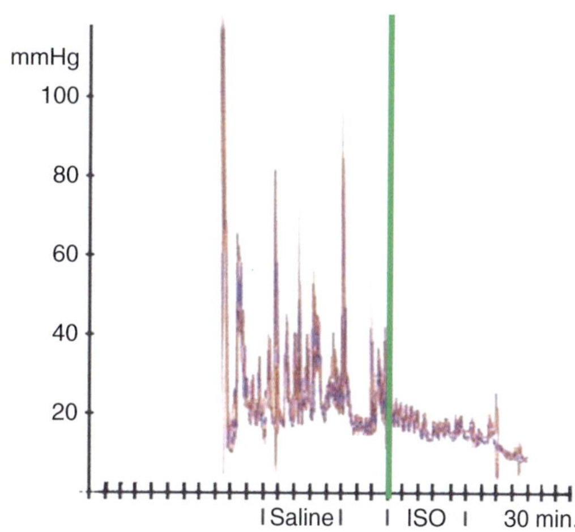

Fig. 3 Pressure profile during saline and isoproterenol irrigation. Left to the green line: typical pressure profile during irrigation with saline during ureterorenoscopy. Pressure peaks to above 100 mmHg (136 cmH_2O) are not unusual. Right to the green line: pressure peaks flattens out due to isoproterenol (0.1 μmol/mL) irrigation due ureteral relaxation. (Adapted from Jung H, Nørby B, Frimodt-Møller PC, Osther PJ. Endoluminal isoproterenol irrigation decreases renal pelvic pressure during flexible ureterorenoscopy: a clinical randomized, controlled study. Eur Urol 2008; 54 (6):1404–1413)

8 Intrarenal Pressure Values During PCNL

In contrast to the retrograde procedures, the percutaneous, antegrade procedures provide relatively better drainage from the collecting system, reducing the risk of pressure increments. Nevertheless, both postoperative infection and sepsis are observed after PNCL as is perioperative elevated IRP. In general, the IRPs during percutaneous procedures are lower than during fURS and sURS and are usually kept below the level for intrarenal backflow [51, 54, 55]. This is obviously attributed to the inherent advantage of the access sheaths securing a wider bridge between the collecting system and the extracorporal space. However, Troxel et al. described IRP up to 59 mmHg and pelvic pressures exceeding 30 mmHg in 8/31 patients undergoing PCNL using a 30 F sheath [56]. A correlation between elevated pressure and postoperative fever could however not be documented. The authors noted that pressure increased most significantly when the nephroscopy sheath was incorrectly positioned in the collecting system and during endoscopy through a narrow infundibulum. Alsyouf and coworkers investigated the IRPs of 20 patients during 26 F nephroscopy vs. 16 F flexible pyeloscopy with percutaneous access. They reported both longer hospitalization and higher pain score in the 26 F nephroscopy group, where IRPs were significantly higher than in the 16 F group (30.3 vs. 12.9 mmHg) [57]. Not surprisingly, a higher outflow is allowed through the access sheath the smaller the endoscope, yielding lower IRP. These findings are confirmed in a review comparing IRPs during PCNL, miniPCNL, and microPCNL [16].

Fluid absorption during PCNL as a result of a continuous high-flow irrigation and following extravasation into the retroperitoneal space has been investigated by different authors. Most frequently, ethanol added to the irrigation fluid is used as a marker to monitor fluid absorption. Malhotra et al. registered fluid absorption in 25 of 32 patients, of whom 28% absorbed a volume in excess of 1 l [58]. Under an irrigation pressure of 60 cmH_2O, Guzelburc and coworkers demonstrated fluid absorption in all 30 included patients, ranging from 13 to 364 mL [17]. Prolongation of the operation led to a significant increase in fluid absorption, which was not seen for a comparable group of fURS patients. The authors suggested that this difference may be due to potentially different mechanisms of backflow (pyelovenous versus pyelolymphatic) in PCNL procedures versus retrograde fURS. However, this theory has not been documented in previous experiments.

Of particular interest is the findings by Gehring, evaluating fluid absorption in 31 PCNL patients [59]. Longer hospitalization and an increased incidence of postoperative complications were documented in 19 patients in whom extravasation and fluid absorption was observed. Gehring's findings were confirmed by Kukreja et al. who strongly recommended to increase focus on keeping IRP and operating time as low as possible during PCNL to avoid fluid absorption and concomitant postoperative complications, especially in patients with compromised cardiorespiratory or renal status and in pediatric patients [46]. Also, fluid absorption was suggested to be associated with both infective and noninfective pyrexia, and the authors proposed staging of the procedure in the presence of perforation or excessive bleeding. This is in accordance with the considerations of Kreydin et al.'s review on risk factors for sepsis after PCNL [11]. In light of the obvious evidence indicating a relationship between elevated IRP and septic complications, also during PCNL procedures, keeping the pressure low and exercise extra caution in case of struvite stones or infected urine is recommended.

9 Ureteral Access Sheaths

For a detailed description of ureteral access sheaths (UASs) and their role in clinical practice, refer to Chap. 4. In this section, we will discuss the role of UASs related to IRP and irrigation. Ureteral access sheath (UAS) usage has unequivocally been shown to reduce IRP during fURS [22, 32, 53, 61–65]. The optimal proportion between the size of the ureteroscope and the diameter of the UAS was investigated by Fang et al. [63]. They concluded that to maintain a low IRP and acceptable flowrate during fURS, the ratio of endoscope-sheath diameter (RESD) should be kept below 0.75. When the RESD exceeded 0.85, which occurred at scope size 9.9 Fr (Olympus URF-V) and 11/13 F UAS, the mean IRP was > 40 cmH_2O at irrigation pressures of 250 cmH_2O. The length of the UAS did not significantly impact the IRP. This is in accordance with findings by Oratis, who concluded that the strongest regulators of IRP during ureteroscopy were the size of the gap between the endoscope and the UAS in addition to the frequency and duration of ureteroscope withdrawals [66]. Based on an in vitro model comparing different ureteroscope and UAS sizes, Sener and coworkers recommended the 10/12 UAS due to an optimal balance between impact on the ureteral wall and irrigant flow and IRP [64]. Indeed, compared to 12/14 or larger sizes, the smaller diameter exerting less strain to the ureteral wall was considered beneficial. Other human studies documented significantly decreased IRPs with the use of UAS, but still the level for intrarenal backflow was surpassed. For example, IRPs of 40 mmHg was found using 12/14 F UAS [53], and Patel et al. deployed a 14/16 sheath to keep the IRP below backflow level [32].

It is an obvious fact that the UAS necessarily has to be bigger than the ureteroscope, and therefore, the strain exercised on the ureteral wall potentially will be greater with UAS usage compared to using the scope alone. This was highlighted in experimental studies, showing upregulation of COX-2 and TNF-α pro-inflammatory mediators in the ureteral wall after UAS insertion, which potentially may be related to fibrosis [10, 67, 68]. Additionally, it was shown in a porcine model that the extent of the histopathological lesion following UAS insertion is often more severe than that observed during endoscopy [69]. Hence, ureteroscopic procedures seeming uneventful at first glance may have caused tissue scarring predisposing for future ureteral malfunction.

Regardless of the above-mentioned disadvantages, the use of UAS has been shown to reduce post-ureteroscopy fever, UTI, and sepsis rates by 28.6%, 18.6%, and 4.3% versus 39.1%, 23.9%, and 15.2% in the non-UAS group, respectively, in a study including 2239 patients [70]. The assumption that UAS reduces infectious complications after ureteroscopy is widespread, although randomized, controlled trials are lacking [71]. However, as irrigation volume and IRP appear to be independent risk factors for postoperative infection, fever, and sepsis in both fURS and PCNL-studies [11, 72], methods to limit pressure increments during endoscopic procedures are highly requested.

Based on these considerations, the UAS may be considered a double-edged sword: on the one hand reducing IRP, and on the other hand increasing strain on the ureteral wall [5]. Indeed, clinical series have documented that severe injuries including the muscular layer of the ureter may occur using larger sized UASs (12/14 Fr and above) [60]; and therefore, it is advisable to use the smallest UAS that is compatible with the ureteroscope used, in order to have sufficient irrigation to insure vision at reasonable IRPs (i.e., RESD < 0.75) [63]. If a larger sized UAS is preferred, for instance for larger and complex stone burdens, pre-stenting should be considered, since pre-stenting has been shown to reduce risk of UAS-induced ureteral injuries sevenfold [60]. This is due to the fact that JJ-stenting results in down-regulation of pacemaker-cell activity, thereby reducing peristalsis and ureteral tone and easing the passage of a larger sized UAS [5].

In conclusion, UASs possess certain advantages as well as potential disadvantages, which makes it of great importance to contemplate its use on an individual patient-to-patient basis and not as a routine procedure.

10 Pharmacological Modulation of the Intrarenal Pressure

Various receptor types are represented in the human ureter and renal pelvis. Both cholinergic and adrenergic innervation has been documented (Table 3) [73, 74]. While β-adrenergic stimulation mediates ureteral smooth muscle relaxation, activation of α-adrenergic receptors is known to cause contraction and increase ureteral peristaltic activity [75]. In everyday clinical practice, the selective α_{1A}- and α_{1D}-adrenergic antagonist Tamsulosin is commonly used to induce relaxation of the ureter in order to facilitate ureteral stone passage. As selective β_2- and β_3-receptors are widely distributed in the human ureter, the effect of different β-adrenergic drugs on upper urinary tract activity has been investigated in

Table 3 Receptors and mediators involved in the regulation of ureteral motility

Ureteral contraction	Ureteral relaxation
Muscarinic receptors	β-Adrenergic receptors
α-Adrenergic receptors	Histamine H_2 receptors
Histamine H_1 receptors	Nitric oxide
Purinergic receptors	K(+) channel openers
Neuronal and non-neuronal bradykinin receptors (intramural ureter)	Adenosine
Rho-kinase pathway	Phosphodiesterases
Neuropeptide Y	VIP
Serotonin	Prostaglandin E_1 and E_2
Substance P	Calcitonine gene-related peptide
Neurokin A	
Prostaglandin F_{2a}	

both human and animal studies. Also, calcium channel blockers are well-known ureteral relaxants, but due to unwanted side effects, drugs such as nifedipine are less frequently used for urinary tract modulation.

Drugs possessing the ability to relax ureteral smooth muscle are potentially capable of reducing IRP which may serve as a clinical benefit during endourological procedures.

Endoluminally administered norepinephrine was in a swine study shown to decrease IRP dose-dependently [76]. Being a potent α-adrenergic stimulator, norepinephrine is not found suitable for human use in the urinary tract. In contrast, endoluminally administered isoproterenol, a non-selective β-agonist, was found effective in reducing IRP significantly in both swine and human studies [39, 52]. Isoproterenol was added in the irrigation fluid in a very low concentration of 0.1 μg/mL during semirigid ureteroscopy in anesthetized pigs. A linear pressure–flow relationship at increasing flow rates from 4 to 33 mL/min was shown. While IRP reached 75 mmHg during saline irrigation, the pressure did not exceed 58 mmHg in pigs receiving isoproterenol irrigation. At high perfusion rates (33 mL/min), isoproterenol was detected systemically indicating intrarenal backflow. No concomitant cardiovascular side effects were detected. In a similar study, the IRP decreased 42% during fURS in pigs without causing any side effects [38]. Isoproterenol was suggested to directly inhibit the ureteral smooth muscle and the local, endoluminal drug administration was assumed beneficial in order to avoid cardiovascular impact. The experimental findings of isoproterenol's effect on IRP led to a clinical, randomized, controlled study including 12 kidney stone patients undergoing fURS. The patients were randomized to either saline or isoproterenol irrigation during ureteroscopic management of the stones, and a significant lower IRP (19 mmHg) was found in patients randomized for isoproterenol compared to the saline group (33 mmHg) [77] (Fig. 3). Moreover, the number of pressure peaks exceeding 50 mmHg, which was frequently observed during stone manipulation, was reduced significantly in the isoproterenol group. No cardiovascular side effects were observed, and isoproterenol could not be detected in blood samples during surgery or postoperatively [50].

Although promising effects on IRP of certain ureteral smooth muscle modulating agents, no drugs have to date been implemented for clinical use with IRP-reducing purposes. The potential cardiovascular toxicity of otherwise potent and qualified IRP reductants make them less appealing for clinical use. Moreover, the clinical implications and advantages of relatively modest pressure reduction during ureteroscopic procedures are not known. Until now, it is unclear whether prolonged, minimal pressure increments are more or less harmful than short, intensive pressure peaks. In other words, the exact relationship between IRP during ureteroscopy and peri- and postoperative complications is not fully investigated. Until it is, a general recommendation must be to keep the IRP as low as possible, taking the clinical, anatomical, and therapeutical circumstances into careful consideration for every individual patient.

The pathophysiological aspects of increased IRP during ureterorenoscopy are summarized in Fig. 4.

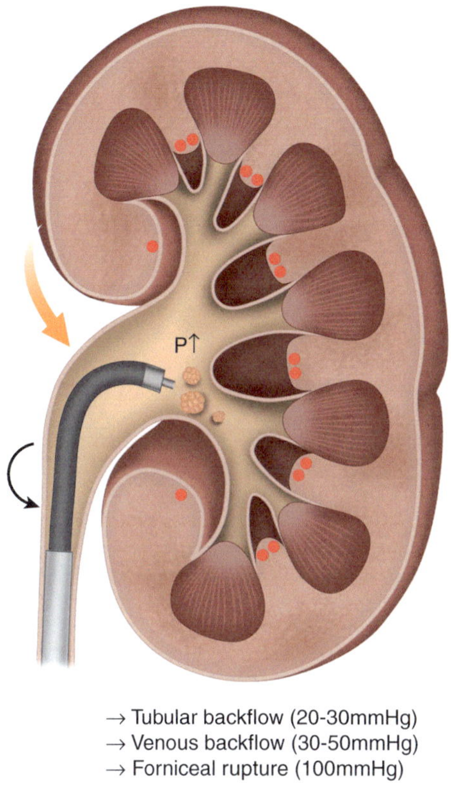

Fig. 4 Pathophysiology of intrarenal pressure rises during flexible ureterorenoscopy (fURS). Introducing the flexible ureteroscope and irrigation results in increased intrarenal pressure that when exceeding threshold levels may result in pyelotubular, venous and lymphatic backflow and forniceal rupture, potentially emerging into septic and hemorrhagic complications. Furthermore, increased pelvic pressure induces strain to the pelvic musculature, which results in increased activity of pacemaker cells at the kidney-pelvic [HCN3-positive cells (red)] and the uretero-pelvic junction [c-kit-positive interstitial cells (blue)], producing contractions at the levels of the calyces, pelvis, and ureter (peristalsis) that may complicate ureteral access with increased risk of ureteral lesions

11 Future Perspectives

Since pyelorenal backflow and intrarenal pressure for the first time gained scientific interest, almost a century has passed. Experimental and clinical studies have been diverse and eventful. The innervation, peristaltic function, and neurogenic and myogenic regulation of the human and animal upper urinary tract have been explored. The mechanisms and variants of intrarenal backflow have been documented. The pressure inside the ureter, renal pelvis, and renal calyces has been studied in detail during normal and pathophysiological conditions. The impact of different kinds of instrumentation and obstruction on renal function and IRP has been elucidated. Several ways to decrease the IRP have been subject to experimental studies.

All these studies contribute to better understanding of the functionality of the upper urinary tract, which is more relevant now than ever before. In a time when subspecialized and technological treatment is in increasing demand, basic research and high-quality clinical studies are essential for further improvement of both diagnostic and therapeutic tools for the benefit of patients.

Ongoing research in the field of pathophysiology and pressure in the upper urinary tract is crucial to ensure optimization of treatment regarding both safety issues and therapeutic outcome. Gaining more knowledge about the irrigation-instrumentation–IRP relationship requires new technology to provide the possibility to measure real-time IRP during ureterorenoscopy. Continuous monitoring of intrapelvic pressure during fURS using a sensor wire was feasible in a human study including four patients [35]. Accurate and easy deployment of pressure sensors may provide valuable perioperative information for the endourologist to take action to reduce rate of postoperative complications. An intelligent pressure controlling system for fURS including an irrigation and suctioning platform and a UAS with a pressure-sensitive tip has also been proposed and seemed safe and efficient in keeping the IRP stable at a predefined value [31].

Until now, the perfect way to keep IRP low while ensuring sufficient vision during ureteroscopy has not been found. Ureteral access sheaths, pharmacological modulation, and vacuum-cleaning/suction systems may all be part of the solution. A thorough and innovative collaboration between scientists, clinicians, and the industry, hopefully, will provide solutions for the future.

References

1. Matlaga BR, Assimos DG. Changing indications of open stone surgery. Urology. 2002;59(4):490–3.
2. Schwalb DM, Eshghi M, Davidian M, Franco I. Morphological and physiological changes in the urinary tract associated with ureteral dilation and ureteropyeloscopy: an experimental study. J Urol. 1993;149(6):1576–85.
3. Jung H, Osther PJ. Intraluminal pressure profiles during flexible ureterorenoscopy. Springerplus. 2015;4:373. https://doi.org/10.1186/s40064-015-1114-4.
4. Tokas T, Herrmann TRW, Skolarikos A, Nagele U. Pressure matters: intrarenal pressures during normal and pathological conditions, and impact of increased values to renal physiology. World J Urol. 2019;37(1):125–31. https://doi.org/10.1007/s00345-018-2378-4.
5. Osther PJS. Risks of flexible ureterorenoscopy: pathophysiology and prevention. Urolithiasis. 2018;46(1):59–67.https://doi.org/10.1007/s00240-017-1018-6.
6. Osther PJ, Pedersen KV, Lildal SK, Pless MS, Andreassen KH, Osther SS, Jung HU. Pathophysiological aspects of ureterorenoscopic management of upper urinary tract calculi. Curr Opin Urol. 2016;26(1):63–9. https://doi.org/10.1097/mou.0000000000000235.
7. Mykoniatis I, Sarafidis P, Memmos D, Anastasiadis A, Dimitriadis G, Hatzichristou D. Are endourological procedures for nephrolithiasis treatment associated with renal injury? A review of potential mechanisms and novel diagnostic indexes. Clin Kidney J. 2020;13(4):531–41. https://doi.org/10.1093/ckj/sfaa020.
8. Lildal SK, Andreassen KH, Baard J, Brehmer M, Bultitude M, Eriksson Y, Ghani KR, Jung H, Kamphuis G, Kronenberg P, Turney B, Traxer O, Ulvik Ø, Osther PJS. Consultation on kidney stones, Copenhagen 2019: aspects of intracorporeal lithotripsy in flexible ureterorenoscopy. World J Urol. 2020;39(6):1673–82. https://doi.org/10.1007/s00345-020-03481-9.
9. Thomsen HS, Dorph S, Larsen S, Talner LB. Intrarenal backflow and renal perfusion during increased intrapelvic pressure in excised porcine kidneys. Acta Radiol Diagn. 1983;24(4):327–36.
10. Boddy SA, Nimmon CC, Jones S, Ramsay JW, Britton KE, Levison DA, Whitfield HN. Irrigation and acute ureteric dilatation—as for ureteroscopy. Br J Urol. 1989;63(1):11–3.
11. Kreydin EI, Eisner BH. Risk factors for sepsis after percutaneous renal stone surgery. Nat Rev Urol. 2013;10(10):598–605. https://doi.org/10.1038/nrurol.2013.183.
12. Yahsi S, Tonyali S, Ceylan C, Yildiz KY, Ozdal L. Intraparenchymal hematoma as a late complication of retrograde intrarenal surgery. Int Braz J Urol. 2017;43(2):367–70. https://doi.org/10.1590/s1677-5538.ibju.2016.0121.
13. Farag M, Timm B, Davis N, Wong LM, Bolton DM, Jack GS. Pressurized-bag irrigation versus hand-operated irrigation pumps during ureteroscopic laser lithotripsy: comparison of infectious complications. J Endourol. 2020;34(9):914–8. https://doi.org/10.1089/end.2020.0148.
14. Mitsuzuka K, Nakano O, Takahashi N, Satoh M. Identification of factors associated with postoperative febrile urinary tract infection after ureteroscopy for urinary stones. Urolithiasis. 2016;44(3):257–62. https://doi.org/10.1007/s00240-015-0816-y.
15. Lechevallier E, Luciani M, Nahon O, Lay F, Coulange C. Transurethral ureterorenolithotripsy using new automated irrigation/suction system controlling pressure and flow compared with standard irrigation: a randomized pilot study. J Endourol. 2003;17(2):97–101. https://doi.org/10.1089/08927790360587423.
16. Tokas T, Skolarikos A, Herrmann TRW, Nagele U. Pressure matters 2: intrarenal pressure ranges during upper-tract endourological procedures. World J Urol. 2019;37(1):133–42. https://doi.org/10.1007/s00345-018-2379-3.
17. Guzelburc V, Balasar M, Colakogullari M, Guven S, Kandemir A, Ozturk A, Karaaslan P, Erkurt B, Albayrak S. Comparison of absorbed irrigation fluid volumes during retrograde intrarenal surgery and percutaneous nephrolithotomy for the treatment of kidney stones larger than 2 cm. Springerplus. 2016;5(1):1707. https://doi.org/10.1186/s40064-016-3383-y.
18. Loftus C, Byrne M, Monga M. High pressure endoscopic irrigation: impact on renal histology. Int Braz J Urol. 2021;47(2):350–6. https://doi.org/10.1590/s1677-5538.ibju.2020.0248.
19. Blew BD, Dagnone AJ, Pace KT, Honey RJ. Comparison of peditrol irrigation device and common methods of irrigation. J Endourol. 2005;19(5):562–5. https://doi.org/10.1089/end.2005.19.562.
20. MacCraith E, Yap LC, Elamin M, Patterson K, Brady CM, Hennessey DB. Evaluation of the impact of ureteroscope, access sheath, and irrigation system selection on intrarenal pressures in a porcine kidney model. J Endourol. 2020;35(4):512–7. https://doi.org/10.1089/end.2020.0838.
21. Proietti S, Dragos L, Somani B, Butticè S, Talso M, Emiliani E, Baghdadi M, Giusti G, Traxer O. In vitro comparison of maximum pressure developed by irrigation systems in a kidney model. J Endourol. 2017;31(5):522–7. https://doi.org/10.1089/end.2017.0005.
22. Noureldin YA, Kallidonis P, Ntasiotis P, Adamou C, Zazas E, Liatsikos EN. The effect of irrigation power and ureteral access sheath diameter on the maximal intra-pelvic pressure during ureteroscopy: in vivo experimental study in a live anesthetized pig. J Endourol. 2019;33(9):725–9. https://doi.org/10.1089/end.2019.0317.
23. Inoue T, Yamamichi F, Okada S, Hamamoto S, Fujisawa M. Change in irrigation flow through a

flexible ureteroscope with various devices in the working channel: comparison between an automatic irrigation pump and gravity-based irrigation. Int J Urol. 2020;27(4):333–8. https://doi.org/10.1111/iju.14197.

24. Lama DJ, Owyong M, Parkhomenko E, Patel RM, Landman J, Clayman RV. Fluid dynamic analysis of hand-pump infuser and UROMAT endoscopic automatic system for irrigation through a flexible ureteroscope. J Endourol. 2018;32(5):431–6. https://doi.org/10.1089/end.2017.0811.
25. Doersch KM, Hart KD, Elmekresh A, Milburn PA, Machen GL, El Tayeb MM. Comparison of utilization of pressurized automated versus manual hand irrigation during ureteroscopy in the absence of ureteral access sheath. Proc (Baylor Univ Med Cent). 2018;31(4):432–5. https://doi.org/10.1080/08998280.2018.1482518.
26. Jefferson FA, Sung JM, Limfueco L, Lu S, Cottone CM, Tapiero S, Patel RM, Clayman RV, Landman J. Prospective randomized comparison of standard hand pump infuser irrigation vs an automated irrigation pump during percutaneous nephrolithotomy and ureteroscopy: assessment of operating room efficiency and surgeon satisfaction. J Endourol. 2020;34(2):156–62. https://doi.org/10.1089/end.2019.0419.
27. Bedke J, Leichtle U, Lorenz A, Nagele U, Stenzl A, Kruck S. 1.2 French stone retrieval baskets further enhance irrigation flow in flexible ureterorenoscopy. Urolithiasis. 2013;41(2):153–7. https://doi.org/10.1007/s00240-012-0540-9.
28. Kruck S, Anastasiadis AG, Gakis G, Walcher U, Hennenlotter J, Merseburger AS, Stenzl A, Nagele U. Flow matters: irrigation flow differs in flexible ureteroscopes of the newest generation. Urol Res. 2011;39(6):483–6. https://doi.org/10.1007/s00240-011-0373-y.
29. Noureldin YA, Farsari E, Ntasiotis P, Adamou C, Vagionis A, Vrettos T, Liatsikos EN, Kallidonis P. Effects of irrigation parameters and access sheath size on the intra-renal temperature during flexible ureteroscopy with a high-power laser. World J Urol. 2020;39(4):1257–62. https://doi.org/10.1007/s00345-020-03287-9.
30. Hein S, Petzold R, Suarez-Ibarrola R, Müller PF, Schoenthaler M, Miernik A. Thermal effects of Ho:YAG laser lithotripsy during retrograde intrarenal surgery and percutaneous nephrolithotomy in an ex vivo porcine kidney model. World J Urol. 2020;38(3):753–60. https://doi.org/10.1007/s00345-019-02808-5.
31. Deng X, Song L, Xie D, Fan D, Zhu L, Yao L, Wang X, Liu S, Zhang Y, Liao X, Liu S, Peng Z, Hu M, Zhu X, Huang J, Liu T, Du C, Guo S, Yang Z, Peng G, Ye Z. A novel flexible ureteroscopy with intelligent control of renal pelvic pressure: an initial experience of 93 cases. J Endourol. 2016;30(10):1067–72. https://doi.org/10.1089/end.2015.0770.
32. Patel RM, Jefferson FA, Owyong M, Hofmann M, Ayad ML, Osann K, Okhunov Z, Landman J, Clayman RV. Characterization of intracalyceal pressure during ureteroscopy. World J Urol. 2020;39(3):883–9. https://doi.org/10.1007/s00345-020-03259-z.
33. Fedrigon D III, Alshara L, Monga M. Comparison of automated irrigation systems using an in vitro ureteroscopy model. Int Braz J Urol. 2020;46(3):390–7. https://doi.org/10.1590/s1677-5538.ibju.2019.0230.
34. De S, Torricelli FC, Sarkissian C, Kartha G, Monga M. Evaluating the automated Thermedx fluid management system in a ureteroscopy model. J Endourol. 2014;28(5):549–53. https://doi.org/10.1089/end.2013.0697.
35. Doizi S, Letendre J, Cloutier J, Ploumidis A, Traxer O. Continuous monitoring of intrapelvic pressure during flexible ureteroscopy using a sensor wire: a pilot study. World J Urol. 2020;39(2):555–61. https://doi.org/10.1007/s00345-020-03216-w.
36. Kiil F. Pressure recordings in the upper urinary tract. Scand J Clin Lab Investig. 1953;5(4):383–4. https://doi.org/10.3109/00365515309094217.
37. Djurhuus JC. Aspects of renal pelvic function. Copenhagen: University of Copenhagen; 1980.
38. Jung HU, Jakobsen JS, Mortensen J, Osther PJ, Djurhuus JC. Irrigation with isoproterenol diminishes increases in pelvic pressure without side-effects during ureterorenoscopy: a randomized controlled study in a porcine model. Scand J Urol Nephrol. 2008;42(1):7–11. https://doi.org/10.1080/00365590701520073.
39. Jakobsen JS, Jung HU, Gramsbergen JB, Osther PJ, Walter S. Endoluminal isoproterenol reduces renal pelvic pressure during semirigid ureterorenoscopy: a porcine model. BJU Int. 2010;105(1):121–4. https://doi.org/10.1111/j.1464-410X.2009.08678.x.
40. Rattner WH. Human ureter and renal pelvis. J Urol. 1957;78(4):359–62. https://doi.org/10.1016/S0022-5347(17)66448-6.
41. Thomsen HS. Pyelorenal backflow. Clinical and experimental investigations. Radiologic, nuclear, medical and pathoanatomic studies. Dan Med Bull. 1984;31(6):438–57.
42. Hinman F. Pyelovenous backflow. J Am Med Assoc. 1926;87(16):1287–93. https://doi.org/10.1001/jama.1926.02680160035011.
43. Stenberg A, Bohman SO, Morsing P, Müller-Suur C, Olsen L, Persson AE. Back-leak of pelvic urine to the bloodstream. Acta Physiol Scand. 1988;134(2):223–34. https://doi.org/10.1111/j.1748-1716.1988.tb08483.x.
44. Jung H, Pless MS, Osther PJS. Anatomic variations and stone formation. Curr Opin Urol. 2018;28(5):420–7. https://doi.org/10.1097/mou.0000000000000519.
45. Pless MS, Williams JC Jr, Andreassen KH, Jung HU, Osther SS, Christensen DR, Osther PJS. Endoscopic observations as a tool to define underlying pathology in kidney stone formers. World J Urol. 2019;37(10):2207–15. https://doi.org/10.1007/s00345-018-02616-3.
46. Kukreja RA, Desai MR, Sabnis RB, Patel SH. Fluid absorption during percutaneous nephrolithotomy: does it matter? J Endourol. 2002;16(4):221–4. https://doi.org/10.1089/089277902753752160.

47. Boccafoschi C, Lugnani F. Intra-renal reflux. Urol Res. 1985;13(5):253–8. https://doi.org/10.1007/bf00261587.
48. Shao Y, Shen ZJ, Zhu YY, Sun XW, Lu J, Xia SJ. Fluid-electrolyte and renal pelvic pressure changes during ureteroscopic lithotripsy. Minim Invasive Ther Allied Technol MITAT. 2012;21(4):302–6. https://doi.org/10.3109/13645706.2011.595419.
49. Wilson WT, Preminger GM. Intrarenal pressures generated during flexible deflectable ureterorenoscopy. J Endourol. 1990;4:135–42.
50. Jung HU, Jakobsen JS, Frimodt-Moeller PC, Osther PJ. Irrigation with isoproterenol during ureterorenoscopy causes no systemic side-effects. Scand J Urol Nephrol. 2008;42(2):158–63. https://doi.org/10.1080/00365590701570631.
51. Doizi S, Uzan A, Keller EX, De Coninck V, Kamkoum H, Barghouthy Y, Ventimiglia E, Traxer O. Comparison of intrapelvic pressures during flexible ureteroscopy, mini-percutaneous nephrolithotomy, standard percutaneous nephrolithotomy, and endoscopic combined intrarenal surgery in a kidney model. World J Urol. 2020;39(7):2709–17. https://doi.org/10.1007/s00345-020-03450-2.
52. Jung H, Norby B, Frimodt-Moller PC, Osther PJ. Endoluminal isoproterenol irrigation decreases renal pelvic pressure during flexible ureterorenoscopy: a clinical randomized, controlled study. Eur Urol. 2008;54(6):1404–13. https://doi.org/10.1016/j.eururo.2008.03.092.
53. Auge BK, Pietrow PK, Lallas CD, Raj GV, Santa-Cruz RW, Preminger GM. Ureteral access sheath provides protection against elevated renal pressures during routine flexible ureteroscopic stone manipulation. J Endourol. 2004;18(1):33–6. https://doi.org/10.1089/089277904322836631.
54. Guohua Z, Wen Z, Xun L, Wenzhong C, Yongzhong H, Zhaohui H, Ming L, Kaijun W. The influence of minimally invasive percutaneous nephrolithotomy on renal pelvic pressure in vivo. Surg Laparosc Endosc Percutan Tech. 2007;17(4):307–10. https://doi.org/10.1097/SLE.0b013e31806e61f4.
55. Landman J, Venkatesh R, Ragab M, Rehman J, Lee DI, Morrissey KG, Monga M, Sundaram CP. Comparison of intrarenal pressure and irrigant flow during percutaneous nephroscopy with an indwelling ureteral catheter, ureteral occlusion balloon, and ureteral access sheath. Urology. 2002;60(4):584–7. https://doi.org/10.1016/s0090-4295(02)01861-7.
56. Troxel SA, Low RK. Renal intrapelvic pressure during percutaneous nephrolithotomy and its correlation with the development of postoperative fever. J Urol. 2002;168(4 Pt 1):1348–51. https://doi.org/10.1097/01.ju.0000030996.64339.f1.
57. Alsyouf M, Abourbih S, West B, Hodgson H, Baldwin DD. Elevated renal pelvic pressures during percutaneous nephrolithotomy risk higher postoperative pain and longer hospital stay. J Urol. 2018;199(1):193–9. https://doi.org/10.1016/j.juro.2017.08.039.
58. Malhotra SK, Khaitan A, Goswami AK, Gill KD, Dutta A. Monitoring of irrigation fluid absorption during percutaneous nephrolithotripsy: the use of 1% ethanol as a marker. Anaesthesia. 2001;56(11):1103–6. https://doi.org/10.1046/j.1365-2044.2001.01962-3.x.
59. Gehring H, Nahm W, Zimmermann K, Fornara P, Ocklitz E, Schmucker P. Irrigating fluid absorption during percutaneous nephrolithotripsy. Acta Anaesthesiol Scand. 1999;43(3):316–21. https://doi.org/10.1034/j.1399-6576.1999.430312.x.
60. Traxer O, Thomas A. Prospective evaluation and classification of ureteral wall injuries resulting from insertion of a ureteral access sheath during retrograde intrarenal surgery. J Urol. 2013;189(2):580–4. https://doi.org/10.1016/j.juro.2012.08.197.
61. Rehman J, Monga M, Landman J, Lee DI, Felfela T, Conradie MC, Srinivas R, Sundaram CP, Clayman RV. Characterization of intrapelvic pressure during ureteropyeloscopy with ureteral access sheaths. Urology. 2003;61(4):713–8.
62. Yoshida T, Inoue T, Abe T, Matsuda T. Evaluation of intrapelvic pressure when using small-sized ureteral access sheaths of ≤ 10/12 F in an ex vivo porcine kidney model. J Endourol. 2018;32(12):1142–7. https://doi.org/10.1089/end.2018.0501.
63. Fang L, Xie G, Zheng Z, Liu W, Zhu J, Huang T, Lu Y, Cheng Y. The effect of ratio of endoscope-sheath diameter on intrapelvic pressure during flexible ureteroscopic lasertripsy. J Endourol. 2019;33(2):132–9. https://doi.org/10.1089/end.2018.0774.
64. Sener TE, Cloutier J, Villa L, Marson F, Butticè S, Doizi S, Traxer O. Can we provide low intrarenal pressures with good irrigation flow by decreasing the size of ureteral access sheaths? J Endourol. 2016;30(1):49–55. https://doi.org/10.1089/end.2015.0387.
65. Wright A, Williams K, Somani B, Rukin N. Intrarenal pressure and irrigation flow with commonly used ureteric access sheaths and instruments. Cent Eur J Urol. 2015;68(4):434–8. https://doi.org/10.5173/ceju.2015.604.
66. Oratis AT, Subasic JJ, Hernandez N, Bird JC, Eisner BH. A simple fluid dynamic model of renal pelvis pressures during ureteroscopic kidney stone treatment. PLoS One. 2018;13(11):e0208209. https://doi.org/10.1371/journal.pone.0208209.
67. Stern JM, Yiee J, Park S. Safety and efficacy of ureteral access sheaths. J Endourol. 2007;21(2):119–23. https://doi.org/10.1089/end.2007.9997.
68. Lildal SK, Nørregaard R, Andreassen KH, Christiansen FE, Jung H, Pedersen MR, Osther PJ. Ureteral access sheath influence on the ureteral wall evaluated by cyclooxygenase-2 and tumor necrosis factor-α in a porcine model. J Endourol. 2017;31(3):307–13. https://doi.org/10.1089/end.2016.0773.

69. Lildal SK, Sørensen FB, Andreassen KH, Christiansen FE, Jung H, Pedersen MR, Osther PJS. Histopathological correlations to ureteral lesions visualized during ureteroscopy. World J Urol. 2017;35(10):1489–96. https://doi.org/10.1007/s00345-017-2035-3.
70. Traxer O, Wendt-Nordahl G, Sodha H, Rassweiler J, Meretyk S, Tefekli A, Coz F, de la Rosette JJ. Differences in renal stone treatment and outcomes for patients treated either with or without the support of a ureteral access sheath: the Clinical Research Office of the Endourological Society Ureteroscopy Global Study. World J Urol. 2015;33(12):2137–44. https://doi.org/10.1007/s00345-015-1582-8.
71. De Coninck V, Keller EX, Rodríguez-Monsalve M, Audouin M, Doizi S, Traxer O. Systematic review of ureteral access sheaths: facts and myths. BJU Int. 2018;122(6):959–69. https://doi.org/10.1111/bju.14389.
72. Zhong W, Leto G, Wang L, Zeng G. Systemic inflammatory response syndrome after flexible ureteroscopic lithotripsy: a study of risk factors. J Endourol. 2015;29(1):25–8. https://doi.org/10.1089/end.2014.0409.
73. Jung HU, Frimodt-Moller PC, Osther PJ, Mortensen J. Pharmacological effect on pyeloureteric dynamics with a clinical perspective: a review of the literature. Urol Res. 2006;34(6):341–50. https://doi.org/10.1007/s00240-006-0069-x.
74. Park YC, Tomiyama Y, Hayakawa K, Akahane M, Ajisawa Y, Miyatake R, Kiwamoto H, Sugiyama T, Kurita T. Existence of a beta3-adrenoceptro and its functional role in the human ureter. J Urol. 2000;164(4):1364–70.
75. Canda AE, Turna B, Cinar GM, Nazli O. Physiology and pharmacology of the human ureter: basis for current and future treatments. Urol Int. 2007;78(4):289–98. https://doi.org/10.1159/000100830.
76. Holst U, Dissing T, Rawashdeh YF, Frokiaer J, Djurhuus JC, Mortensen J. Norepinephrine inhibits the pelvic pressure increase in response to flow perfusion. J Urol. 2003;170(1):268–71. https://doi.org/10.1097/01.ju.0000069824.13258.14.
77. Jung H, Nørby B, Frimodt-Møller PC, Osther PJ. Endoluminal isoproterenol irrigation decreases renal pelvic pressure during flexible ureterorenoscopy: a clinical randomized, controlled study. Eur Urol. 2008;54(6):1404–13. https://doi.org/10.1016/j.eururo.2008.03.092.

Double J Stents in Flexible Ureteroscopy: Rationale and Indications of Ureteric Stenting Before and After Flexible Ureteroscopy

Georgios Tsampoukas and Noor Buchholz

Abstract

Flexible ureteroscopy is the cornerstone of diagnosis and treatment of multiple upper urinary tract pathologies, including intrarenal and ureteric stones and renal pelvic tumors. Retrograde ureteral and intrarenal surgery requires excellent knowledge of the surgical equipment, familiarization with the collecting system anatomy, and advanced endoscopic skills. However, the optimal surgical strategy lies in the hands of the operating urologist. The clinical dilemma of pre- and postoperative stenting is quite common in clinical practice and remains a matter of debate.

In most instances, the surgeon must balance the obvious benefits of stenting against well-known and significant stent-related side effects such as infection, stent-related lower urinary tract symptoms, pain, and discomfort for the patient.

Pre-stenting has benefits, but it may not always be possible due to clinical or other limitations, e.g., cost or availability. However, it can facilitate the operating steps, reduce surgical time, and increase the chances for a successful outcome. Similarly, postoperative stenting is not considered to be mandatory, but it is strongly recommended in complicated cases, although there is a lack of consensus of what constitutes a complicated ureteroscopy. There is a definitive agreement though on mandatory stenting in cases of any kind of ureteric violation or injury.

Keywords

Flexible ureteroscopy · Double J stent · Ureteral sheath

G. Tsampoukas (✉)
Scientific Office, U-merge (Urology in Emerging Countries), Athens, Greece

Department of Urology, The Great Western Hospital NHS Trust, Swindon, UK
e-mail: gt@u-merge.com

N. Buchholz
Scientific Office, U-merge (Urology in Emerging Countries), Athens, Greece

1 Introduction

In 2019, a worldwide survey organized by European Association of Urology young academic urologists (EAU-YAU) and uro-technology (EAU-ESUT) groups examined the current surgical practice in flexible ureteroscopy (fURS). The survey revealed the wide variety in operative strategies among urologists, and the absence of a consensus regarding the role of pre- and postoperative stenting. However, more than 50% of the participants responded that they use a double J (DJ) stent before and after an fURS in the majority of their cases. This number increased when a ureteral access sheath (UAS) was used [1]. Whereas there can be no doubt that both pre- and

G. Zeng et al. (eds.), *Flexible Ureteroscopy*, https://doi.org/10.1007/978-981-19-2936-6_11

postoperative DJ stenting have benefits, the indication to stent should meet appropriate surgical criteria. Any such decision should take into consideration the anatomical peculiarities, the objectives of the procedure, the expectations of the patients, the financial implications, and the usage of additional equipment. Because clear benefits and harms of stenting are still controversially discussed, there is no generally recommended approach to be followed [2].

2 Rationale, Indications, and Alternatives

To date, the American Urological Association (AUA) and International Endourological Society (IES) both recommend against the routine preoperative placement of a DJ before ureteroscopy (URS) for renal or ureteral calculi [3]. From the surgical point of view, preoperative stenting will facilitate the passage of the flexible ureteroscope or a UAS by passively dilating the ureter. Also, when no DJ has been used before retrograde intrarenal surgery, there is a potential risk of ureteral injury due to primary instrumentation and the usage of UAS. Therefore, preoperative stenting seems to offer efficient dilatation of the ureter, helps to avoid ureteral edema or injury when UAS is used, and reduces pain secondary to residual stone fragments or clot passage [4]. In a multicenter retrospective study with 727 participants, preoperative ureteral stenting increased the success rate of a 12/14 Fr UAS placements in comparison to nonstented cases. Although the clinical outcomes of the operation (stone-free rates, operative time, complication rates) were unaffected in this study, preoperative stenting did assist the surgeons to finish the procedure successfully without the need of a secondary procedure [5].

Regarding timing, a 5- to 10-day preoperative stenting is recommended by some urologists prior to fURS, with the consecutive use of a wide UAS (14/16 Fr). This strategy, called "Freiburg FURS technique," is associated with excellent "immediate" stone-free rates (SFR) of 96.7% [6]. The beneficial effect of preoperative stenting on treatment outcomes of kidney stones was also shown in a large study conducted by the Clinical Research Office of the Endourological Society (CROES). In this study of 1622 participants from multiple countries, preoperative stent placement increased the SFR along with a borderline significant decrease in intraoperative complications [7].

Traditionally, when narrow or tortuous ureters are encountered, segmental or full-length dilatation with balloons, semirigid URS, or serial dilators will be performed. Both the condition being encountered and the instrumentation may lead to tearing of the ureteric wall which, in turn, may lead to impaired vision by bleeding, false passage, or later stricture formation [8]. Aggressive manipulations of the ureter should be avoided and the use of a DJ for pre-stenting in such cases has found its way into the EAU guidelines [9].

However, infrastructural and socio-economic factors of a given health system in a given society may make it difficult to apply pre-stenting. In countries where patients travel long distances to have one single procedure, pre-stenting and a 1- to 2-week wait may be impractical and unaffordable. Pre-dilatation techniques such as a first-look semirigid ureteroscopy will still have to be applied [10].

Postoperative stenting reduces the pressure in the collecting system and reduces pain associated with the passage of small stone fragments or clots. However, DJ stents have their own short-term side effects such as stent-related infections, lower urinary tract symptoms (LUTS), and patient discomfort. Ureteral stents have been found independently responsible for significant pain after fURS, affecting the domains of general health, working, and sexual activity [11]. The EAU guidelines do not recommend postoperative stenting after an uncomplicated URS; however, there is no consensus mentioned on what actually constitutes an uncomplicated URS [9]. In our practice, obscuring bleeding which gives the surgeon a bad time to continue, it is reliable enough to build the indication for stenting. In general, in his decision for a postoperative DJ, the surgeon must weigh the balance between benefits and possible stent-related side effects.

The decision of postoperative stenting depends also on the pre-stented status of the ureter. In a retrospective study of 70 pre-stented patients who underwent uncomplicated fURS with the use of UAS, there was no statistically significant difference between the stented and non-stented group postoperatively in terms of emergency department visits, urinary tract infections, development of renal colic and readmission rate [12]. Pre-stenting is associated with better pain scores after fURS without postoperative DJ [13]. Therefore, postoperative stenting might not be necessary in pre-stented cases of uncomplicated fURS.

In other cases, postoperative stenting is advisable though to facilitate the healing of the ureteral mucosa and to reduce the risk of renal colic because of residual stones or clots. Although the severity of stent-related symptoms may vary, a-blockers have been proven useful in the management of the side effects, by reducing morbidity and increasing tolerability [14].

As an alternative to a DJ stent, a short-term ureteral catheter can be used. In a randomized (but not-blinded) study of 141 pre-stented patients undergoing fURS for kidney stones with or without UAS, a short-term catheter (5-Fr, 70 cm) for only 6 h post-operatively was found to be superior to a DJ (7-Fr, 26 cm) for 5 days in terms of pain, quality of life, and stent-related urinary symptoms. Patients' recovery and return to work was quicker, and most patients would prefer a ureteral catheter in the future [15].

In our clinical practice, we consider the use of a sizeable (12 Fr or more) UAS a strong indication for post-operative DJ, regardless of preoperative pre-stenting, as the possibility of a renal colic due to clot passage and secondary ureteric edema is significant. However, we attempt to keep the indwelling time as short as possible; 1 week is usually an efficient and well-tolerated time period.

In conclusion, the use of DJ before and after fURS is widespread. Yet, there is no consensus or guidelines on the specific indications.

Preoperative stenting is a less invasive method to dilate narrow and tortuous ureters, but it requires a delayed main procedure. This may not be feasible and affordable in all circumstances. There is emerging evidence that pre-stented patient may not require a postoperative stent which may, if proven over time, partially offset the disadvantages of pre-stenting.

In cases of invasive treatment of the ureter (dilatation, UAS, injury), postoperative stenting is mandatory to prevent obstruction and later stricture formation. The same is true for complicated URS to prevent stone fragments or blood clots from obstructing the ureter. However, a consensus on what constitutes a complex URS is needed.

In any case, the urologist must balance the obvious benefits of stenting against well-known significant stent-related side effects such as infection, stent-related LUTS, pain, and discomfort for the patient.

References

1. Pietropaolo A, et al. Worldwide survey of flexible ureteroscopy practice: a survey from European Association of Urology sections of young academic urologists and uro-technology groups. Cent Eur J Urol. 2019;72(4):393–7. https://doi.org/10.5173/ceju.2019.0041.
2. Ordonez M, et al. Ureteral stent versus no ureteral stent for ureteroscopy in the management of renal and ureteral calculi. Cochrane Database Syst Rev. 2019;2(2):CD012703. https://doi.org/10.1002/14651858.CD012703.pub2.
3. Assimos D, Crisci A, et al. Preoperative JJ stent placement in ureteric and renal stone treatment: results from the Clinical Research Office of Endourological Society (CROES) Ureteroscopy (URS) Global Study. BJU Int. 2016a;117(4):648–54. https://doi.org/10.1111/bju.13250.
4. Traxer O, Thomas A. Prospective evaluation and classification of ureteral wall injuries resulting from insertion of a ureteral access sheath during retrograde intrarenal surgery. J Urol. 2013;189(2):580–4. https://doi.org/10.1016/j.juro.2012.08.197.
5. Yuk HD, et al. The effect of preoperative ureteral stenting in retrograde intrarenal surgery: a multicenter, propensity score-matched study. BMC Urol. 2020;20(1):147. https://doi.org/10.1186/s12894-020-00715-1.
6. Miernik A, et al. Standardized flexible ureteroscopic technique to improve stone-free rates. Urology. 2012;80(6):1198–202. https://doi.org/10.1016/j.urology.2012.08.042.

7. Assimos D, Krambeck A, et al. Surgical management of stones: American Urological Association/Endourological Society Guideline, Part II. J Urol. 2016b;196(4):1161–9. https://doi.org/10.1016/j.juro.2016.05.091.
8. Ulvik Ø, Harneshaug J-R, Gjengstø P. Ureteral strictures following ureteroscopic stone treatment. J Endourol. 2020;35(7):985–90. https://doi.org/10.1089/end.2020.0421.
9. Türk C, et al. EAU guidelines on urolithiasis 2018. Eur Urol. 2019. https://doi.org/10.1159/000049803.
10. Doizi S, Traxer O. Flexible ureteroscopy: technique, tips and tricks. Urolithiasis. 2018;46(1):47–58. https://doi.org/10.1007/s00240-017-1030-x.
11. Bosio A, et al. How bothersome double-J ureteral stents are after semirigid and flexible ureteroscopy: a prospective single-institution observational study. World J Urol. 2019;37(1):201–7. https://doi.org/10.1007/s00345-018-2376-6.
12. Astroza G, et al. Is a ureteral stent required after use of ureteral access sheath in presented patients who undergo flexible ureteroscopy? Cent Eur J Urol. 2017;70(1):88–92. https://doi.org/10.5173/ceju.2016.919.
13. Torricelli FC, et al. Flexible ureteroscopy with a ureteral access sheath: when to stent? Urology. 2014;83(2):278–81. https://doi.org/10.1016/j.urology.2013.10.002.
14. Dellis AE, et al. Role of α-blockers in the treatment of stent-related symptoms: a prospective randomized control study. Urology. 2014;83(1):56–62. https://doi.org/10.1016/j.urology.2013.08.067.
15. Bach P, et al. Short-term external ureter stenting shows significant benefit in comparison to routine double-J stent placement after ureterorenoscopic stone extraction: a prospective randomized trial—the Fast Track Stent Study (FaST). Int J Urol. 2018;25(8):717–22. https://doi.org/10.1111/iju.13711.

Flexible Ureteroscopy for Large Renal Stones

Guohua Zeng and Wei Zhu

Abstract

The treatment of large renal stones is challenging for endourologists. Due to the advent of new and more efficient endourological equipment, flexible ureteroscopy (f-URS) has become an attractive option even in case of larger stones, offering the advantage of a reduced invasiveness, if compared to percutaneous approaches. In this chapter, we discuss how to treat large renal stones by f-URS and advise urologists seeking to gain more experience with the procedure.

Keywords

Flexible ureteroscopy · Large stones · Complex stones · Staghorn

1 Introduction

f-URS was first used to treat small kidney stones. Because of its minimally invasive nature, over the last few years, it has been more and more used to treat also larger renal stones. The recent technological advancements, such as the availability of thinner scopes and instruments with an optimized vision, have also rendered f-URS more appealing even in case of larger renal stones. In comparison to the percutaneous nephrolithotomy (PCNL), f-URS has the advantages of fewer complications, less morbidity, easier renal function preservation, and shorter hospital stays. Sometimes, when patients are counseled about the potential complications of PCNLs, they may ask whether a safer option is available and may option for f-URS even though they are told that a staged treatment will be required, especially if the stone burden is high.

2 Indications and Contraindications

f-URS is not recommended as a first-line treatment option in case of large renal stones (≥2 cm) according to recent guidelines. f-URS can be considered in case of:

- Patients for whom PCNL is contraindicated, such as uncorrected bleeding disorders, use of anticoagulants, or with unfavorable anatomy.
- Patients with solitary kidneys who present bleeding diathesis.
- Patients with psychogenic fear of invasive procedures.
- Patient's preference.
- Obese patients with high anesthetic risk, especially if prone PCNL is offered.

G. Zeng (✉) · W. Zhu
Department of Urology, The First Affiliated Hospital of Guangzhou Medical University, Guangzhou, China

G. Zeng et al. (eds.), *Flexible Ureteroscopy*, https://doi.org/10.1007/978-981-19-2936-6_12

Contraindications

- Severe hydronephrosis.
- Large staghorn stones with large stone volume.
- Uncontrolled urinary tract infection.

3 Current Results and Comparison with PCNL

Although not supported by high evidence due to the absence of prospective randomized studies, it appears that in selected patients with large renal stones, f-URS may represent an acceptable option with low morbidity (Figs. 1 and 2). In case of 2–3 cm renal stones, Lin et al. [1] confirmed that the stone-free rate of a single-stage f-URS is not inferior than PCNL. In case of patients with stones larger than 3 cm, a multi-stage f-URS can also provide an adequate stone-free rate and a lower complication rate compared to PCNL. A study from Giusti et al. [2] found that the success rate of f-URS was 87.7% if the stone diameter was larger than 2 cm. Bryniarski et al. [3] compared the efficacy of f-URS and PCNL in the treatment of renal stones larger than 2 cm. The results showed that the success rates were 94% in the PCNL group and 75% in the f-URS group. Similarly, Akman et al. [4] also found that the success rate of f-URS was 73.5% compared to 91.2% of the PCNL cohort in case of 2–4 cm renal stones.

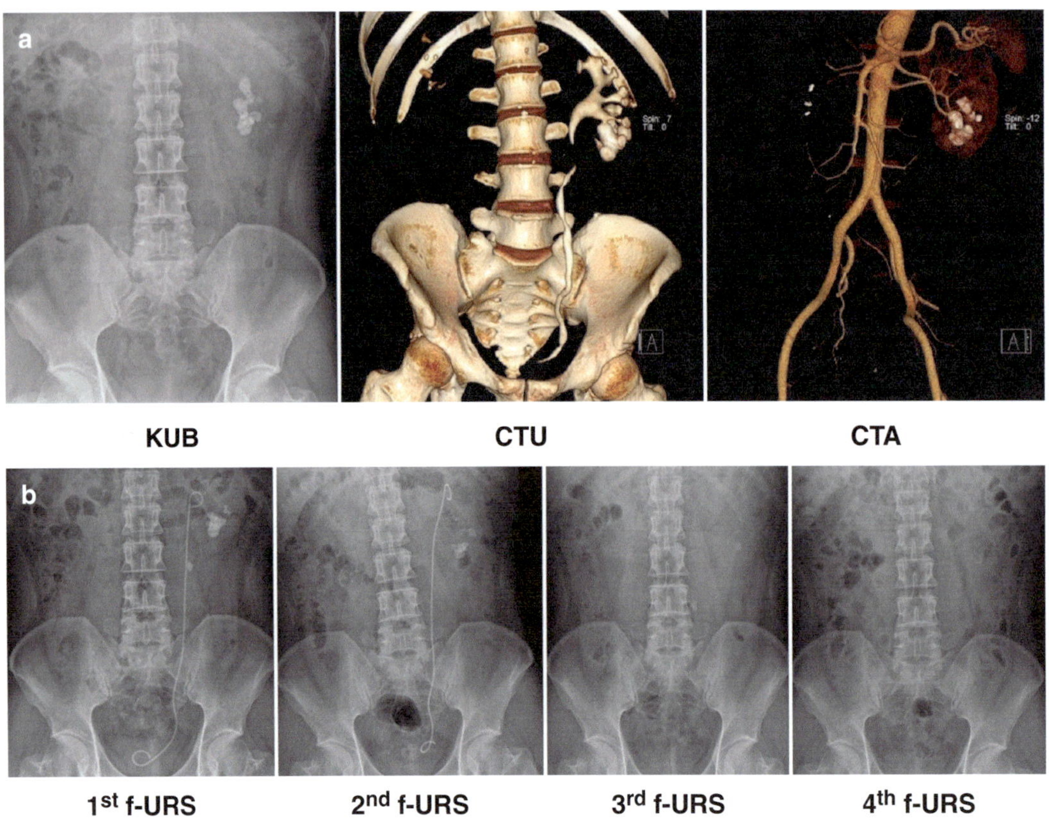

Fig. 1 Staghorn stones in solidary kidney were treated by multiple sessions f-URS. (**a**) Preoperative KUB and CT scans; (**b**) Postoperative KUB after each session f-URS

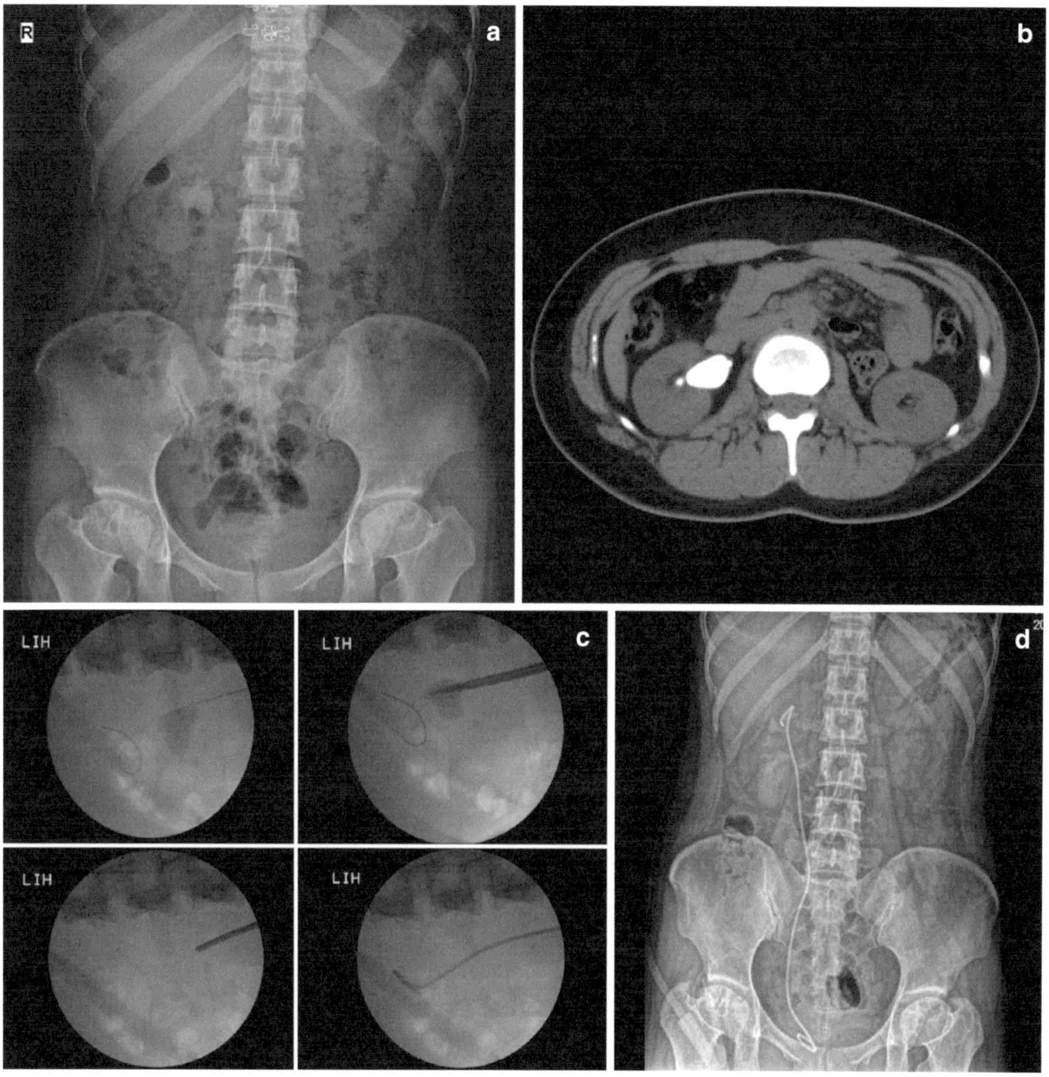

Fig. 2 f-URS treated large stone in patient who used anticoagulants. (**a**) Preoperative KUB showed a 3.5 cm large stone in the right kidney; (**b**) Preoperative CT scan; (**c**) Fluoroscopic images during the operation; (**d**) Postoperative KUB

4 Limitations of f-URS in the Treatment of Large Stones

A disadvantage of f-URS in the treatment of large renal stones is that multiple stages may be necessary. Consequently, f-URS would incur in a significantly longer treatment period, the need of more hospitalizations/anesthesia and higher costs. However, on the other side, it offers a lower invasiveness. Breda et al. [5] reported performances of flexible ureteroscopies in the treatments of 2–2.5 cm stones, showing an average need of 2.3 sessions per case. Moreover, staged f-URSs were deemed to be safe and tolerable for patients with large renal stones. A study from Niwa et al. reported that this approach was not associated with severe complications, such as ureteral stricture or infections [6].

5 How to Improve the Surgical Technique

Several strategies can be used to optimize the fragmentation and shorten the operation time. The first strategy is called "the popcorn method." All the fragments are located in a single calyx, with the laser fiber placed in the middle of the fragments without targeting any particular stone. This allows to save a lot of time and, at the same time, to obtain <4 mm fragments. Repositioning the stone fragments in a favorable calix is a second important method. In fact, the flexible scope should be kept as straight as possible during the fragmentation, avoiding strains on the deflection mechanism and minimizing the risk of damaging the scope while lasering. Most importantly, this maneuver significantly affects the stone-free rate, making the stone targeting during laser lithotripsy easier and more effective. In addition, in case of larger renal calculi, the risk of scope rupture is high. Therefore, utilization of disposable single-use ureteroscopes might be a valid option for these cases [7].

The placement of a ureteral access sheath with a wide inner caliber may also help to shorten the operation time. In fact, it is postulated that wider ureteral access sheaths improve stone-free rates and operative times after f-URS by improving the vision and allowing passage of wider scopes. Additionally, basketing and retrieval of larger fragments becomes easier and faster. A wider caliber also provides a better irrigation, favoring at the same time a passive wash out of small fragments and dust, maintaining the intra-renal pressure low.

In a study by Shvero et al. [8], the authors evaluated associations between different ureteral access sheaths and chances of achieving a stone-free status after f-URS. They found a trend toward a higher stone-free rate in the 12–14 F ureteral access sheath group in comparison to the 9.5–11.5 F ureteral access sheath group (85.7% vs. 73.5%, $p = 0.056$). Tracy et al. [9] carried out a retrospective study comparing outcomes of f-URS utilizing 12–14 F or 14–16 F ureteral access sheath. In this case, authors failed to find any difference in terms of stone-free rates. However, patients in the 14–16 F ureteral access sheath group had a significantly larger stone burden compared to patients in 12–14 F ureteral access sheath group; therefore, a bias could be involved. Despite a larger stone burden, it was found that 14–16 F ureteral access sheaths allowed a quicker operation, reported as up to 30% faster with similar stone-free rates. Thus, especially in case of large stones, wider ureteral access sheaths might be a better choice [9].

f-URS may also be utilized in combination with a percutaneous approach. This strategy is called endoscopic combined intrarenal surgery (ECIRS). It has been proposed as an efficient surgical treatment to overcome the disadvantages of f-URS or PCNL alone. ECIRS can achieve high stone-free rates with a low morbidity. In fact, in several studies, ECIRS is mainly associated with low-grade complications according to the Clavien–Dindo classification. Most of the times, this approach allows to clear the stone using only a single access, reducing the need of multiple punctures. Stone-free rates are reported >80%, ranging from 61 to 97%. Operative times also have to be considered, being longer for ECIRS compared to f-URS but often shorter than PCNLs (being as low as 70 min, including patient positioning). It is credible that in a single-access ECIRS, the integrated use of flexible nephroscopy and flexible retrograde ureteroscopy might represent an effective strategy to achieve a stone-free status in a single session [10].

6 How to Improve Discharge of Stone Fragments After Flexible Ureteroscopy

Residual stones and "Steinstrasses" represent possible complications after f-URS. They may be serious events and might lead to infections and obstruction of the urinary tract. In most cases, the stone fragments eventually pass out of the body spontaneously, but the process can be excruciatingly painful, especially in patients with large stone burdens. To improve the stone fragments clearance, a novel and noninvasive device called External Physical Vibration

Lithecbole (EPVL) was designed. Several articles have proved that EPVL is a safe, simple, effective, and noninvasive method for residual fragments removal after flexible ureteroscopy with high levels of evidence [11–15]. Wu et al. [11] showed that EVPL, as a supplement to f-URS, was more effective than f-URS alone regarding stone clearance speed, stone-free rate, and patient compliance. With the aim of maximizing the performances, Zhang et al. [14] found that the best time to deliver EPVL is 3 days after f-URS, maintaining at the same time a very low risk of complications. This auxiliary procedure provides an additional tool to treat efficiently large stones by f-URS.

7 Future Perspectives

Recently, a vacuum-assisted ureteral access sheath was introduced and considered as a new way to improve the efficacy of f-URS. The sheath has an oblique draining tube that is connected to a negative pressure aspirator. The obtained effect is the suction of fragments while dusting/fragmenting. Using a vacuum-assisted ureteral access sheath has the potential benefit of removing the tiny fragments and dust while lithotripsy is carried out. The continuous irrigation combined with an active suction guarantees a clear vision and shortens the procedure. Lai et al. [16] confirmed that using a vacuum-assisted ureteral access sheath can improve surgical efficiency with lower early postoperative pain when treating 2–4 cm renal stones.

Thulium fiber laser is a promising technology that offers several advantages over Holmium:YAG laser and may expand the boundaries of laser lithotripsy. The advantages of thulium fiber laser include a smaller size of the fiber with a faster dusting, leading to a more efficient operation. Some studies showed that thulium fiber laser was 1.5–4 times faster than Holmium:YAG laser, when lithotripsy was performed on calcium oxalate or uric acid stones [17]. The development of laser lithotripsy may be combined with a vacuum-assisted ureteral access sheath to break up large stones for an easier removal.

8 Summary

Generally, when treating large renal stones, our goals include a stone-free collecting system and a preserved renal function. PCNL is still the recommended first-line treatment option for stones larger than 2 cm. f-URS is usually considered as monotherapy or as part of ECIRS only if PCNL is not doable. The optimal treatment strategy should be individualized according to the patient's circumstances. In order to do so, a closer look at the advantages and disadvantages of each option is necessary. Currently, the motivation and knowledge of patients influence the final treatment choice. Consequently, a detailed and frank counseling is of paramount importance to inform patients about minimal invasiveness, the eventual need of a staged procedure, and outcomes of the surgeon and the center.

References

1. Lin C-F, Wu C-T, Huang S-S, Chen W-H, Wu LS-H, Lin C-C. Safety and efficacy of staged retrograde intrarenal surgery for large stone burden of renal stones in selected patients: a single-center experience. Urol Sci. 2017;28:94–6. https://doi.org/10.1016/j.urols.2016.11.003.
2. Giusti G, Proietti S, Luciani LG, Peschechera R, Giannantoni A, Taverna G, et al. Is retrograde intrarenal surgery for the treatment of renal stones with diameters exceeding 2 cm still a hazard? Can J Urol. 2014;21:7207–12.
3. Bryniarski P, Paradysz A, Zyczkowski M, Kupilas A, Nowakowski K, Bogacki R. A randomized controlled study to analyze the safety and efficacy of percutaneous nephrolithotripsy and retrograde intrarenal surgery in the management of renal stones more than 2 cm in diameter. J Endourol. 2012;26:52–7. https://doi.org/10.1089/end.2011.0235.
4. Akman T, Binbay M, Ozgor F, Ugurlu M, Tekinarslan E, Kezer C, et al. Comparison of percutaneous nephrolithotomy and retrograde flexible nephrolithotripsy for the management of 2–4 cm stones: a matched-pair analysis. BJU Int. 2012;109:1384–9. https://doi.org/10.1111/j.1464-410X.2011.10691.x.
5. Breda A, Ogunyemi O, Leppert JT, Lam JS, Schulam PG. Flexible ureteroscopy and laser lithotripsy for single intrarenal stones 2 cm or greater—is this the new frontier? J Urol. 2008;179:981–4. https://doi.org/10.1016/j.juro.2007.10.083.
6. Niwa N, Matsumoto K, Ohigashi T, Komatsuda A, Katsui M, Bessyo H, et al. Clinical outcomes of ret-

rograde intrarenal surgery as a primary treatment for staghorn calculi: a single-center experience. Clin Med Insights Urol. 2019;12:1179561119854772. https://doi.org/10.1177/1179561119854772.

7. Ventimiglia E, Godínez AJ, Traxer O, Somani BK. Cost comparison of single-use versus reusable flexible ureteroscope: a systematic review. Turk J Urol. 2020;6:S40.
8. Shvero A, Herzberg H, Zilberman D, Mor Y, Winkler H, Kleinmann N. Is it safe to use a ureteral access sheath in an unstented ureter? BMC Urol. 2019;19:1. https://doi.org/10.1186/s12894-019-0509-x.
9. Tracy CR, Ghareeb GM, Paul CJ, Brooks NA. Increasing the size of ureteral access sheath during retrograde intrarenal surgery improves surgical efficiency without increasing complications. World J Urol. 2018;36:971–8. https://doi.org/10.1007/s00345-018-2204-z.
10. Cracco CM, Scoffone CM. Endoscopic combined intrarenal surgery (ECIRS)—tips and tricks to improve outcomes: a systematic review. Turk J Urol. 2020;46:S46–57. https://doi.org/10.5152/tud.2020.20282.
11. Wu W, Yang Z, Xu C, Gu X, Yang S, Liao S, et al. External physical vibration lithecbole promotes the clearance of upper urinary stones after retrograde intrarenal surgery: a prospective, multicenter randomized controlled trial. J Urol. 2017;197:1289–95. https://doi.org/10.1016/j.juro.2017.01.001.
12. Long Q, Zhang J, Xu Z, Zhu Y, Liu L, Wang H, et al. A prospective randomized controlled trial of the efficacy of external physical vibration lithecbole after extracorporeal shock wave lithotripsy for a lower pole renal stone less than 2 cm. J Urol. 2016;195:965–70. https://doi.org/10.1016/j.juro.2015.10.174.
13. Tao R, Tang Q, Zhou S, Jia C, Lv J. External physical vibration lithecbole facilitating the expulsion of upper ureteric stones 1.0–2.0 cm after extracorporeal shock wave lithotripsy: a prospective randomized trial. Urolithiasis. 2020;48:71–7. https://doi.org/10.1007/s00240-018-1100-8.
14. Zhang Y, Xu C, Wang Y, Wang R, Wu W, Yan J, et al. When is the best time to perform external physical vibration lithecbole (EPVL) after retrograde intrarenal surgery (RIRS): a multi-center study based on randomized controlled trials. Urolithiasis. 2019;48(6):533–9. https://doi.org/10.1007/s00240-019-01175-5.
15. Wu W, Yang Z, Tang F, Xu C, Wang Y, Gu X, et al. How to accelerate the upper urinary stone discharge after extracorporeal shockwave lithotripsy (ESWL) for <15 mm upper urinary stones: a prospective multi-center randomized controlled trial about external physical vibration lithecbole (EPVL). World J Urol. 2018;36:293–8. https://doi.org/10.1007/s00345-017-2123-4.
16. Lai D, He Y, Li X, Chen M, Zeng X. RIRS with vacuum-assisted ureteral access sheath versus MPCNL for the treatment of 2–4 cm renal stone. Biomed Res Int. 2020;2020:e8052013. https://doi.org/10.1155/2020/8052013.
17. Traxer O, Keller EX. Thulium fiber laser: the new player for kidney stone treatment? A comparison with Holmium:YAG laser. World J Urol. 2020;38:1883–94. https://doi.org/10.1007/s00345-019-02654-5.

Around Endoscopic Combined IntraRenal Surgery (ECIRS) in 80 Papers

Cesare Marco Scoffone and Cecilia Maria Cracco

Abstract

The acronym ECIRS means Endoscopic Combined IntraRenal Surgery and indicates a comprehensive endourologic treatment of large and/or complex urolithiasis consisting in the combined antegrade and retrograde approach to the collecting system performed with both rigid and flexible endoscopes. ECIRS was explored in the late 1980s in the United States, standardized and popularized in Italy since 2005, and only recently—more than 30 years after its first appearance—is becoming widespread all over the world. Like Jules Verne, in this chapter, we performed "a journey around ECIRS in 80 papers." Nothing better than the literature published from 1988 until nowadays can tell us about birth, growth, and maturation of ECIRS in the different parts of the world, with multifaceted interpretations of the role of retrograde flexible ureteroscopy performed in the context of PNL. In the end, the emerging concept of all the published literature on ECIRS is that the contribution of simultaneous retrograde flexible ureteroscopy substantially improves safety and efficacy of PNL, covering a dual role: diagnostic (integrating the preoperative knowledge on the static anatomy of the collecting system and urolithiasis with real-time intraoperative elements of dynamic anatomy) and active (with the through-and-through guidewire, the Endovision renal puncture, and dilation also sparing radiation exposure, the possibility to reach calyces challenging to access through the single lower pole percutaneous tract, the ability to finally explore the collecting system looking for residual fragments).

Keywords

Percutaneous nephrolithotomy · PCNL · Retrograde intrarenal surgery · RIRS · ECIRS · Endoscopic combined intrarenal surgery

1 Introduction

The acronym ECIRS means Endoscopic Combined IntraRenal Surgery and indicates a comprehensive endourologic treatment of large and/or complex urolithiasis, consisting in the combined antegrade and retrograde approach to the collecting system performed with both rigid and flexible endoscopes. More specifically, ECIRS combines Retrograde IntraRenal Surgery (RIRS) and percutaneous nephrolithotomy (PNL), aiming at the improvement of the one-step efficacy and overall safety of the procedure.

Jules Verne wrote in 1872 his novel *Around the World in 80 Days*; similarly, we are now embarking on a journey around ECIRS in 80

C. M. Scoffone (✉) · C. M. Cracco
Department of Urology, Cottolengo Hospital, Torino, Italy

G. Zeng et al. (eds.), *Flexible Ureteroscopy*, https://doi.org/10.1007/978-981-19-2936-6_13

papers. Nothing better than the literature published along more than 20 years can tell us about birth, growth, and maturation of ECIRS in different parts of the world, with multifaceted interpretations of the role of retrograde flexible ureteroscopy performed in the context of PNL and several clinical applications.

§ 1988: The First ECIRS *ante-litteram* for Stone Treatment

About 33 years ago, *Lehman and Bagley* in the United States reported for the very first time the use of a combined antegrade and retrograde endoscopic approach in the reverse lithotomy position (four times in three patients) in women suffering from massive renal and ureteral calculi [1].

§ 1993: Variations in Patient Positioning for PNL and the Concept of the Two-Team Simultaneous Approach

Always in the United States, 5 years afterwards, *Grasso, Nord, and Bagley* described a modified flank roll position (15 cases) in alternative to the prone split-leg position (111 cases), allowing safe and efficient simultaneous antegrade and retrograde endoscopy for staghorn stones. Two skilled endoscopists used to work together from either end of the urinary tract, employing various combinations of endoscopes and lithotrites and increasing the efficiency of the procedure [2].

§ 1995: The First Endovision Puncture and the First Through-and-Through Guidewire

After a couple of years, in continuity with the school of thoughts of D. Bagley, *Grasso and colleagues* performed in the prone split-leg position the percutaneous puncture of selected calyces under retrograde flexible ureteroscopic control (absolutely the first description of the Endovision renal puncture), in seven patients with minimally dilated collecting systems, narrow infundibula, and complex stone burdens [3]. The pioneering concept of the relevance of the anatomy of the collecting system containing the stones was also clearly stated for the first time.

Always *Grasso and coauthors* used the same combined strategy for accessing five calyceal diverticula containing stones in four patients, with the first description of the through-and-through guidewire [4].

§ 1997: The Combined Treatment of a Tight Recurrent Ureteral Stricture

In Italy, *Scarpa and coworkers* reported the case of a woman with a severe ureteral stricture, requiring a combined endoscopic approach in the prone split-leg position, with transillumination from above guiding the recanalization from below [5]. A decade already passed since the first report of the combined approach, and this was only the fifth publication.

§ 2000: The Combined Treatment of Urinary Diversion-Associated Pathologies

In the United States, *Delvecchio and colleagues* (group of G. Preminger) described the efficiency of the combined approach in order to treat urinary diversion-associated pathologies in five patients [6].

§ 2003: The Key Role of Retrograde Flexible Ureteroscopy During PNL

In the United States, *Landman and coauthors* described the favorable outcomes of the combined antegrade and retrograde approach for the treatment of nine patients with staghorn calculi, in the prone split-leg position as usual.

In particular, the use of a 12–14 F ureteral access sheath advanced up to the ureteropelvic junction instead of the ureteral catheter was felt as a key choice, allowing retrograde dilation of the collecting system with the obturator in place, through-and-through wire placement, easy stone fragments' drainage, decreased intrarenal pressures due to better irrigation outflow, a rapid and atraumatic retrograde passage of the flexible ureteroscope. In practice, the role of retrograde ureteroscopy was that of an additional access site without the associated risks of complications, being crucial for the visualization of calyces challenging to access through the single lower pole 30 F percutaneous tract and their treatment [7].

Once again in the United States, ureteroscopically assisted percutaneous renal access in the prone split-leg position was gained in three difficult cases. *Kidd and Conlin* described in detail the valuable contribution of this technique, not affecting either procedural time or complication rates [8].

§ 2004: The Active Role of Retrograde Flexible Ureteroscopy During PNL: "pass the ball" (But Respect the Ureter)

In the United Kingdom, *Undre* et al. (group of A. Patel) employed "a synchronous bidirectional technique," combining the use of flexible instruments through antegrade and retrograde approaches for the treatment of branched calculi in a lateral position. They described a case of "pass the ball," using the ureteroscope to move calculi from difficult calyces within reach of the nephroscope introduced through a single percutaneous access. For the very first time, the authors underlined the importance of decreasing the possibility of iatrogenic ureteral injury, avoiding multiple passages through the ureter in order to remove stone fragments [9].

§ 2005: The Combined Approach Reduces the Number of Percutaneous Tracts Required to Treat Complex Urolithiasis

In a joint study between the United States (group of G. Preminger) and the United Kingdom (group of A. Patel), *Marguet and coauthors* presented their early experience in managing seven cases of complex renal calculi using a combined ureteroscopic and percutaneous approach, effectively reducing the number of access tracts required with the related morbidity. In particular, a 7.5 F flexible ureteroscope was introduced into a 12–14 F ureteral access sheath and employed in order to relocate stones in an unfavorable location relative to the 30 F access tract and fragment them within easy reach of the single nephrostomy tract [10].

§ 2006: Endoscopic Guidance Not Only as Salvage Approach but on a Routine Planned Basis

In the United States, *Khan and colleagues* (group of R. Clayman) routinely placed a 12 F access sheath in 12 patients undergoing PNL for complex stone burdens, beneficial for spontaneous passage of stone fragments during percutaneous lithotripsy, as well as for providing ureteroscopic access for diagnostic and therapeutic maneuvers in concert with antegrade endoscopy in prone position (being the ureteroscope readily visible on fluoroscopy, dilating with retrograde irrigation the targeted calyx, confirming endoscopically the entry of the needle into the collecting system, accessing calyces that cannot be attained readily through the percutaneous tract) [11].

§ 2007: The Innovative Galdakao-Modified Supine Valdivia Position Offers Anesthesiologic Advantages and Optimally Supports ECIRS

A joint study between Italy (group of R. Scarpa) and Spain described for the first time an alternative patient position optimally supporting the simultaneous antegrade and retrograde access for stone treatment. *Ibarluzea and coworkers* described in detail the supine Valdivia position associated with the modified lithotomy position of the lower limbs, later named Galdakao-modified supine Valdivia position, allowing easy retrograde access during PNL and minimizing the anesthesiologic problems due to the traditional prone position [12].

In the United Kingdom, *Papatsoris* et al. commented such paper in a Letter to the Editor, describing a similar position, the lateral modified lithotomy position, for the combined antegrade and retrograde access to the collecting system in complex endourological cases, also underlining its anesthesiological advantages [13].

§ 2008: Two Scopes are Better Than One Irrespective of the Position: The First Consistent ECIRS Series

We are 20 years after the first published combined approach, with only 12 papers on this topic.

In the United States, *Borin* wrote a case report, describing again the benefits of the combined retrograde approach in terms of safety and efficacy, the possibility to insert a through-and-through guidewire, to have a single percutaneous access, to perform an Endovision puncture and retrograde laser lithotripsy simultaneously to prone PNL for staghorn calculi [14].

In the same year in the United States, *Patel and coauthors* wrote another case report, using ECIRS in the prone split-leg position not only as salvage procedure but also as a welcome integration to PNL [15]. The retrograde flexible ureteroscope provided a radiopaque target for the renal puncture, aided the accurate placement of the puncture needle in the desired calyx, facilitated wire advancement, and reduced radiation exposure.

In the United Kingdom, *Papatsoris and coworkers* reported the efficacy and safety of the simultaneous antegrade and retrograde access (called the Barts technique) to manage complex and demanding cases in their supine-modified position (20 patients), and notably under combined ultrasound and fluoroscopic guidance [16].

In Italy, *Scoffone and colleagues* (school of R. Scarpa) for the first time used the acronym ECIRS, i.e., Endoscopic Combined IntraRenal Surgery, reporting the favorable outcomes of this combined antegrade and retrograde approach using both rigid and flexible scopes performed on 127 consecutive patients arranged in the Galdakao-modified supine Valdivia position, the first consistent series ever published [17].

§ 2009: The Ureteroscopic Access During PNL Minimizes the Trauma to the Collecting System: The First Comparative Study

In the United States, *Sountoulides and coauthors* (group of R. Clayman) reported the results of 51 endoscopic-assisted PNL for urolithiasis, comparing them to standard PNL. Success rates were improved as well as safety because of the constant endoscopic control of all the percutaneous steps, while the need for multiple percutaneous tracts was reduced. Therefore, the authors claimed that these advantages well balance increased operative times and costs [18].

§ 2010: Dead Calm Year for Publications on ECIRS

One paper was published during this year, authored by the usual Italian group of R. Scarpa. *Scoffone* et al. [19] stressed the standardization as well as the versatility of the endoscopic combined approach. Admittedly, the debate was more concentrated on pros and cons of the Galdakao-modified supine Valdivia position compared to the traditional prone one rather than on those of ECIRS compared to the traditional rigid-only antegrade PNL, which in our opinion were much more crucial.

§ 2011: Patient Positioning for ECIRS Draws More Attention Than ECIRS Itself

In Italy, *Cracco and Scoffone* went on supporting ECIRS performed in the Galdakao-modified supine Valdivia position as a new way of affording PNL, exploiting the full array of endourological equipment and allowing a personalized approach to urolithiasis [20, 21]. The latter paper [21] was the one introduced in the EAU (European Association of Urology) guidelines on Urolithiasis since 2016.

In Morocco, *Lezrek and coworkers* performed ECIRS in the split-leg modified lateral position, underlining the optimal retrograde access to the upper urinary tract during PNL [22].

§ 2012: The First Prospective Study and Video on ECIRS and the First Minimally Invasive ECIRS in Solitary Kidneys

In France, *Hoznek and colleagues* produced a video on ECIRS step-by-step performed in the Galdakao-modified supine Valdivia position, and performed a prospective study on 47 patients operated with this safe and effective approach [23].

In China, 20 patients with staghorn calculi in solitary kidneys underwent single-tract minimally invasive (18–20 F) PNL and RIRS combination in the Galdakao-modified supine Valdivia position. *Lai and coworkers* demonstrated that minimally invasive ECIRS did not affect renal function at both short- and long-term follow-up, being safe, effective, and feasible through a single miniaturized access tract [24].

§ 2013: The Consolidated American and Italian Experiences and the First Asian Steps

About 25 years have passed since the first paper on ECIRS, and 25 papers have been published on the topic. In 2013 one paper from the United States, one from Hong Kong, and one from Italy were additionally published [25–27].

In a retrospective study, *Isac and colleagues* (group of M. Monga) compared endoscopic-guided (62 patients) and fluoroscopic-guided (96 patients) renal access for PNL, concluding that endoscopic-guided access was safe and effective, and additionally decreases fluoroscopy time, need for multiple tracts, risk of early termination of PNL, need for secondary procedures [25].

Kan et al. shared their initial experience with supine PNL, comparing 25 supine and 35 prone PNL (in a prospective but non-randomized study), and prospectively evaluating 11 additional ECIRS, reporting the ability to incorporate simultaneous ureteroscopic lithotripsy as an additional benefit [26].

Scoffone et al. described in a published abstract [27] a multimodal approach conceived in order to minimize the risk of infectious complications of ECIRS, identifying pre- (like negative urine culture and management of any indwelling urinary catheter), intra- (like antibiotic prophylaxis and low intrarenal pressures), and postoperative (like early identification of initial urosepsis) criteria.

§ 2014: The First Textbook on ECIRS and Its First Application for the Management of Encrusted Ureteral Stents

In 2014, some papers dealing with ECIRS underlined the different fields of application of this technique [28–33].

In Japan, *Hamamoto and coworkers* in a retrospective nonrandomized study compared 60 mini-ECIRS performed in the prone split-leg position with 19 mini-PNL (18 F) and 82 conventional 30 F PNL as monotherapies, obtaining better stone-free rates, shorter surgical times, and limited complication rates with mini-ECIRS [28]. In another paper published in the same year, the same authors underlined safety and one-step efficiency of this hybrid surgery for the management of large renal calculi [29].

One more time in Japan, *Isero* et al. wrote a case report, describing the use of miniaturized ECIRS in the prone split-leg position for a single-session removal of an encrusted ureteral stent [30].

In Spain, *Nuño de la Rosa and coauthors* published a retrospective study comparing 98 supine PNL and 73 ECIRS in the Galdakao-modified supine Valdivia position, concluding that the additional use of flexible ureteroscopy/nephroscopy in supine PNL improves the success rate with a single access in most cases [31].

In the United States, *Sivalingam and colleagues* published the results of an Internet survey administered to all Endourological Society members, stating that only 10% used the supine position and 4% the lateral decubitus, while only 12% used the combined approach for PNL [32].

Scoffone, Hoznek, and Cracco from Italy and France were editors and authors of a book [33] dealing with all the aspects of ECIRS, "a new way of interpreting PNL," including the historical point of view, the rationale, pros and cons of the technique, all the technical aspects (instrumentation, accessories, devices, organization of the operating room, patient positioning, contribution of the scrub nurse, urologic team), and new applications (like micro-ECIRS), with the contribution of a number of distinguished endourologists from all over the world.

§ 2015: The Asian Contribution to ECIRS Miniaturization and Its First Pediatric Use

In 2015, ECIRS became progressively more widespread and popular in Asia, in particular in its miniaturized version.

Cracco and Scoffone from Italy reported a decreased radiation exposure for Endovision-assisted ECIRS [34].

Kuroda and colleagues from Japan identified preoperative predictors of ECIRS outcomes analyzing the results of 329 procedures, namely stone surface areas and number of involved calyces, developing a classification table for predicting success rates after ECIRS in the modified Valdivia position [35].

Shah et al. from China implemented 13 F ultramini-PNL in 22 patients with a retrograde ureteral access sheath and retrograde flexible ureteroscopy in a 45° semi-supine combined lithotomy position, appreciating the low intrarenal pressures, the simple removal of stone fragments, and the easy reach of otherwise inaccessible calyces from the percutaneous tract [36].

Taguchi and coauthors from Japan again reported for the first time 18 F mini-ECIRS in the prone split-leg position in a 2-year-old boy [37].

§ 2016: The First Time of ECIRS in a Multicentric Review of the Literature and in a Randomized Controlled Trial

Two case reports were published in Italy by *Benincasa and coworkers* [38, 39], two rare cases of hydroperitoneum, and one case of salvage ECIRS performed in embolized kidney.

Ghani and coworkers from the United States, Canada, and various European countries wrote a literature review on PNL, dedicating a subsection to the advantages of ECIRS [40].

Inoue and coauthors from Japan reported the positive outcomes of 41 patients with large renal stones treated with mini-ECIRS in the modified Valdivia position, obtaining the access under wideband Doppler ultrasound guidance [41].

Manikandan and coauthors from India reported their results using ECIRS in 43 patients suffering from simultaneous renal and ureteral calculi arranged in the Galdakao-modified supine Valdivia position [42].

Tabei et al. from Japan identified risk factors of developing systemic inflammation response syndrome after ECIRS, adding the number of involved calyces larger than four, stone surface area > 500 mm^2, and a history of febrile urinary tract infection to female sex, diabetes, staghorn calculi, prior PNL, preoperative positive urine culture, preoperative use of a nephrostomy tube, and operation time [43]. The paper was followed by an editorial comment by *Scoffone and Cracco* from Italy, clearly indicating all the pre-, intra-, and postoperative elements minimizing the risk of infectious complications of ECIRS [44].

Wen and coworkers from China published the first randomized controlled trial comparing 34 minimally invasive PNL in prone position and 33 ECIRS in the Galdakao-modified supine Valdivia position for partial staghorn calculi, obtaining significantly higher one-step stone-free rates and comparable safety [45].

§ 2017: The First Systematic Review on ECIRS and Its Increasing Use in Latin America

Cracco et al. from Italy, Germany, Greece, Denmark, and the United States wrote a systematic review demonstrating the benefits of the adjunct of antegrade and retrograde flexible scopes to the traditional rigid-only PNL in terms of efficacy and safety [46].

Huang and colleagues from Taiwan treated 13 patients with large proximal ureteral stones in the Galdakao-modified supine Valdivia position using ECIRS with semi-rigid ureterolithotripsy. The authors observed that this approach created an open, low-pressure system reducing both absorption of irrigation fluid into the circulation and the risk of ureteral injury [47].

Kwon and coauthors from Korea combined 15 F miniaturized ECIRS performed on one side and retrograde intrarenal surgery on the other side in 26 patients in a single session and bilateral stones [48].

Manzo and coworkers from Brazil and Mexico investigated PNL practice patterns in Latin America, discovering that endourology-trained and non-trained urologists used ECIRS in 45.2% and 32.1%, respectively, in the Valdivia supine and Galdakao-modified supine Valdivia positions in 33% and 25%, respectively [49].

Yamashita et al. from Japan confirmed increasing stone size as independent predictor for residual stones after 81 ECIRS but not an increasing number of involved calyces; female gender and increasing Hounsfield units of the stones were significantly associated with perioperative complications [50].

§ 2018: ECIRS is Used for the Management of Difficult Cases of Ureteral and Renal Stones

In 2018, 30 years have passed since the first paper on ECIRS, and 50 publications have been written on the topic. During this year, the Asian contribution was relevant, with some innovative applications.

Chen and coauthors from Taiwan recognized the role of the combined approach in the Galdakao-modified supine Valdivia position for the treatment of large ureteral stones with severe ureteral tortuosity in eight patients, avoiding preoperative ureteral stenting, respecting the ureter, creating an open low-pressure system reducing the absorption of irrigation fluids, and increasing the degree of stone clearance in a single procedure [51].

Inoue and coworkers from Japan used ultra-minimally invasive (8.5–9.5 F) ECIRS in a 2-year-old boy suffering from large bilateral cystine kidney stones, in the Barts modified Valdivia position [52].

Jung and colleagues from Korea described in detail ECIRS and reported their experience in 30 patients arranged in the Galdakao-modified supine Valdivia position. They recognized that retrograde flexible ureteroscopy performed during PNL contributed to the washout mechanism of the stone fragments, improved safety by reducing the number of percutaneous tracts, afforded difficult anatomies of the collecting system consequently increasing the one-step stone-free rates [53].

Leng et al. from China presented their experience of combined single-tract minimally invasive 18F PNL and flexible ureteroscopic lithotripsy in the absence of ureteral access sheath for staghorn stones in oblique supine lithotomy position in 44 patients, comparing them with 43 minimally invasive PNL without the retrograde access. Improved stone-free rates, reduced operative time and length of hospital stay, and decreased complications were reported [54].

Scoffone and Cracco from Italy summarized in an invited review the evolution of ECIRS along the years, especially highlighting its role in tailoring the procedure on the patient, the dynamic anatomy of the collecting system, and the urolithiasis [55].

Suarez-Ibarrola and coauthors from Germany employed ECIRS in the Galdakao-modified supine Valdivia position for the treatment of a complete staghorn stone in a patient with a single functional kidney and renal insufficiency [56].

§ 2019: ECIRS Appears for the First Time in the Most Comprehensive Textbook in the Field of Endourology

Year after year, an increasing number of publications on ECIRS appeared.

Gökce and coworkers from Turkey employed ECIRS in 137 patients and observed that the retrograde approach was more effective than the antegrade one to reach all calyces detecting residual fragments, improving the stone-free rates and decreasing the need for second look surgeries [57].

Keoghane and colleagues from the United Kingdom used ECIRS for the treatment of complex ureteric strictures, removing the need for a long-term nephrostomy thanks to the rendezvous technique [58].

Schulster and coauthors from the United States reviewed 110 ECIRS, comparing final combined endoscopic assessment for residual fragments with postoperative CT scans and concluding that ECIRS accurately predicts clinical stone-free status, obviating the need for additional early postoperative X-ray exposure [59].

Scoffone and Cracco from Italy summarized all the intraoperative advantages of performing retrograde flexible ureteroscopy before and during PNL, additionally recognizing its role in improving the mini-invasiveness of the procedure [60]. During the same year, a chapter on patient positioning, supine position, and the rationale of ECIRS written by the same authors was published on the fourth edition of the *Smith's Textbook of Endourology* [61].

Tanaka et al. from Japan reported hemothorax following mini-ECIRS, in spite of endoscopic and US-guided access and of the miniaturized approach, probably caused by the supracostal puncture [62].

Ulker and Celik from Turkey described the usefulness of ECIRS in the removal of 18 forgotten heavily encrusted stents in a single session [63].

§ 2020: The Golden Year for the Publications on ECIRS

During this year, 13 papers on ECIRS were published, more than ever before.

Axelsson et al. from all over the world underlined the role of retrograde flexible ureteroscopy in preventing fragments during lithotripsy from draining into the ureter, acknowledged its role in reducing the need for multiple accesses and described its benefits during PNL [64].

Cracco and Scoffone from Italy wrote a systematic review on ECIRS, detailing all the tips and tricks to improve PNL outcomes in terms of efficacy and safety [65].

Doizi and coauthors from France compared for the first time intrapelvic pressures during flexible ureteroscopy, miniaturized, and standard PNL and ECIRS in a kidney model, concluding that intrarenal pelvic pressures are significantly lower with an increasing working sheath diameter [66].

Gómez-Regalado and coworkers from Mexico (and Italy also involved) described the safe and effective use of ECIRS for the treatment of a staghorn stone in a crossed fused renal ectopia [67].

Miyai and colleagues from Japan wrote a case report of a patient with a complete ureteral iatrogenic stenosis, successfully managed with a combined approach [68].

Santiapillai and Agrawal from the United Kingdom reported the case of an intra-renal cyst treated by means of ECIRS after abandoning the planned and attempted laparoscopic deroofing during the same surgical session [69].

Soedarman et al. from Indonesia wrote a case report on a complex stone burden treated by means of endoscopic-guided percutaneous nephrolithotomy in the prone split-leg position [70].

Taguchi et al. from Japan reported the results of a pilot single-center trial investigating the clinical safety and feasibility of robot-assisted fluoroscopy-guided ECIRS for the treatment of 19 patients suffering from large renal stones [71].

Turco and coauthors from Italy reported the use of ECIRS for the treatment of two cases of urolithiasis developed on a permanent suture migrated into the calyceal system after conservative renal surgical procedures [72].

Usui and colleagues from Japan compared 77 standard ECIRS (24 F) and 77 mini-ECIRS (16.5 F) for renal stones, concluding that miniaturization maintains similar stone-free rates without increasing perioperative complications, tends to reduce postoperative pain and bleeding-related complications [73].

Veys and coworkers from Belgium, Canada, and the United States report their positive experience with ultrasound-guided ECIRS on Thiel-embalmed cadavers as training model [74].

Wang et al. from China reported the use of ECIRS in the prone split-leg position for the removal of an encrusted ureteral stent [75].

Yeow and coauthors from Singapore and Italy described two cases of migrated embolization coils with stones/bleeding treated by means of ECIRS [76].

§ 2021: ECIRS Hangs in There in Spite of SARS-CoV-2 Pandemic

Birowo et al. from Indonesia wrote a case report on an X-ray-free ECIRS in the Galdakao-modified supine Valdivia position for a complex ureteral stone, highlighting the good results in terms of stone-free rate (also visually assessed) in the absence of significant complications, with lower anesthesiological and radiation risks [77].

Chung et al. from Korea described in 171 patients a technique with two guidewires passing through the nephrostomy and exiting through the urethra, in order to overcome the renal hypermobility typical of the supine positions [78].

Tawfeek et al. from Egypt adopted once again ECIRS in order to manage neglected calcified stents in patients with complex renal stones [79].

Zhao and coauthors from China compared 66 ECIRS and 74 mini-ECIRS patients in the Galdakao-modified supine Valdivia position, concluding that for medium and severe complex nephrolithiasis, ECIRS has higher stone-free rates in the single session and low morbidity compared to miniaturized ECIRS [80].

2 Conclusions

ECIRS is an innovative way of affording PNL, embracing all the endourologic armamentarium and combining both antegrade and retrograde approaches. The Galdakao-modified supine Valdivia position optimally supports ECIRS, but of course the combined approach is possible also in prone-modified and flank positions.

ECIRS was born in the late 1980s in the United States and popularized 20 years afterwards in Europe, especially in Italy, becoming more widespread all over the world only recently, not only for the treatment of complex or large renal stones, but also for that of encrusted stents, ureteral calculi, and strictures. Currently feasibility, safety, and efficacy of ECIRS are widely recognized, as well as its anesthesiological and radiological advantages.

The emerging concept of all the published literature on ECIRS (Fig. 1) is that the contribution of simultaneous retrograde flexible ureteroscopy is essential and plays a dual role: diagnostic (integrating the preoperative knowledge on the static anatomy of the collecting system and urolithiasis with real-time intraoperative elements of dynamic anatomy of both lower and upper tract), and active (with the through-and-through guidewire, the Endovision renal puncture and dilation also

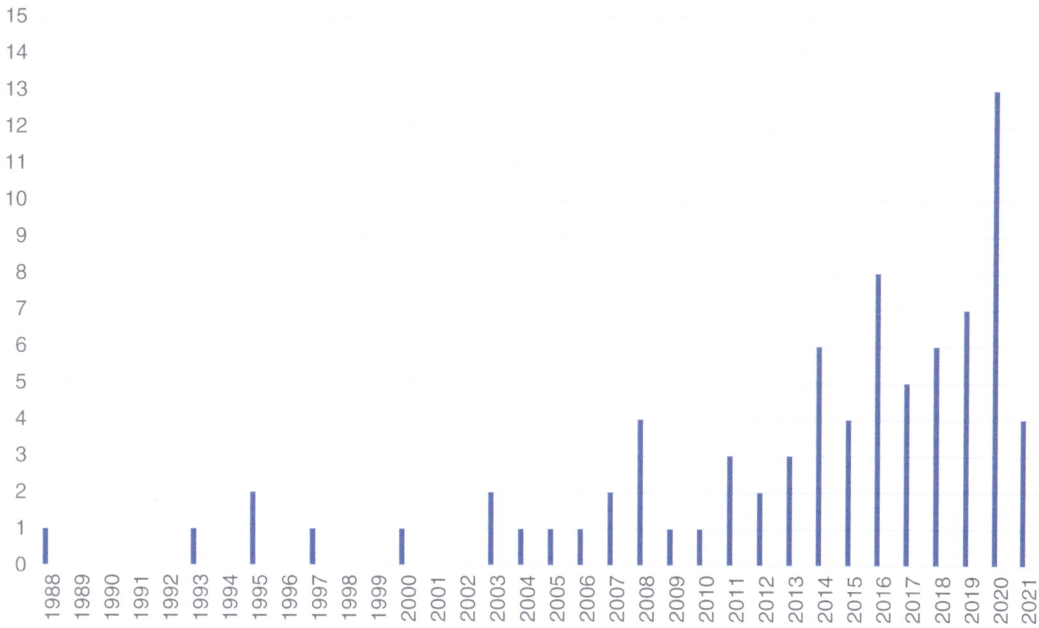

Fig. 1 Number of publications per year on ECIRS from 1988 until 2021 (first quarter)

sparing radiation exposure, the possibility to reach calyces challenging to access through the single percutaneous tract, the ability to finally explore the whole collecting system looking for residual fragments).

In conclusion, ECIRS is here to stay, representing a consistent innovation in percutaneous surgery and a valuable tool in order to personalize surgery, tailoring all the intraoperative choices on the patient, the urolithiasis, and the anatomy of the collecting system.

References

1. Lehman T, Bagley DH. Reverse lithotomy: modified prone position for simultaneous nephroscopic and ureteroscopic procedures in women. Urology. 1988;32:529–31.
2. Grasso M, Nord R, Bagley DH. Prone split leg and flank roll positioning: simultaneous antegrade and retrograde access to the upper urinary tract. J Endourol. 1993;7(4):307–10.
3. Grasso M, Lang G, Taylor FC. Flexible ureteroscopically assisted percutaneous renal access. Tech Urol. 1995;1:39–43.
4. Grasso M, Lang G, Loisides P, Bagley D, Taylor F. Endoscopic management of the symptomatic caliceal diverticular calculus. J Urol. 1995;153:1878–81.
5. Scarpa RM, Cossu FM, De Lisa A, Porru D, Usai E. Severe recurrent ureteral stricture: the combined use of an anterograde and retrograde approach in the prone split-leg position without X-rays. Eur Urol. 1997;31:254–6.
6. Delvecchio FC, Kuo RL, Iselin CE, Webster GD, Preminger GM. Combined antegrade and retrograde endoscopic approach for the management of urinary diversion-associated pathology. J Endourol. 2000;14:251–6.
7. Landman J, Venkatesh R, Lee DI, Rehman J, Ragab M, Darcy M, Sundaram CP. Combined percutaneous and retrograde approach to staghorn calculi with application of the ureteral access sheath to facilitate percutaneous nephrostolithotomy. J Urol. 2003;169:64–7.
8. Kidd CF, Conlin MJ. Ureteroscopically assisted percutaneous renal access. Urology. 2003;61:1244–5.
9. Undre S, Olsen S, Mustafa N, Patel A. "Pass the ball!" simultaneous flexible nephroscopy and retrograde intrarenal surgery for large residual upper-pole staghorn stone. J Endourol. 2004;18:844–7.
10. Marguet CG, Springhart WP, Tan YH, Patel A, Undre S, Albala DH, et al. Simultaneous combined use of flexible ureteroscopy and percutaneous nephrolithotomy to reduce the number of access tracts in the management of complex renal calculi. BJU Int. 2005;96:1097–100.

11. Khan F, Borin JF, Pearle MS, McDougall EM, Clayman RV. Endoscopically guided percutaneous renal access: "seeing is believing". J Endourol. 2006;20:451–5.
12. Ibarluzea G, Scoffone CM, Cracco CM, Poggio M, Porpiglia F, Terrone C, et al. Supine Valdivia and modified lithotomy position for simultaneous anterograde and retrograde endourological access. BJU Int. 2007;100:233–6.
13. Papatsoris AG, Masood J, Saunders P. Supine Valdivia and modified lithotomy position for simultaneous anterograde and retrograde endourologic access. BJU Int. 2007;100:1192.
14. Borin JF. Prone retrograde laser lithotripsy facilitates endoscope-guided percutaneous renal access for staghorn calculi: two scopes are better than one. J Endourol. 2008;22:1881–3.
15. Patel MB, Mason BM, Hoenig DM. Retrograde endoscopic-assisted percutaneous renal access: a novel "lasso" technique to achieve rapid secure access to the collecting system. J Endourol. 2008;22(4):591–6.
16. Papatsoris AG, Zaman F, Panah A, Masood J, El-Husseiny T, Buchholz N. Simultaneous anterograde and retrograde endourologic access: "the Barts technique". J Endourol. 2008;22:2665–6.
17. Scoffone CM, Cracco CM, Cossu M, Grande S, Poggio M, Scarpa RM. Endoscopic combined intrarenal surgery in Galdakao-modified supine Valdivia position: a new standard for percutaneous nephrolithotomy? Eur Urol. 2008;54:1393–403.
18. Sountoulides PG, Kaufmann OG, Louie MK, Beck S, Jain N, Kaplan A, et al. Endoscopy-guided percutaneous nephrostolithotomy: benefits of ureteroscopic access and therapy. J Endourol. 2009;23:1649–54.
19. Scoffone CM, Cracco CM, Poggio M, Scarpa RM. Endoscopic combined intrarenal surgery for high burden renal stones. Arch Ital Urol Androl. 2010;82:41–2.
20. Cracco CM, Scoffone CM, Scarpa RM. New developments in percutaneous techniques for simple and complex branched renal stones. Curr Opin Urol. 2011;21:154–60.
21. Cracco CM, Scoffone CM. ECIRS (endoscopic combined intrarenal surgery) in the Galdakao-modified supine Valdivia position: a new life for percutaneous surgery? World J Urol. 2011;29:821–7.
22. Lezrek M, Ammani A, Bazine K, Assebane M, Kasmaoui EH, Qarro A, et al. The split-leg modified lateral position for percutaneous renal surgery and optimal retrograde access to the upper urinary tract. Urology. 2011;78:217–20.
23. Hoznek A, Rode J, Ouzaid I, Faraj B, Kimuli M, de la Taille A, et al. Modified supine percutaneous nephrolithotomy for large kidney and ureteral stones: technique and results. Eur Urol. 2012;61:164–70.
24. Lai D, He Y, Dai Y, Li X. Combined minimally invasive percutaneous nephrolithotomy and retrograde intrarenal surgery for staghorn calculi in patients with solitary kidney. PLoS One. 2012;7:e48435.
25. Isac W, Rizkala E, Liu X, Noble M, Monga M. Endoscopic-guided versus fluoroscopic-guided renal access for percutaneous nephrolithotomy: a comparative analysis. Urology. 2013;81(2):251–6.
26. Kan RW, Fu KK, Wong BT, Ho KL, Yiu MK. Percutaneous nephrostomy, nephrolithotomy and combined ureteroscopic lithotripsy using the supine approach. Hong Kong Med J. 2013;19(2):142–9.
27. Scoffone CM, Cracco CM. Multimodal strategy for the prevention of infectious complications of percutaneous surgery: our experience. J Endourol. 2013;27(S1):A86.
28. Hamamoto S, Yasui T, Okada A, Taguchi K, Kawai N, Ando R, et al. Endoscopic combined intrarenal surgery for large calculi: simultaneous use of flexible ureteroscopy and mini-percutaneous nephrolithotomy overcomes the disadvantages of percutaneous nephrolithotomy monotherapy. J Endourol. 2014;28(1):28–33.
29. Hamamoto S, Yasui T, Okada A, Takeuchi M, Taguchi K, Shibamoto Y, et al. Developments in the technique of endoscopic combined intrarenal surgery in the prone split-leg position. Urology. 2014;84:565–70.
30. Isero T, Hamamoto S, Koiwa S, Kamiya H, Hashimoto Y, Yasui T, Iwase Y, Kohri K. Combined endoscopic surgery in the prone-split leg position for successful single-session removal of an encrusted ureteral stent: a case report. J Med Case Reports. 2014;8:128.
31. Nuño de la Rosa I, Palmero JL, Miralles J, Pastor JC, Benedicto A. A comparative study of percutaneous nephrolithotomy in supine position and endoscopic combined intrarenal surgery with flexible instrument. Actas Urol Esp. 2014;38(1):14–20.
32. Sivalingam S, Cannon ST, Nakada SY. Current practices in percutaneous nephrolithotomy. J Endourol. 2014;28(5):524–7.
33. Scoffone CM, Hoznek A, Cracco CM. Supine percutaneous nephrolithotomy and ECIRS. 1st ed. Paris: Springer; 2014.
34. Cracco CM, Scoffone CM. Assessing radiation exposure during endoscopic combined IntraRenal surgery (ECIRS). J Endourol. 2015;29(S1):A314.
35. Kuroda S, Ito H, Sakamaki K, Tabei T, Kawahara T, Terao H, Fujikawa A, Makiyama K, Yao M, Matsuzaki J. Development and internal validation of a classification system for predicting success rates after endoscopic combined intrarenal surgery in the modified Valdivia position for large renal stones. Urology. 2015;86(4):697–702.
36. Shah AK, Xu K, Liu H, Huang H, Lin T, Bi L, et al. Implementation of ultramini percutaneous nephrolithotomy for treatment of 2–3 cm kidney stones: a preliminary report. J Endourol. 2015;29:1231–6.
37. Taguchi K, Hamamoto S, Okada A, Mizuno K, Tozawa K, Hayashi Y, et al. First case report of staghorn calculi successfully removed by mini-endoscopic combined intrarenal surgery in a 2-year boy. Int J Urol. 2015;22:978–80.

38. Benincasa A, Nicolosi F, Falsaperla M, Saita A. Hydroperitoneum: a rare complication performing endoscopic combined intrarenal surgery. J Endourol Case Rep. 2016;2(1):55–8.
39. Benincasa A, Nicolosi F, Lughezzani G, Buffi NM, Casale P, Hurle R, et al. Safety and feasibility of salvage endoscopic intrarenal surgery in embolized kidney. J Endourol Case Rep. 2016;2:127–30.
40. Ghani KR, Andonian S, Bultitude M, et al. Percutaneous nephrolithotomy: update, trends, and future directions. Eur Urol. 2016;70:382–90.
41. Inoue T, Kinoshita H, Okada S, Hamamoto S, Taguchi M, Murota T, Matsuda T, SMART Study Group. Wideband Doppler ultrasound-guided mini-endoscopic combined intrarenal surgery as an effective and safe procedure for management of large renal stones: a preliminary report. Urology. 2016;95:60–6.
42. Manikandan R, Mittal JK, Dorairajan LN, Mishra AK, Sreerag KS, Verma A. Endoscopic combined intrarenal surgery for simultaneous renal and ureteral stones: a retrospective study. J Endourol. 2016;30(10):1056–61.
43. Tabei T, Ito H, Usui K, Kuroda S, Kawahara T, Terao H, et al. Risk factors of systemic inflammation response syndrome after endoscopic combined intrarenal surgery in the modified Valdivia position. Int J Urol. 2016;23(8):687–92.
44. Scoffone CM, Cracco CM. Editorial comment to risk factors of systemic inflammation response syndrome after endoscopic combined intrarenal surgery in the modified Valdivia position. Int J Urol. 2016;23(8):692–3.
45. Wen J, Xu G, Du C, Wang B. Minimally invasive percutaneous nephrolithotomy versus endoscopic combined intrarenal surgery with flexible ureteroscope for partial staghorn calculi: a randomized controlled trial. Int J Surg. 2016;28:22–7.
46. Cracco CM, Knoll T, Liatsikos EN, Osther PJ, Smith AD, Scarpa RM, Scoffone CM. Rigid-only versus combined rigid and flexible percutaneous nephrolithotomy: a systematic review. Minerva Urol Nefrol. 2017;69(4):330–41.
47. Huang TY, Feng KM, Lo IS. Percutaneous nephrolithotomy: update, trends, and future directions for simultaneous supine percutaneous nephrolithotomy and retrograde ureterolithotripsy in the Galdakao-modified supine Valdivia position for large proximal ureteral calculi. Eur Urol. 2017;71(5):837–8.
48. Kwon O, Park J, Cho MC, Son H, Jeong H, Cho SY. Feasibility of single-session endoscopic combined intrarenal surgery for ipsilateral large renal stones and retrograde intrarenal surgery for contralateral renal stones: initial experience. Int J Urol. 2017;24(5):377–82.
49. Manzo BO, Lozada E, Vicentini FC, Sanchez FJ, Manzo J. Differences in the percutaneous nephrolithotomy practice patterns among Latin American urologists with and without endourology training. Int Braz J Urol. 2017;44:512–23.
50. Yamashita S, Kohjimoto Y, Iba A, Kikkawa K, Hara I. Stone size is a predictor for residual stone and multiple procedures of endoscopic combined intrarenal surgery. Scand J Urol. 2017;51(2):159–64.
51. Chen YC, Chen HW, Lo IS, Li CC, Shih PM, Huang TY. Management of large ureteral stone with severe ureteral tortuosity: a novel technique of "straightening" against the tortuous ureter using simultaneous supine percutaneous nephrolithotomy and retrograde semirigid ureterolithotripsy. Int J Urol. 2018;25(10):896–7.
52. Inoue T, Watanabe M, Shimada S, Kinoshita H, Matsuda T. Successful ultra-minimally invasive endoscopic intrarenal surgery for 2-year-old boy with bilateral cystine kidney stones over 2 cm. J Endourol Case Rep. 2018;4(1):101–4.
53. Jung AD, Kim JC, Ahn HK, Kwon JH, Han K, Han WK, et al. Real-time simultaneous endoscopic combined intrarenal surgery with intermediate-supine position: washout mechanism and transport technique. Investig Clin Urol. 2018;59:348–54.
54. Leng S, Xie D, Zhing Y, Huang M. Combined single-tract of minimally percutaneous nephrolithotomy and flexible ureteroscopy for staghorn calculi in oblique supine lithotomy position. Surg Innov. 2018;25(1):22–7.
55. Scoffone CM, Cracco CM. Invited review: the tale of ECIRS (endoscopic combined IntraRenal surgery) in the Galdakao-modified supine Valdivia position. Urolithiasis. 2018;46(1):115–23.
56. Suarez-Ibarrola R, Obaid MA, Miernik A. Modified salvage endoscopic combined intrarenal surgery in a single functional kidney with refractory staghorn stone. Urol Case Rep. 2018;17(23):13–4.
57. Gökce MI, Gülpinar O, Ibis M, Kubilay E, Süer E. Retrograde vs. antegrade flexible nephroscopy for detection of residual fragments following PNL: a prospective study with computerized tomography control. Int Braz J Urol. 2019;45:581–7.
58. Keoghane SR, Deveril SJ, Woodhouse J, Shennoy V, Johnston T, Osborn P. Combined antegrade and retrograde access to difficult ureters: revisiting the rendezvous technique. Urolithiasis. 2019;47(4):383–90.
59. Schulster M, Small AC, Silva MV, Abbott JE, Davalos JG. Endoscopic combined intrarenal surgery can accurately predict high stone clearance rates on post-operative CT. Urology. 2019;133:46–9.
60. Scoffone CM, Cracco CM. The role of retrograde flexible ureteroscopy during percutaneous surgery: trick or treat? In: Autorino R, Liatsikos E, Porpiglia F, editors. New technologies and techniques in minimally invasive urologic surgery. An ESUT collection. Torino: Minerva Medica; 2019. p. 148–54.
61. Scoffone CM, Cracco CM. In: Smith A, Preminger G, Kavoussi L, Badlani G, editors. Patient positioning, the supine position and the rationale of ECIRS, Chapter 11. Hoboken, NJ: Wiley-Blackwell; 2019.
62. Tanaka Y, Taguchi K, Hamamoto S, Ota Y, Oda R, Yokota K, Ando R, Okada A, Tozawa K, Nakanishi R, Yasui T. Hemothorax during miniaturized endoscopic

combined intrarenal surgery under ureteroscope-assisted ultrasound-guided access. IJU Case Rep. 2019;2(5):257–60.
63. Ulker V, Celik O. Endoscopic single-session management of encrusted, forgotten ureteral stents. Medicina (Kaunas). 2019;55(3):58.
64. Axelsson TA, Cracco C, Desai M, Hasan MN, Knoll T, Montanari E, et al. Consultation on kidney stones, Copenhagen 2019: lithotripsy in percutaneous nephrolithotomy. World J Urol. 2020;39(6):1663–70. https://doi.org/10.1007/s00345-020-03383-w.
65. Cracco CM, Scoffone CM. Endoscopic combined intrarenal surgery (ECIRS)—tips and tricks to improve outcomes: a systematic review. Turk J Urol. 2020;46(Suppl.1):S46–57.
66. Doizi S, Uzan A, Keller EX, De Coninck V, Kamkoum H, Barghouthy Y, Ventimiglia E, Traxer O. Comparison of intrapelvic pressures during flexible ureteroscopy, mini-percutaneous nephrolithotomy, standard percutaneous nephrolithotomy, and endoscopic combined intrarenal surgery in a kidney model. World J Urol. 2020;39(7):2709–17. https://doi.org/10.1007/s00345-020-03450-2.
67. Gómez-Regalado F, Manzo BO, Figueroa-Garcia A, Sanchez-Lopez H, Basulto-Martinez M, Cracco CM, Scoffone CM. Efficacy of the endoscopic combined intrarenal surgery for the treatment of a staghorn calculus in crossed fused renal ectopia. J Endourol Case Rep. 2020;6(3):205–8.
68. Miyai T, Kawahara T, Kuroda S, Yasui M, Uemura H. Complete ureteral stenosis after ureteroscopic lithotripsy successfully managed using a simultaneous retrograde and antegrade flexible ureteroscopic approach. Clin Case Rep. 2020;9(1):246–50.
69. Santiapillai J, Agrawal S. Combined flexible URS and percutaneous 'through and through' puncture of an intra-renal cyst with internalisation of drainage, to treat calyceal obstruction and recurrent stones. Urol Case Rep. 2020;30:101125.
70. Soedarman S, Rasyid N, Birowo P, Atmoko W. Endoscopic-guided percutaneous nephrolithotomy (EPSL) with prone split-leg position for complex kidney stone: a case report. Int J Surg Case Rep. 2020;77:668–72.
71. Taguchi K, Hamamoto S, Kawase K, Hattori T, Okada T, Chaya R, Nagai T, Kato T, Okada A, Yasui T. The first case report of robot-assisted fluoroscopy-guided renal access during endoscopic combined intrarenal surgery. J Endourol Case Rep. 2020;6(4):310–4.
72. Turco M, Guiggi P, Tiezzi A, Boni A, Paladini A, Mearini E, Cochetti G. Endoscopic combined intrarenal surgery for stone formation after previous laparoscopic and open renal surgery. J Endourol Case Rep. 2020;6(2):60–3.
73. Usui K, Komeya M, Taguri M, Kataoka K, Asai T, Ogawa T, et al. Minimally invasive versus standard endoscopic combined intrarenal surgery for renal stones: a retrospective pilot study analysis. Int Urol Nephrol. 2020;52(7):1219–25.
74. Veys R, Verpoort P, Van Haute C, Wang ZT, Chi T, Tailly T. Thiel-embalmed cadavers as a novel training model for ultrasound-guided supine endoscopic combined intrarenal surgery. BJU Int. 2020;125(4):579–85.
75. Wang D, Sun H, Chen L, Liu Z, Zhang D, Yu D, Ding D. Endoscopic combined intrarenal surgery in the prone-split leg position for successful single session removal of an encrusted ureteral stent: a case report. BMC Urol. 2020;20(1):37.
76. Yeow Y, Ortega-Polledo LE, Basulto-Martínez M, Saitta G, Rapallo I, Proietti S, Gaboardi F, Giusti G. Endourologic treatment of late migration of embolization causing nephrolithiasis in two patients. J Endourol Case Rep. 2020;6(4):278–82.
77. Birowo P, Raharia PAR, Atmoko W, Rasyid N. X-ray-free endoscopic combined intrarenal surgery for complex proximal ureteral stone: a case report. Res Rep Urol. 2021;4:121–5.
78. Chung JW, Ha H, Park DJ, Ha YS, Lee JN, Chun SY, et al. Efficacy and safety of modified tract dilation technique using simultaneous pulling of proximal and distal ends of a guidewire for percutaneous nephrolithotomy in supine modified position. Investig Clin Urol. 2021;62(2):186–94.
79. Tawfeek AM, Elmoazen M, Saafan A, Higazy A, Radwan A, Gad HH. Simultaneous antegrade and retrograde endourological approach in Galdakao-modified supine Valdivia position for the management of missed stents associated with complex renal stones: a non-randomized pilot study. Int Urol Nephrol. 2021;53(2):211–7.
80. Zhao F, Li J, Tang L, Li C. A comparative study of endoscopic combined intrarenal surgery (ECIRS) in the Galdakao-modified supine Valdivia (GMSV) position and minimally invasive percutaneous nephrolithotomy for complex nephrolithiasis: a retrospective single-center study. Urolithiasis. 2021;49(2):161–6.

Flexible Ureterorenoscopy in the Treatment of Childhood Stone Disease

Hüseyin Kocatürk, Mehmet Sefa Altay, Fevzi Bedir, and Kemal Sarica

Abstract

Incidence of urolithiasis in pediatric patients is increasing, and similar to the regional variability in adults, the prevalence varies in different parts of the world being endemic in developing countries such as Turkey, Iran, Pakistan, and the Far East. Metabolic problems are more common in children than adults and they increase the risk of disease recurrence in this specific population. Although the majority of stones in pediatric patients are idiopathic, secondary causes such as congenital urinary system anomalies, metabolic abnormalities, or neurological diseases are common in this specific population. For this reason, anatomical and stone-related factors (composition, size, and location) are important in decision-making for pediatric stone treatment. Similar to adult population, the introduction of small-sized endoscopic equipment into urology practice along with the improvement of optical systems has increased the use of flexible ureteroscopes also in children for the management of upper tract stones. Based on the currently available guidelines, use of flexible ureteroscopy is recommended as a therapeutic option in renal stones smaller than 15 mm, particularly hard and large stones, resistance to SWL.

Keywords

Children · Flexible ureteroscopy · Urolithiasis

As a worldwide endemic health problem, urolithiasis can be diagnosed in all age groups, but the incidence has been found to be lower in children than in adults. Although the prevalence has been reported to vary between 10 and 15% (5–9% in Europe, 12% in Canada, and 13–15% in the USA) in adult population [1, 2], the incidence of the disease in pediatric patients is limited. Regarding this issue, of all the cases treated for urinary stones, only 1–3% are children with a marked variation of incidence in developed and developing countries. While the disease has been reported to be rather rare in some countries, like Scandinavia and USA; it is still an endemic problem in developing ones such as Turkey, Iran, Pakistan, and the Far East. Stones occur in children of all ages and do not disproportionately affect any age group [1, 3, 4].

Additionally, in contrast to adult patients, there is a lack of well-conducted epidemiological studies concerning the actual prevalence of the pediatric stone disease [3]. Taking the asymptomatic course of the disease in this specific pop-

H. Kocatürk (✉) · M. S. Altay · F. Bedir
Department of Urology Health Sciences University, Erzurum Regional Training and Research Hospital, Erzurum, Turkey

K. Sarica
Department of Urology, Faculty of Medicine, Biruni University, Istanbul, Turkey

G. Zeng et al. (eds.), *Flexible Ureteroscopy*, https://doi.org/10.1007/978-981-19-2936-6_14

ulation, stones may be overlooked and the true prevalence may be higher than the data reported so far [3, 5]. Pediatric stone disease is endemic in Turkey, Pakistan, and some South Asian, African, and South American countries, and recent studies show that the prevalence is also rising in the Western world [2, 4]. Predisposing factors for urolithiasis in children include genetic and metabolic abnormalities (hypercalciuria, hyperoxaluria, hypocitraturia, hyperuricosuria, and cystinuria), diet, environmental factors, anatomical characteristics, and certain drugs (such as excess vitamin C and D, and furosemide) [6]. The age at onset of urolithiasis in children also varies, but the majority of patients are aged 5–15 years. Urinary tract stones in children do not generally cause very severe pain as they do in adults, although 70–80% emerge symptomatically with flank or abdominal pain. Hematuria is seen in 10–32% and accompanying urinary tract infection in 4–20% [3].

Due to the recurring nature of the disease, requiring frequent interventions, regular and close follow-up visits with thorough metabolic work-up evaluations with stone composition assessments at every attack are highly important. Despite the idiopathic etiology of stone formation in the majority of adult patients, an underlying cause such as congenital urinary tract anomaly, metabolic abnormality, or neurological disease may be present in kids suffering from stone formation. In light of these facts stated and, given the high risk of recurrent stone formation particularly in this specific population, it should be kept in mind that all children suffering from stone disease should be evaluated in detail to determine the possible underlying causes and to help planning the proper management strategies. Through these efforts, future stone formation and/or growth may be controlled in an attempt to limit the morbidity of the disease. Long-term postoperative follow-up is needed, especially after using recently developed and established technical innovations for the management of urinary stones in children. Regarding the medical as well as the surgical management of stone-forming children, clinicians have to choose the appropriate treatment on the basis of the results of metabolic evaluation and stone analysis as well as the frequency of stone events [6–8]. It is very clear that through these crucial approaches the adverse effects of both stone disease and the interventions on the growing kidneys of the children could be prevented.

Technological advancements and miniaturization of endourologic instruments along with the increasing experience of the surgeons have significantly altered the surgical management of pediatric stone disease. Although the management of urinary system stones in children may vary depending on personal experience and technical possibilities, the use of techniques such as shock wave lithotripsy (ESWL), flexible ureterorenoscopy (FURS), retrograde ureterolithotripsy, mini percutaneous nephrolithotomy (miniperc), micro percutaneous nephrolithotomy (microperc), and ultramini percutaneous nephrolithotomy are regarded as safe, effective, and minimally invasive [9–11]. In other words, the vast majority of the pediatric stones can be managed with either ESWL, PNL, or URS, or a combination of these modalities where open surgery is currently needed in a limited percent of all cases. Like in adults, accumulated experience did clearly show that the stone (location, composition, and size) as well as the patient (BMI, anatomy of the collecting system, and the presence of obstruction with or without infection) are the crucial factors to be considered for a well-planned stone removal procedure which will result in high stone-free rates with minimal or no complications [9, 11–17].

In general, relatively small stones (<4–5 mm) could be anticipated to pass spontaneously, but the likelihood of spontaneous passage for larger stones is low. On the other hand, again, accumulated experience so far has clearly shown that the majority of stones of size less than 2 cm might be well disintegrate with ESWL therapy, and successful outcomes with higher stone-free rates can be achieved. Percutaneous surgery can also be performed for kidney stones in children, although very few patients require surgery. Complete stone-free status must be achieved to the greatest possible extent in the surgical techniques applied, because only 20–25% of residual stones can be passed spontaneously [18–20].

1 Management of Renal Stones in Pediatric Cases with Flexible Ureteroscopy

With increasing experience of RIRS in adults, increasing number of cases have been reported regarding the successful application of flexible ureterorenoscopy in the management of stones in the kidneys in children. Adoption of techniques used in the adult population and the use of a 6.9 Fr flexible ureteroscope along with ureteral access sheaths have facilitated access to the entire pediatric urinary tract. The development of small-scale endoscopic equipment and the entry into clinical use of nitinol-type equipment, together with improved laser technology, have led to an increase in endourological interventions in pediatric stone disease [21]. Improved optic systems, the inclusion of active deflexion, and the development of a functional working channel in particular have increased the use of flexible ureteroscopes for therapeutic and diagnostic purposes in the upper urinary tract. The working length of current flexible ureteroscopes ranges between 54 and 70 cm, with tip diameters of approximately 4.9–7.5 Fr and a midshaft diameter of 7.5–9.0 Fr, and the retinal unit can be entered without active dilation in the majority of cases (Fig. 1). In addition, improved access sheaths permit both ease of manipulation and a reduction of pressure in the kidney (Fig. 2). The majority of ureteroscopes have a 0° visual field. In some flexible ureteroscopes, a 9° visual field is provided in order to assist early visualization of the working tools on exiting the working channel. The use of smaller diameter ureteroscopes has been linked to a decrease in ureteral complication rates. Although flexible ureteroscopes can be employed in the treatment of other urinary tract diseases in children, they are more practicable in both ureteral and kidney stones [22–24].

As stated above, in light of technological advancements and also the experience gained from adult applications, flexible ureteroscopic lithotripsy has recently been increasingly applied to treat upper urinary stones in infants and children because of its advantages, such as practical natural access to the upper urinary tract, less likelihood of trauma, established repeatability, uneventful recovery, limited complications, and well-accepted safety and efficacy [25].

Currently, with the help of this approach, treatment of lower pole calculi also became possible in an efficient manner that would have previously required SWL or PNL [26, 27]. Regarding the management of renal stones with this method

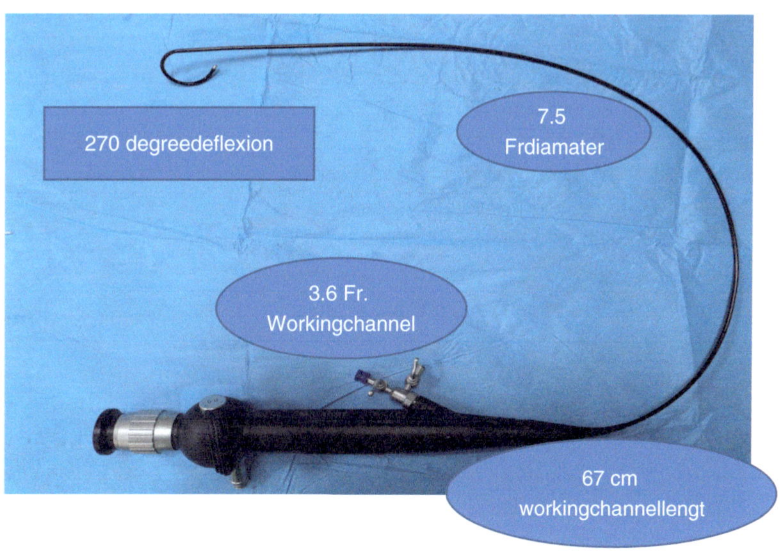

Fig. 1 A flexible ureterorenoscope (Karl Storz, Tuttlingen, Germany)

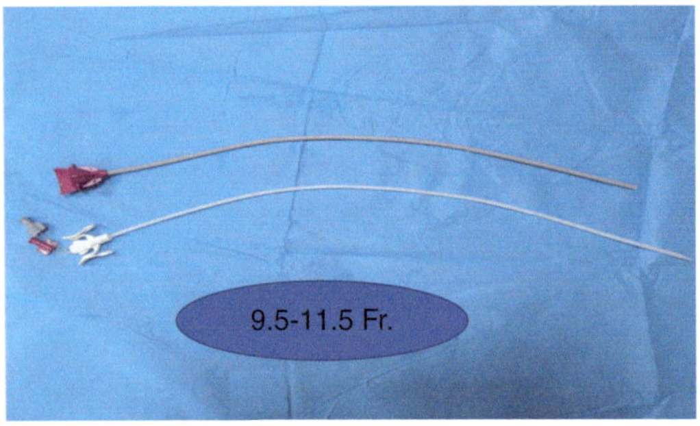

Fig. 2 The ureteral access sheath

in children, Cannon et al. reported a 76% stone-free rate in 21 children with lower pole calculi with a mean stone diameter of 12.2 cm. After a mean follow-up of 11.4 months, they reported no major complications [28]. Again, by performing 52 URS procedures for intrarenal calculi, Tanaka et al. demonstrated that flexible ureterorenoscopic management of renal stones is safe and effective with an initial stone-free rate of 50% after the first session. They reported the stone-free rate to increase to 58% during a mean follow-up period of 246 days. Predictors for further treatment in this study were younger age and preoperative stone size >6 mm. Re-treatment was not necessary if the stone size ≤6 mm [29]. Although the number of cases treated are limited, other authors did also report safe and successful use of this method even in pre-school-aged children [30–34].

Current relative contraindications to ureteroscopic management of stones in children include large and complex stones, anatomical anomalies making retrograde access difficult and previous endoscopic failure.

Although SWL has been reported to be the most reasonable option in the management of calculi of size less than 20 mm, one study reported similar stone-free rates between retrograde intrarenal surgery (RIRS) and ESWL. However, RIRS was found to be more successful than ESWL in stones larger than 2 cm. In addition, RIRS achieves success rates of 78–91%, irrespective of the stone composition. RIRS is also more effective in the lower pole calyx [22, 35–38].

Due to the use of smaller instruments such as mini, ultramini and micro nephroscopes in the last decade, PNL began to be applied more commonly than ever in the minimal invasive management of medium- and large-sized stones in children. The indication range has broadened with equipment miniaturization, and with the inclusion of even medium-sized stones (10–20 mm), higher stone-free rates have been achieved in pediatric patients, with fewer complications. However, based on the accumulated experience and reported data in the literature, it is clear that PNL in any form is more invasive than RIRS, and it can lead to more serious complications because of the fragility of the developing renal parenchyma in children, the small calibration of the pelvicalyceal system, and mobile kidney. For this reason, percutaneous approaches need to be recommended for the treatment of larger and more complex kidney stones in this population. Related with this issue, RIRS has been described as a better option than micro-PNL and mini-PNL in stones 10–20 mm in size due to its low radiation exposure, short hospital stay, and high stone-free rates [37, 39]. RIRS has also been reported to entail lower stone-free rates than PNL in stones larger than 20 mm, but a similar stone-free rate in smaller stones, with lower complication rates. The main advantage of F-URS over PNL is that it is much less invasive, with a minimal risk of bleeding and a shorter hospital stay. Additionally, the use of an appropriate sized ureteral sheath permits greater access to the kidney with higher stone-free and lower complication rates. However, like in adult cases if it is not possible to insert the ureteral sheath on the first attempt in pediatric cases, depending on the age of the child and the size of the pediatric ureter, passive dilation of the ureter could be established with the insertion of a DJ stent in case of large or hard stones requiring the use of a ureteral sheath [35, 37–40].

In conclusion, the use of F-URS is recommended as a therapeutic option in preference to ESWL in case of renal stones smaller than 10 mm in size, especially hard stone, and as an alternative to ESWL in large stones. Stone-free rates achieved with PNL are better than those with RIRS as the stone size increases, but complication rates are higher.

References

1. Pathan SA, Mitra B, Bhutta ZA, Qureshi I, Spencer E, Hameed AA, Nadeem S, Tahir R, Anjum S, Cameron PA. A comparative, epidemiological study of acute renal colic presentations to emergency departments in Doha, Qatar, and Melbourne, Australia. Int J Emerg Med. 2018;11:1.
2. Sarica K. Pediatric urolithiasis: etiology, specific pathogenesis and medical treatment. Urol Res. 2006;24:1–6.
3. Clayton DB, Pope JC. The increasing pediatric stone disease problem. Ther Adv Urol. 2011;3(1):3–12.
4. Kroovand RL. Pediatric urolithiasis. Urol Clin N Am. 1997;12:173–7.
5. Schwarz RD, Dwyer NT. Pediatric kidney stones: long-term outcomes. Urology. 2006;67:812–6.
6. Nicoletta JA, Lande MB. Medical evaluation and treatment of urolithiasis. Pediatr Clin North Am. 2006;53:479–91.
7. Tasian GE, Ross ME, Song L, Sas DJ, Keren R, Denburg MR, et al. Annual incidence of nephrolithiasis among children and adults in South Carolina from 1997 to 2012. Clin J Am Soc Nephrol. 2016;11(3):488–96.
8. Sarica K, Erturhan S, Yurtseven C, Yagci F. Effect of potassium citrate therapy on stone recurrence and regrowth after extracorporeal shockwave lithotripsy in children. J Endourol. 2006;20:875–9.
9. Sarica K, Sahin C. Contemporary minimally invasive surgical management of urinary stones in children. Eur Urol Suppl. 2017;16(1):2–7.
10. Ganpule AP, Bhattu AS, Desai M. PCNL in the twenty-first century: role of Microperc, Miniperc, and Ultraminiperc. World J Urol. 2015;33:235–40.
11. Schultz-Lampel D, Lampel A. The surgical management of stones in children. BJU Int. 2001;87:732–40.
12. Lahme S. Shockwave lithotripsy and endourological stone treatment in children. Urol Res. 2006;34:112–7.
13. Erdenetsesteg G, Manohar T, Singh H, Desai MR. Endourologic management of pediatric urolithiasis: proposed clinical guidelines. J Endourol. 2006;20:737–48.
14. Li J, Yu H, Zhou P, Pan H, Li R, Wang Y, Song C, Lou Y, Zhu J. Application of flexible ureteroscopy combined with holmium laser lithotripsy and their therapeutic efficacy in the treatment of upper urinary stones in children and infants. Urol J. 2019;16(4):343–6.
15. Androulakakis PA. Treatment of renal stones in children. Eur Urol Update Ser. 1992;1:50–4.
16. Dogan HS, Tekgül S. Management of pediatric stone disease. Curr Urol Rep. 2007;8:163–73.
17. Bartosh SM. Medical management of pediatric stone disease. Urol Clin N Am. 2004;31:575–87.
18. Dincel N, Resorlu B, Unsal A, Tepeler A, Silay MS, Armağan A, et al. Are small residual stone fragments insignificant in children? J Pediatr Surg. 2013;48(4):840–4.
19. El-Assmy A, El-Nahas AR, Harraz AM, El Demerdash Y, Elsaadany MM, El-Halwagy S, et al. Clinically insignificant residual fragments: is it an appropriate term in children? Urology. 2015;86(3):593–8.
20. Radmayr C, Bogaert G, Dogan HS, Nijman JM, Silay MS, Stein R, et al. Urinary stone disease. Guidelines on paediatric urology. 2020. https://uroweb.org/guideline/paediatric-urology. Accessed 05 Sept 2020.
21. Xiao J, Wang X, Li J, Wang M, Han T, Zhang C, Du Y, Hao G, Tian Y. Treatment of upper urinary tract stones with flexible ureteroscopy in children. Can Urol Assoc J. 2019;13(3):E78–82.
22. Günaydın B, Öztorun K, Sılay MS. Çocuklarda üreterorenoskopi ve retrograde intrarenal cerrahi: Teknik, endikasyonlar ve komplikasyonları. In: Mutlu N, editor. Çocukluk Çağı Üriner Sistem Taş Hastalığı. 1. Baskı. Ankara: TürkiyeKlinikleri; 2020. p. 51–4.
23. Basillote JB, Lee DI, Eichel L, Clayman RV. Ureteroscopes: flexible, rigid, and semirigid. Urol Clin N Am. 2004;31(1):21–32.
24. Dave S, Khoury AE, Braga L, Farhat WA. Single-institutional study on role of ureteroscopy and retrograde intrarenal surgery in treatment of pediatric renal calculi. Urology. 2008;72(5):1018–21.
25. Li J, Xiao J, Han T, Tian Y, Wang W, Du Y. Flexible ureteroscopic lithotripsy for the treatment of upper urinary tract calculi in infants. Exp Biol Med (Maywood). 2017;242(2):153–9.
26. Straub M, Gschwend J, Zorn C. Pediatric urolithiasis: the current surgical management. Pediatr Nephrol. 2010;25:1239–44.
27. Wu H-Y, Docimo SG. Surgical management of children with urolithiasis. Urol Clin N Am. 2004;3:589–94.
28. Cannon GM, Smaldone MC, Wu H, et al. Ureteroscopic management of lower-pole stones in a pediatric population. J Endourol. 2007;21:1179–82.
29. Tanaka ST, Makari JH, Pope JC, Adams MC, Brock JW III, Thomas JC. Pediatric ureteroscopic management of intrarenal calculi. J Urol. 2008;180:2150–3.
30. Lesani OA, Palmer JS. Retrograde proximal rigid ureteroscopy and pyeloscopy in prepubertal children: safe and effective. J Urol. 2006;176:1570–3.
31. Corcoran AT, Smaldone MC, Mally D, et al. Flexible ureteroscopy for proximal stones in pediatric patients: how complete access simplifies the surgical approach. J Endourol. 2007;21:A84.
32. Smaldone MC, Cannon GM Jr, Wu HY, et al. Is ureteroscopy first line treatment for pediatric stone disease? J Urol. 2007;178:2128.
33. Minevich E, Defoor W, Reddy P, et al. Ureteroscopy is safe and effective in prepubertal children. J Urol. 2005;174:276.
34. Unsal A, Resorlu B. Retrograde intrarenal surgery in infants and pre-school age children. J Pediatr Urol. 2011;46:2195–9.
35. Chen Y, Deng T, Duan X, Zhu W, Zeng G. Percutaneous nephrolithotomy versus retrograde intrarenal surgery for pediatric patients with upper urinary stones: a systematic review and meta-analysis. Urolithiasis. 2019;47(2):189–99.

36. Mokhless IA, Abdeldaeim HM, Saad A, Zahran AR. Retrograde intrarenal surgery monotherapy versus shock wave lithotripsy for stones 10 to 20 mm in preschool children: a prospective, randomized study. J Urol. 2014;191(5 Suppl):1496–9.
37. Saad KS, Youssif ME, Hamdy SA, Fahmy A, El Din Hanno AG, El-Nahas AR. Percutaneous nephrolithotomy vs retrograde intrarenal surgery for large renal stones in pediatric patients: a randomized controlled trial. J Urol. 2015;194(6):1716–20.
38. Tekgül S. Percutaneous nephrolithotomy vs retrograde intrarenal surgery for upper tract calculi in children: which is a better option for which stone condition? J Urol. 2015;194(6):1529–30.
39. Baş O, Dede O, Aydoğmus Y, Utangaç M, Yıkılmaz TN, Damar E, et al. Comparison of retrograde intrarenal surgery and micro-percutaneous nephrolithotomy in moderately sized pediatric kidney stones. J Endourol. 2016;30(7):765–70.
40. Lu P, Song R, Yu Y, Yang J, Qi K, Tao R, et al. Clinical efficacy of percutaneous nephrolithotomy versus retrograde intrarenal surgery for pediatric kidney urolithiasis: a PRISMA-compliant article. Medicine. 2017;96(43):e8346.

Flexible Ureteroscopy in Special Situations

Yazeed Barghouthy and Olivier Traxer

Abstract

In the last two decades, the share of flexible ureteroscopy (fURS) in the treatment of stone disease has increased dramatically, while the share of total treatments for percutaneous nephrolithotomy (PCNL) remained static and the share for extracorporeal shockwave lithotripsy and open surgery fell (Geraghty et al. J Endourol, 31(6):547–556, 2017). This is the result of substantial improvements in equipment, whether it be the endoscopes or laser technologies. Accordingly, the indications for the performance of fURS have increased considerably, and it has become the first-line modality in cases where it was previously impossible to perform, such as urinary diversions or anomalous kidneys.

Keywords

Flexible ureteroscopy · Diverticular stones Encrusted stents · Urinary diversions Pregnancy · Obesity · Ectopic · Horseshoe Transplanted · Kidney

Y. Barghouthy · O. Traxer (✉)
GRC n°20, Groupe de Recherche Clinique sur la Lithiase Urinaire, Sorbonne Université, Hôpital Tenon, Paris, France

Service d'Urologie, Sorbonne Université, AP-HP, Hôpital Tenon, Paris, France
e-mail: olivier.traxer@aphp.fr

In the last two decades, the share of flexible ureteroscopy (fURS) in the treatment of stone disease has increased dramatically, while the share of total treatments for percutaneous nephrolithotomy (PCNL) remained static and the share for extracorporeal shockwave lithotripsy and open surgery fell [1]. This is the result of substantial improvements in equipment, whether it be the endoscopes or laser technologies. Accordingly, the indications for the performance of fURS have increased considerably, and it has become the first-line modality in cases where it was previously impossible to perform, such as urinary diversions or anomalous kidneys.

In the next chapter, we will present the use of flexible ureteroscopy in special scenarios that need specific considerations, and the different approaches needed for a successful intervention will be highlighted.

1 Diverticular Stones

Calyceal diverticula of the kidney are non-secretory, urothelial-lined cavities, mostly found in the upper and mid-calyceal groups of the renal collecting system. These cavities are filled with urine that passively originates in the adjacent collecting system [2]. The prevalence of calyceal diverticula is approximately 4.5/1000 intravenous pyelograms. In one large review, calyceal diverticula were more common in female patients (63%) than in males (37%) and were equally

G. Zeng et al. (eds.), *Flexible Ureteroscopy*, https://doi.org/10.1007/978-981-19-2936-6_15

present in the left and right side. Average diverticulum size across the series was 1.72 cm and ranged from 0.5 to 7.5 cm [3].

Different types and classification systems of calyceal diverticula exist, the simpler of which differentiates between type I (communication with a minor calyx or infundibulum) and type II (communication with a major calyx or the renal pelvis) [4].

While many calyceal diverticula are asymptomatic, others may present complications requiring intervention. Persistent flank pain—present in approximately 50% of cases—accounts for the most common complaint. Other manifestations include diverticular stones, recurrent infections, and hematuria related to the diverticulum.

Diverticular stones, present in 10–50% of cases [5, 6], are primarily the result of urinary stasis due to a stenotic diverticular neck (see Fig. 1). Nonetheless, many patients with diverticular stones have underlying metabolic factors, promoting stone formation. Treatment of these factors is mandatory to prevent recurrence [7].

1.1 Management of Diverticular Stones

Management of diverticular stones with ESWL, although an attractive option due to its noninvasive nature, has low success rates [8], mainly due to the difficulty to evacuate fragments through a stenotic opening.

PCNL has been shown to achieve the best results for diverticular stone management [9, 10]. Nevertheless, PCNL in this scenario has certain limitations [11]. First, the puncture to achieve access to the diverticulum can pose a difficult challenge due to the upper pole position of many diverticula. Second, the ability to pass a guidewire through the opening of the diverticulum to the renal pelvis is usually impossible by the presence of a stone blocking the opening or the difficulty to negotiate the guidewire into the renal pelvis. Third, many diverticula have a small space not allowing the introduction of the nephroscope into the diverticular space for stone fragmentation.

With the remarkable advance in endoscopic equipment, facilitating access and manipulation even in small and difficult spaces, flexible ureteroscopy, allowing for retrograde intrarenal surgery (RIRS), has become a standard alternative for the management of diverticular stones, thus bypassing many of the limitations stated above for the standard treatments.

1.2 Endoscopic Management

Preoperative preparation, with the appropriate imaging and endoscopic tools, is a key to the success in managing these cases. Precise evaluation of the anatomy is made possible with CT urography, which shows the exact location of the diverticula, stone burden, and relation to other organs. A high index of suspicion is also important for identifying diverticular stones.

Before surgical treatment, it is important to bear in mind the different differential diagnoses to diverticular stones on preoperative imaging. These can include hydrocalyces or calyceal stones secondary to infundibular stenosis, submucosal stones caused by medullary sponge kidney, stones engulfed in a tissular matrix after previous procedures, and more rarely, renal milk of calcium cysts (a colloidal suspension of calcium salts occurring in calyceal cysts and diverticula) [12].

The presence of a sterile urine culture is mandatory, and antibiotic prophylaxis is required. Certain patients with recurrent positive cultures might need continuous, large spectrum antibiotic prophylaxis in the preoperative setting.

The cooperation of the anesthetic team is essential. Ventilation with low tidal volumes and respiratory rates facilitates the performance of the procedure by reducing renal mobility during respirations [13].

After positioning the patient in lithotomy and performance of a cystoscopy, a retrograde pyelography is performed (Fig. 1a), with the image acquired serving as a baseline for the rest of the procedure. A 0.038-in. safety guidewire is inserted into the renal pelvis. Access to the collecting system with a flexible ureteroscope along-

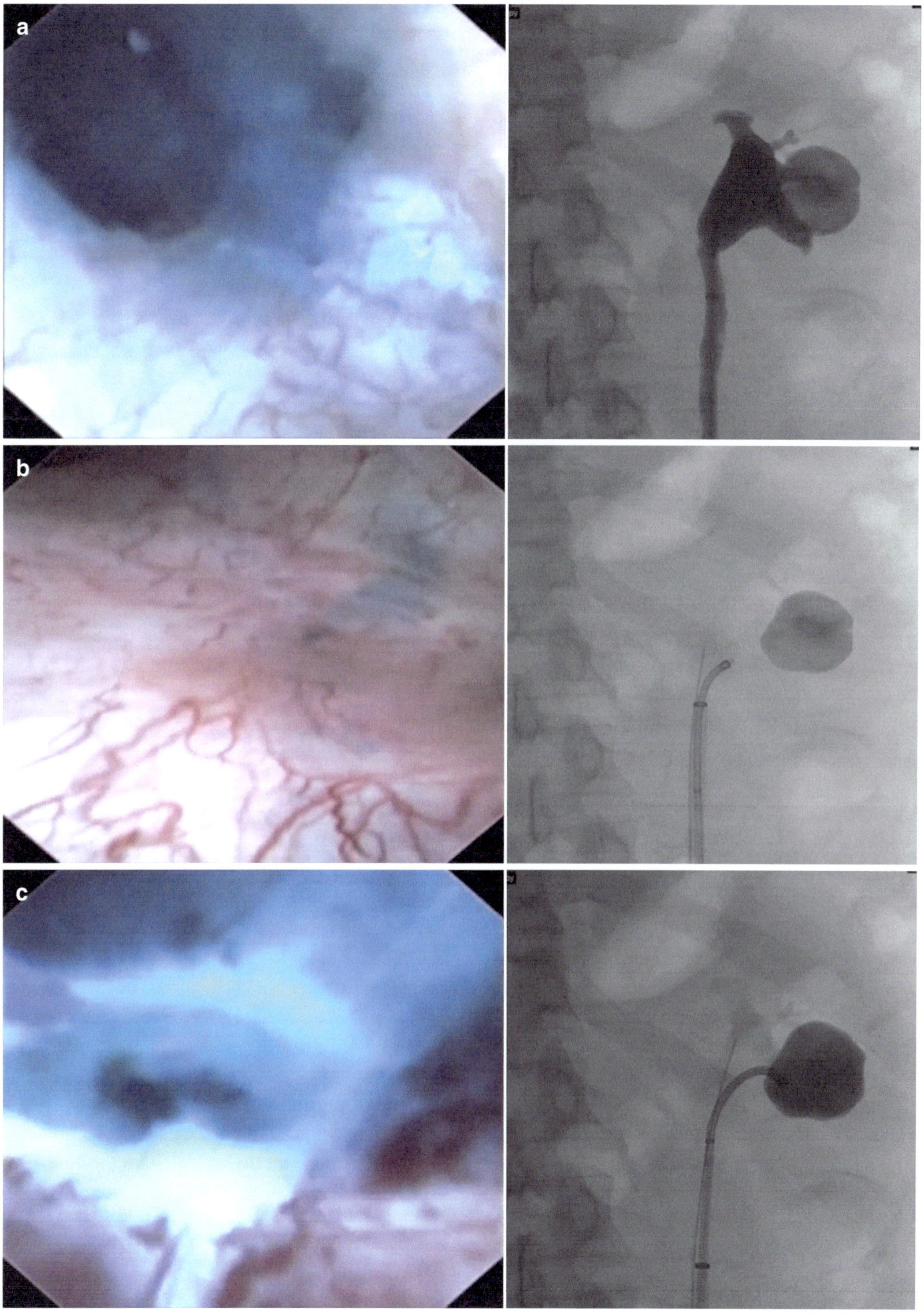

Fig. 1 Diverticular stone management: endoscopic and corresponding fluoroscopic views. From top to bottom: (**a**) blue dye contrast injection into the collecting system. (**b**) Identification of diverticular neck. (**c**) Neck incision by laser and access into diverticulum. (**d**) Fragmentation of diverticular stone. (*Courtesy of Dr Saeed bin Hamri- with permission- video available on Twitter/@ sbinhamrii*)

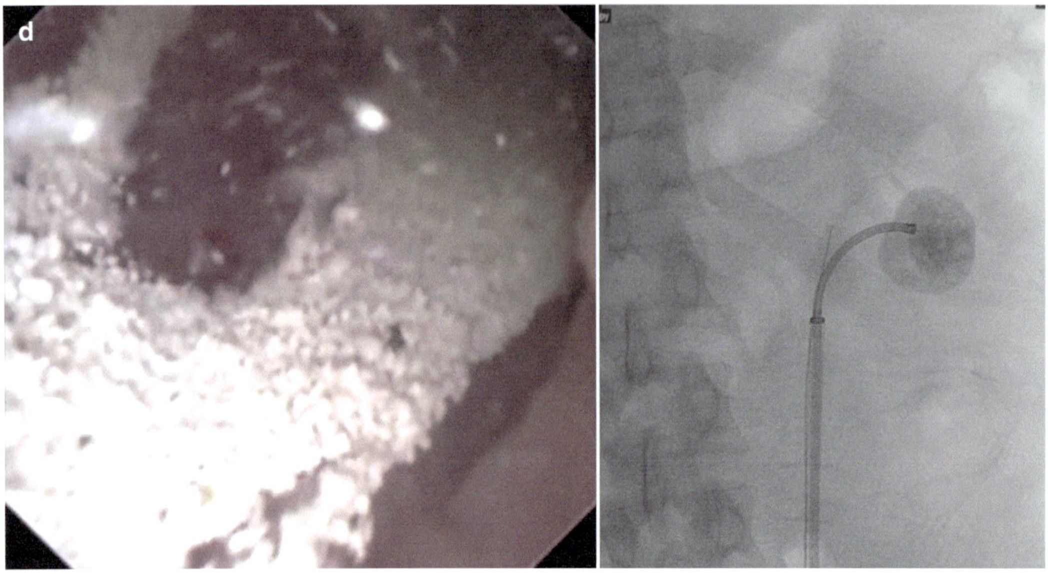

Fig. 1 (continued)

side the safety wire can be attempted, especially if a stent was placed previously and the ureter seems accommodating. If that is not possible, the ureteroscope can be railroaded up into the renal pelvis, over a second 0.038-in. working wire, under fluoroscopic guidance. In cases where resistance is encountered, and the ureteroscope cannot be advanced up into the ureter, a double-J stent is left in place, allowing the narrow ureter to passively dilate for 1–2 weeks, before another attempt is undertaken.

In our institution, we prefer the use of digital endoscopes for these procedures, which gives an optimal image quality while maintaining excellent maneuverability of the ureteroscope, both valuable assets for accurate and effective performance of the procedure. The two leading digital endoscopes available today are the Flex-X[c] (Karl Storz) and the URF-V3 (Olympus). New-generation disposable endoscopes, with better quality imaging, offer a good alternative in difficult cases, especially where risk of breakage of the endoscope might be high.

The endoscopic image quality can play a crucial role in localization of the diverticular opening, usually pinhole-sized and barely visible, located anywhere from the fornix of the calyx to the infundibulum (Fig. 1b). Intra-operative fluoroscopy, enhanced by the injection of diluted contrast, can aid in directing the tip of the endoscope toward the location of the diverticular stone, while the surgeon inspects endoscopically any mucosal site, suggesting the presence of the diverticular opening.

In cases in which the diverticular opening is not easily localized, the "blue spritz" technique can be easily utilized. This technique entails the injection of a readily available colored dye solution, in the presumed location of diverticular opening. After irrigating the system, droplets of blue dye solution, trapped in the diverticulum, start dripping out through the narrow opening, thus helping to identify the site of the diverticulum. A minor modification involves injection of a 50:50 mixture of methylene blue and iodine contrast. This allows for fluoroscopic guidance of the previous steps and further helps to localize the diverticular opening [14].

Once the opening is identified, a working 0.038-in. guidewire is introduced through the working channel and coiled in the diverticulum to guard the access. The endoscope is pulled out and re-introduced alongside the working wire. Two options exist to access the cavity of the diverticulum and treat the stones. If the opening neck is short, then laser incision is performed, and the ureteroscope is introduced into the cavity (Fig. 1c). Use of a small laser fiber (e.g., 200 μm) is advised to limit the effect on endoscope deflection. An alternative option is balloon dilation, preferred in cases where the neck is long, preferred over a laser incision, which would raise the risk of bleeding or extravasation [15]. Upon entry into the diverticular cavity, the stones can be treated as in normal cases, with laser dusting, fragmentation, and basketing, preferably with a zero-tip basket to reduce trauma to the mucosa and inadvertent hematuria affecting visibility (Fig. 1d). Careful inspection of the mucosa for suspicious lesions is mandatory, and the decision to fulgurate the mucosa is usually taken for recurrent cases rather than in the primary intervention.

At the end of the procedure, an indwelling double-J stent is left in place, preferably with the upper loop inside the diverticular space, to facilitate the evacuation of stone fragments or other debris and prevent the early restenosis of the diverticular opening. A urinary catheter is usually left in place for 1 day, depending on the complexity of the procedure. Postoperative imaging is mandatory to decide on the need for re-treatment.

Potential adverse effects include urinary infection, bleeding from the infundibular vessels during laser incision of the diverticular neck, and urinary extravasation due to perforation of the thin layer of cortex above the diverticulum. This is usually identified intra-operatively by fluoroscopy showing contrast perirenal extravasation. In this case, the safest option would be to abort the procedure, drain the collecting system with an indwelling stent, and performing a second look in 2 weeks. If the surgeon chooses to complete the procedure, the use of low irrigation pressure is highly recommended.

1.3 Treatment Selection

Different factors are considered when choosing the best management option for diverticular stones [16]. These include the location of the diverticula, its anterior or posterior aspect, stone burden, the presence of associated symptoms, concomitant anomalies, and finally, surgeon's experience and available equipment.

In large stones, specifically >12 mm in size, we suggest the following algorithm for treatment selection (Fig. 2):

The results for flexible ureteroscopy in the management of diverticular stones are generally satisfactory, with previous reviews reporting a high stone-free rates of 73–90% [15].

Despite the fact that these numbers are lower than the results of the percutaneous approach in the treatment of diverticular stones, fURS has the advantage of being less invasive with lower complication rates than PCNL, presenting a fair compromise for many surgeons and patients alike. The patient should be nonetheless aware of the possibility of repeat procedures to achieve a stone-free status.

Endoscopic combined intra-renal surgery (ECIRS) is the preferred option in cases of large stone burden, lower pole stones, or large diverticula requiring ablation of the cavitary urothelial lining. A combination of flexible ureteroscopy with ESWL is also an option in certain centers.

Laparoscopic surgery has also been utilized for large diverticula difficult to manage endoscopically, or simultaneous with other anomalies requiring surgical repair [17].

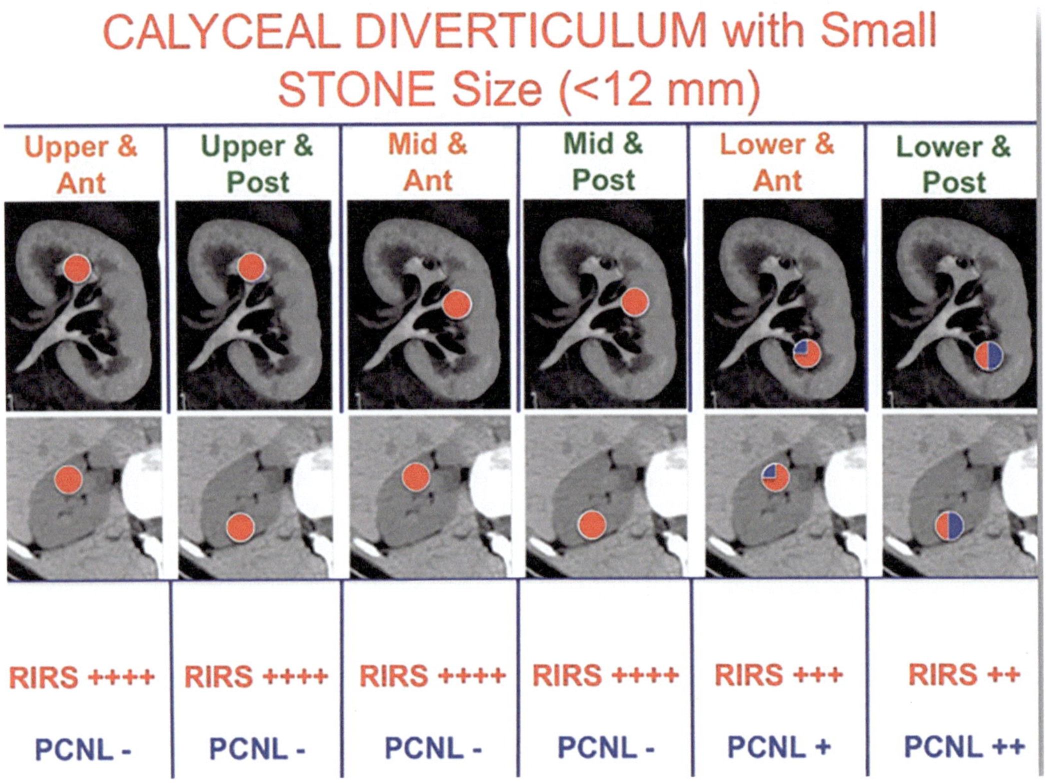

Fig. 2 Guide to treatment choice for renal diverticular stones larger than 12 mm. (*Image from O. Traxer on Twitter*)

2 Horseshoe, Pelvic, and Transplanted Kidneys

2.1 Horseshoe Kidneys

Horseshoe kidneys present multiple challenges for the performance of flexible ureteroscopy, owing to their unique location and orientation. The most common renal fusion abnormality, with an estimated prevalence of 0.25%, horseshoe kidneys are the result of incomplete cephalad migration and malrotation of the two fused kidneys, due to the entrapment of the isthmus under the inferior mesenteric artery [18].

While the lower urinary system and lower ureter are usually normal, the course of the upper ureter is aberrant in horseshoe kidneys. Below the insertion of the ureter into the UPJ, it passes over the fused lower poles, where it is susceptible to compression by the vessels supplying the isthmus and the lower poles. This might give rise to ureteral obstruction leading to urinary stasis, hydronephrosis, and stone formation, the incidence of which is evaluated between 20% and as high as 60% [19]. Most stones are composed of calcium oxalate, with the medially situated, posterior lower pole calyx the most common site for stone formation, followed by the renal pelvis [9].

2.2 Flexible Ureteroscopy in Horseshoe Kidney

Preoperative planning with CT urography and, if possible, 3D reconstruction images is indispensable. Careful mapping of all calyces and stones should be prepared before the procedure starts, and all images and diagrams must be available to the surgeon in the operative room. Antibiotic prophylaxis is the rule as in usual practice.

The procedure should begin with insertion of a 0.038-in guidewire through the ureter and performance of a retrograde uretero-pyelogram. The images obtained should be compared with the preoperative imagery and kept for further reference.

Access of the ureteroscope through the ureterovesical junction is usually straightforward, and the ureter is usually shorter due to the lower position of the kidneys. In case of a tortuous ureter, the use of a hydrophilic stiff guidewire and UAS can straighten the ureter, facilitate the access with the ureteroscope, and improve its deflection in the kidney.

Next, the ureter classically has a high insertion into an elongated ureteropelvic junction (UPJ). Thus, access to the lower poles—where stones are often found—can be challenging, and the urologist needs to work with an almost constant deflection. The use of nitinol baskets can help place lower pole stones in an easier-to-reach site, such as the renal pelvis or the upper pole calyces.

The axis of the horseshoe kidney is more horizontal than usual, the renal pelvis is more anterior, and the calyces point either dorso-medially or dorso-laterally. For these reasons, the orientation in the collecting system and the calyceal spaces is not intuitive, and it can be a challenging task even for experienced endourologists, especially if hydronephrosis is also present. The position of the bubble on the endoscopic field will point to the 12 o'clock position, and this is always a helpful tool for orientation.

Moreover, stone fragmentation in a horseshoe kidney can result in accumulation of fragments in the dependent portions of the kidney, the removal of which is necessary to reduce recurrence rates.

To avoid the strain and the possible breakage on the endoscope, a single-use ureteroscope should be considered, if a challenging case is anticipated. A ureteral stent should always be left in place to help evacuate residual fragments, and to improve drainage in these kidneys.

The use of fURS for these cases is becoming more popular with the evolution of new basketing equipment and endoscopes with better secondary deflection. In addition, new laser technology, allowing more efficient dusting techniques, with smaller fibers allowing for better endoscope deflection, also helps in rendering even difficult cases stone-free.

Few studies with small cohorts have been published regarding the performance of fURS in horseshoe kidneys. Molimard et al. (2010) published their results in 17 patients, with an average stone burden of 16 mm, treated consecutively with fURS. The mean number of procedures was 1.5 per patient and the mean operative time was 92 min. About 88.2% of patients were successfully treated using only flexible ureteroscopy [20].

Despite the promising improvements with fURS, horseshoe kidneys are considered challenging cases due to the anatomic reasons stated above, and many surgeons still regard PCNL as the classical treatment option in horseshoe kidneys, especially for a large stone burden. Indeed, the lower position of the kidney, the anterior rotation of the renal pelvis, and the horizontal axis of the kidney, all make access through the upper pole calyces a relatively safe option. However, even with these conditions favoring the percutaneous approach, the length of the puncture tract often exceeds the length of the rigid nephroscope. Thus, if PCNL is performed in horseshoe kidneys, flexible ureteroscopy can play an essential complementary role, as part of an endoscopic combined intra-renal surgery (ECIRS).

Therefore, the patient should always be informed regarding this option before surgery even if fURS is planned, and the surgeon should also be prepared to conversion to PCNL with the appropriate technical setup available in the operation room.

Last but certainly not least, prevention of stone recurrence with a full metabolic evaluation is indispensable in these patients due to underlying metabolic abnormalities in many patients, responsible for stone formation in the first place [21].

2.3 Ectopic Kidneys

The most common site of ectopic kidneys is the pelvis, reported in approximately 1/1000 births [22]. Other rare sites are the abdomen and the thorax. The pelvic kidney, more common on the left than on the right side, is retroperitoneal, with posterior access usually blocked by the bony pelvis, and interposing intestinal loops precluding percutaneous access through the anterior abdominal wall.

Flexible ureteroscopy is the least invasive and thus the preferable first treatment option. Access through the UVJ might be challenging due to an ectopic orifice. This obstacle can be overcome by searching the jet of blue dye in the bladder mucosa after IV injection of methylene blue, in the absence of allergy or contra-indication (e.g., G6PD deficiency).

The ureter might have a tortuous course that might complicate the insertion of the endoscope. This is usually overcome by using a hydrophilic stiff guidewire or a UAS that can help straighten the ureter, thus facilitating the passage of the ureteroscope. Flexible ureteroscopy with holmium laser and basketing can then be performed with reported good results [23].

An alternative to flexible ureteroscopy is PCNL, with percutaneous access acquired through US or CT guidance. If this is not possible, laparoscopic-assisted PCNL procedures can be performed. In these procedures, laparoscopy can guide the percutaneous puncture of the kidney and mobilize intervening organs or bowel loops away from the puncture needle's tract.

2.4 Transplantation Kidneys

Urolithiasis in transplanted kidneys is relatively rare with an incidence between 0.2 and 4.4% [24]. Due to the substantial risks involved, management in these cases should preferably take place in experienced centers.

Risk factors for stone formation in transplanted kidneys are metabolic abnormalities, presence of foreign bodies (nonabsorbable suture material, forgotten stents), papillary necrosis, and recurrent infection.

The most common anatomical position for transplanted kidneys entails having the donor's left kidney placed into the recipient's right iliac fossa, with the kidney rotated 180° on its axis. Thus, the renal pelvis is oriented medially, the posterior calyces point anteriorly, and, vice versa, the anterior calyces point posteriorly.

These are important points to remember during flexible ureteroscopy, or during PCNL, where an anterior percutaneous approach through the abdominal wall is similar to the posterior approach in native kidneys.

ESWL is a possible primary treatment option for stones less than 15 mm in transplanted kidneys [25]. However, the serious consequences of potential complications such as steinstrasse and the good results of flexible ureteroscopy, make the latter the preferred option in many centers.

2.5 Technique

During cystoscopy, identification of the ureteral orifice can be challenging and is achieved by careful inspection of the mucosa in the presumed area of ureteral insertion. If the ureteral insertion was done by an extra-vesical approach (i.e., Lich Gregoir) as is in the majority of cases, the orifice will usually be located supero-laterally, in the right upper bladder wall. Use of a 70° cystoscope can be helpful.

Blind repeated attempts to introduce the guidewire into a presumed orifice in the mucosal wall should be discouraged, since the resulting hematuria can obscure vision and delay the procedure. In certain cases, IV injection of methylene blue can help in identifying the ureteral orifice.

Once the orifice is identified, a guidewire is introduced gently under fluoroscopic guidance, and a pyelogram is performed, with care to avoid high instillation pressure of contrast to reduce the risk for infection. In case of difficult insertion of the guidewire, angled tip guidewires, or angled catheters, such as a Kumpe or cobra catheter, can prove extremely helpful [26].

Ureteral obstruction, whether intrinsic or extrinsic, occurs in up to 10% of renal transplant recipients, and blind instrumentation can thus risk perforation or even avulsion, hence the importance of identifying these cases early with a uretero-pyelogram.

As mentioned before for pelvic kidneys, insertion of the ureteroscope through the tortuous and redundant ureter can be facilitated through the insertion of a hydrophilic stiff guidewire. Certain endourologists advocate exchanging the hydrophilic safety wire for an Amplatz extra-stiff wire to reduce the risk of inadvertent wire withdrawal and loss of access to the ureter, in addition to support the allograft ureter. The use of a UAS can also straighten the ureter, reduce the fluid pressure in the collecting system, and facilitate repeated passage of the flexible ureteroscope; however, attention must be given to the length of the UAS used, and its insertion must be done with great care, due to the risk of traumatic injury to the ureteral wall or orifice [27, 28].

Once access to the collecting system is achieved, flexible ureteroscopy can then be performed as for a normal kidney, with keeping in mind the mirror image of the calyceal system in the transplanted kidney from that of the normal kidney.

In a comprehensive review including 101 cases from 11 studies, an SFR of 100% in five studies and 60–91% in four studies with an overall complication rate of 12.9%, of which 10 were Clavien 1 and three Clavien ≥ 3. The authors concluded that posttransplant urolithiasis a safe and effective procedure for posttransplant urolithiasis [29].

If access of the endoscope and completion of the procedure is not possible, the retrograde access can guide a percutaneous approach, which is usually facilitated by the superficial position of the transplanted kidneys. Antegrade access in this case is usually safely established into the lower pole, with the skin puncture performed as caudal as possible to avoid intraperitoneal content.

The surgeon must remember that entrance is through the anterior calyces of the transplanted kidney, thus puncturing through the papilla might be harder, and instead puncturing of the infundibulum may occur, increasing the risk of hemorrhagic complications (e.g., pseudoaneurysm and AV fistula). In addition, puncture and subsequently dilation of the access tract might be more difficult due to the scar tissue around the graft.

3 Management of Encrusted Stents

Ureteral stents are routinely used in endoscopic surgery for the drainage of the urinary system. In lithotripsy, ureteral double-J stents or urinary catheters are inserted to prevent postoperative obstruction by edema or residual fragments. In urinary system reconstructive surgery and diversion procedures, they are used to maintain the patency of the ureter and minimize urinary leaks.

Since their introduction, urinary stents have gone through significant development in material composition, coating materials, and designs, resulting in a wide range of different stents responding to various clinical indications and with different biocompatibility and tolerability profiles [30].

Despite the central role stents play in endourological surgery, their use is not devoid of side effects and potential complications, such as irritative urinary symptoms, hematuria, and pain.

Moreover, previous studies have shown that in contact with urine, ureteral stents are rapidly covered by a bacterial film (biofilm) and by mineral and/or organic encrustations [31].

Stent encrustation can potentially give rise to new stones and even lead to obstruction of the urine drainage. In one study, the main composition of the encrustations was calcium oxalate monohydrate and dihydrate, carbapatite, and protein matrix [32]. The FeCal classification proposed by Acosta-Miranda et al. is used to describe the location and the degree of encrustation of each calcified stent [33].

The rate of stent encrustation is primarily dependent on the duration of contact with urine, which can be prolonged in cases of forgotten stents. This situation is usually caused by patients' poor compliance or misinformation regarding the need and timing for stent retrieval after an intervention, leading to their belated presentation with significantly incrusted stents. Some patients are also left with retained stents due to comorbidities outweighing the importance of stent retrieval. In addition, encrustation is also affected by patient factors such as a history of stone formation or pregnancy for example.

Stent material composition also plays a role, with several studies suggesting that silicone stents might have significantly fewer mineral encrustations and biofilm development in kidney stone formers, compared to other materials including polyurethane stents [34].

Surgical intervention in these cases is essential due to the serious consequences to the urinary system, including recurrent infections, loss of renal function, and in extreme cases, urothelial dysplasia and even development of squamous cell carcinoma due to the constant irritation of the mucosa.

Management has traditionally involved multistaged procedures and combined retrograde and antegrade approaches, with PCNL playing a central role in cases with large encrustation or stone burden in the renal pelvis. More recently, endoscopic combined intra-renal surgery (ECIRS) has gained popularity for more complex cases. However, with the advance of endoscopic and laser equipment, multiple publications highlighted the role of flexible ureteroscopy in the treatment of encrusted stents, even in complex cases.

In the next segment, we will present the technique of managing encrusted stents in a stepwise approach, using only flexible ureteroscopy.

3.1 Preoperative Considerations

Preoperative CT urography must be obtained before surgery to evaluate the anatomy and the stone burden in the collecting system (Fig. 3b). If doubt exists, renal scan must be performed to evaluate the basal function of the ipsilateral renal parenchyma. This examination is also important for its medicolegal value. Urinary culture results must be verified, and antibiotic prophylaxis must be noted, if needed starting 48 h before surgery. This is especially critical in these cases due to the high rate of contaminated urine and the risk for serious infections postoperatively.

General anesthesia is preferred in all cases. The surgeon must be prepared on a technical and organizational level, to the potential need of a combined retrograde and antegrade approach if the procedure cannot be completed solely retrogradely. The patient must also be informed regarding this scenario.

3.2 Procedure Technique

After appropriate antibiotic prophylaxis and installation of the patient in a lithotomy position, cystoscopy is performed to evaluate the inferior

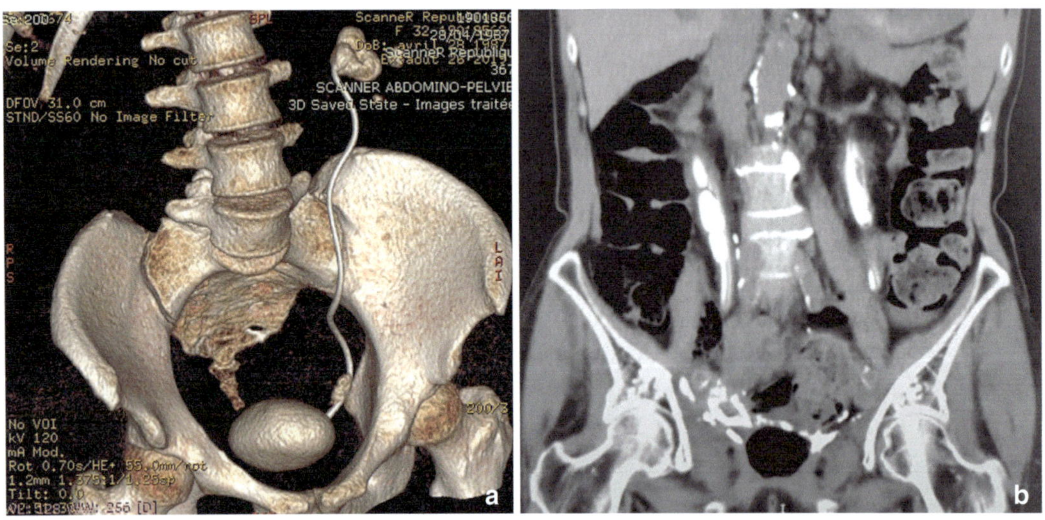

Fig. 3 (**a**) 3D reconstruction image of an incrusted stent in the left kidney, lower ureter, and bladder. (**b**) CT image in coronal view demonstrating bilateral encrusted stents

loop of the stent. The first step is insertion of a 0.038-in. safety guidewire into the collecting system, under fluoroscopic guidance, alongside the encrusted stent. Fragmentation of the encrustations or stone engulfing the inferior stent loop is performed cystoscopically with laser energy (e.g., Ho:YAG laser). To reduce the oscillations of the laser fiber, it is introduced through a 35-cm segment of 5 F ureteral catheter, cut with simple scissors. In certain situations, the stone burden in the bladder is so large, it necessitates fragmentation with an ultrasonic or mechanical lithotripter, inserted into the bladder by a nephroscope through the urethra in females or percutaneously through a working channel in the supra pubic area in males.

After the inferior loop is freed from encrustations, the next step involves liberating the intra ureteral portion of the stent. This segment is usually less prone to encrustation than the bladder or renal pelvis, due to the function of the ureter as a conduit of urine and thus the shorter contact duration between the stent and the urine. The presence of the indwelling ureteral stent allows for sufficient ureteral distension, and subsequently enough space to accommodate a flexible ureteroscope, introduced into the ureter alongside the stent under direct vision. To facilitate this step, the distal loop of the stent is exteriorized through the urethral orifice and fixed by a stitch to the skin, to maintain a gentle traction on the stent. This is achievable usually only in female patients due to the length of the urethra in males. If insertion of a flexible ureteroscope is not successful, the use of a semirigid ureteroscope can be a good alternative. The ureteroscope is introduced as proximal as possible alongside the encrusted stent.

If the renal pelvis is reached, the procedure is continued as usual for retrograde intra-renal surgery, and the encrustations engulfing the proximal loop are fragmented, thus uncoiling the loop and removing the stent entirely. In most cases, however, it is impossible to advance the ureteroscope all the way up to the renal pelvis, due to encrustations in the ureteral portion. In these cases, the encrustations are fragmented and the double-J stent is cut using the Ho:YAG laser cutting setting (10 Hz–1.0 J). The free, cut portion of the stent can be removed with a forceps to create space and allow further progression of the ureteroscope, until the arrival to the renal segment of the encrusted stent. This step is usually repeated twice, depending on the length of the ureter and burden of encrustations around the stent.

When the ureter is emptied from encrustations and stent segments, the mucosa needs to be inspected carefully, and if found intact, a ureteral access sheath (UAS) can be inserted, thus allowing the continuation of the procedure in the upper portion of the collecting system with low intrapelvic pressure. In addition, the UAS protects the ureteral wall from injury during removal of the proximal loop.

When the renal pelvis is reached, the encrustations and any concomitant stones can be fragmented, and the final upper portion of the stent can be removed with a basket or endoscopic forceps (Fig. 4).

The surgeon must avoid working with elevated intrapelvic pressures, to reduce fluid extravasation, which is extremely important given the high risk of contaminated urine due to the presence of biofilm on the encrusted stents.

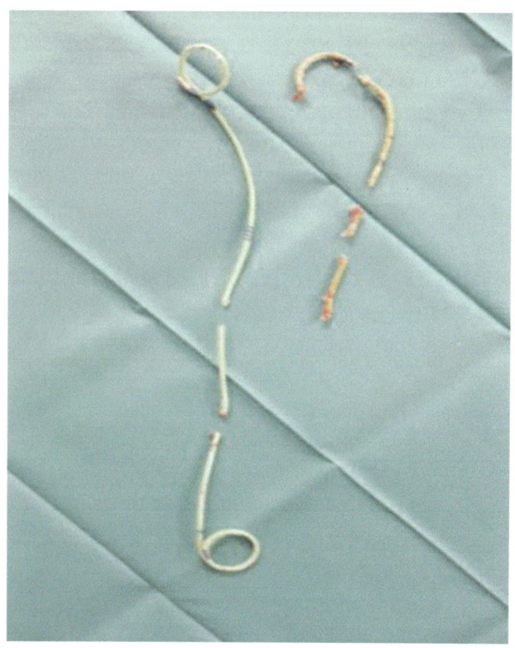

Fig. 4 Cut segments after procedure to extract encrusted stents

Due to the complexity and length of these procedures, they can be performed in a multi-stage approach. A new double-J ureteral stent can be placed until the next session in tandem with the encrusted stent, to prevent obstruction by edema or residual fragments.

Thomas et al. reported their results with this technique. In their study including 51 patients with a mean indwelling time of 10.4 months and grade 5 encrustations according to the FeCa classification in 80% of patients, removal of the encrusted stent was possible in 98% of patients through flexible ureteroscopy, with a mean operative time of 110 min and mean hospital stay was 2.33 days [35].

The principal complication to this procedure is pyelonephritis, and in some cases bacteremia and sepsis. This is especially relevant in the treatment of encrusted stents since biofilm is present in virtually all retained stents. The use of UAS and working in the minimal possible irrigation pressure can lower the risk for infection. Postoperative antibiotic therapy should be considered for all patients, especially in patients with struvite stones, and monitoring is essential for early management in case of sepsis. Another possible important complication is injury to the ureteral wall due to the extensive use of laser energy in a limited luminal working space.

Flexible ureteroscopy thus is an important tool in the management of retained encrusted stents, offering a less-invasive option than PCNL. Nonetheless, cases with a large stone burden might require a combined endoscopic approach (ECIRS) with PCNL to avoid multiple procedures.

4 Obese Patients

Obesity is a major healthcare problem with increasing prevalence worldwide [36], aggravated by accompanying conditions such as hypertension, hyperlipidemia, diabetes mellitus, cardiovascular disease, in addition to gout and obstructive sleep apnea. The relative risk of these comorbidities increases significantly with the BMI of the patient, and thus presents significant anesthetic and operative challenges in this patient population [37].

Moreover, obese patients present multiple lithogenic factors increasing the risk of kidney stone disease [38]. These include insulin resistance accompanied by a low urinary pH, lower urinary citrate levels, in addition to a high caloric intake, and metabolic sequels of previous bariatric surgeries. These factors among others increase the risk of urinary stones, principally calcium oxalate (both mono- and di-hydrate) and uric acid stones [39].

Diagnosis of stones might be affected by the lower yield of sonography in obese patients, making CT a better diagnostic tool in these patients. The management of stones in obese patients presents certain limitations of the standard treatment options.

ESWL might be less effective in obese patients, and increasing abdominal circumference and visceral fat is related to decreasing stone-free rates after SWL [40, 41]. Moreover, targeting of the stone might be harder due to the increased skin to stone distance and higher prevalence of uric acid in obese patients [42].

PCNL might pose an anesthetic difficulty due to the need to ventilate a patient with smaller functional residual capacity of the lungs, in a flank or prone position. In addition, patient positioning on the table is more challenging and requires more time and personnel. PCNL in an obese patient can also necessitate extra-long puncturing needles and access sheaths to reach the collecting system (Fig. 5), while this equipment might not be readily available in every center.

With the improvement of ureteroscopy in recent decades, flexible ureteroscopy has become a preferred option in obese patients, presenting multiple advantages in comparison with ESWL and PCNL. These include a higher success rate than ESWL, easier positioning in lithotomy than flank or prone positions in PCNL and absence of a kidney puncture.

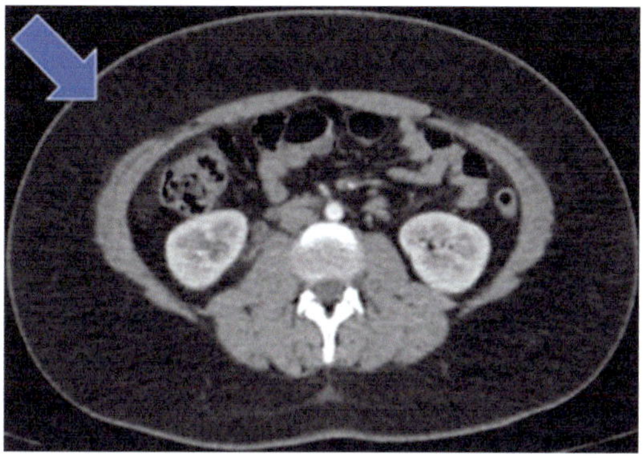

Fig. 5 CT image in an obese patient, arrow showing abdominal wall fat content. (*From O. Traxer twitter account*)

4.1 Preoperative Considerations

Multidisciplinary evaluation is essential in this patient population, due to the possible presence of associated comorbidities, especially cardiopulmonary diseases, and obstructive sleep apnea. These conditions carry potential anesthetic risks, and any concern regarding intubation (e.g., LMA vs. intubation) or ventilation of a patient in the lithotomy position must be discussed with the anesthetist preoperatively, with higher ventilation pressures sometimes needed to compensate for a restricted respiratory capacity.

Blood pressure and glycemic control must be maintained to avoid perioperative complications. Prophylaxis to deep vein thrombosis with compression stockings and possibly subcutaneous heparin is also essential. Postoperative monitoring is also important and must be discussed with the anesthetist and the patient beforehand.

4.2 Technical Considerations

The presence of a fluoroscopy table in the operation room, able to withstand the overweight patient, must be verified before the patient arrives to the surgery room. In rare cases, the use of two tables might be necessary to accommodate a patient with severe morbid obesity (BMI > 40 kg/m^2).

Special attention should be drawn to the appropriate positioning and padding of the patient, to avoid the risk of nerve compression and crush injuries, which may even lead to rhabdomyolysis in extreme conditions. Access to the urethral meatus might not be straightforward as in normal conditions, and the pannus or adjacent skin folds might require special positioning.

While the different steps of flexible ureteroscopy are performed in a similar fashion to nonobese patients, the use of fluoroscopy during the procedure deserves special attention. The operator must be aware of the larger scatter of radiation, due to the larger body mass of the patient [43]. Thus, despite the lower quality of the image due to the patient's habitus, overuse of fluoroscopic imaging must be avoided to limit radiation exposure of the operating team.

Given the limitations and risks of the other treatment modalities as stated above, several studies have shown that fURS is an excellent option for the treatment of *most* stones in obese patients, with operative times, an important indicator of surgical complexity, reported to be comparable among the obese and nonobese patients [44, 45]. As for large stones (>2 cm), fURS might also be an alternative, to avoid the risks of PCNL, even at the cost of a multi-staged approach. In complex cases with a large stone burden, endoscopic combined intra-renal surgery (ECIRS) is an excellent option, in which flexible URS guides the percutaneous calyceal puncture and contributes to the fragmentation of the stones.

5 Flexible Ureteroscopy in Urinary Diversions

Urinary diversions, whether for oncological or reconstructive functional reasons, constitute another subset of challenging cases in endoscopic surgery. They are usually divided into continent (orthotopic or non-orthotopic neobladder) or non-continent diversions (e.g., Bricker, Wallace) [46]. Regardless of the type of diversion, retrograde ureteroscopy may be indicated for the treatment of nephrolithiasis, surveillance, and diagnosis of suspected malignancies or the treatment of ureteric strictures. For these reasons, acquaintance with the endoscopic approach to the diverted urinary system is mandatory.

Stone formation in patients with urinary diversion is a multifactorial process and includes dehydration, metabolic disturbances like chronic metabolic acidosis, hypocitraturia, hypercalciuria, and enteric hyperoxaluria [47, 48]. In addition, chronic bacterial colonization with urease-producing bacteria can lead to the formation of struvite stones. The presence of foreign bodies like sutures, exposed staples, in addition to the urinary stasis within a chronically refluxing dilated system, also constitutes a risk factor for stone formation.

PCNL was long considered the most straightforward approach to treat stones or obstructions in the diverted upper urinary system. This is especially true for neobladder cases and non-orthotopic diversions (e.g., Indiana pouch), due to the extremely difficult retrograde access. However, with the improvements in ureteroscopes, allowing better maneuvering and deflection of the endoscope, and better endoscopic imaging, more experience is being gained with flexible ureteroscopy, offering a less-invasive alternative to PCNL.

5.1 Technical Aspects

Preoperative evaluation of the anatomy with CT urography and 3D reconstruction images is imperative, assuming no allergies to contrast exist and renal function allows for the injection of IV contrast material. In any doubt regarding the surgical anatomy, previous medical records must be inspected. Antibiotic prophylaxis is also mandatory due to the high risk of infectious complications.

The patient should be informed regarding the different approaches for treatment and the possibility of combined antegrade and retrograde endoscopic surgery. The surgeon must also be prepared with the equipment for both approaches available in the operation theater.

In patients with *ileal conduit*, the procedure begins with a flexible cystoscope through the conduit (conduitoscopy). Use of the flexible cystoscope also allows for simultaneous suction of mucus which might obscure vision. Injection of contrast material and fluoroscopy helps to find the right orientation, which can be difficult to achieve in elongated redundant conduits. Injection of contrast can suggest the site of the ureteral orifice through passive reflux into the ureter. Patients with Bricker's anastomosis will have two independent ureteral orifices, toward the proximal end of the conduit. Patients with the less common Wallace anastomosis will classically have a single-joint orifice for the two ureters at the proximal end of the ileal loop. If identification of the orifices is impossible, IV administration of methylene blue or indigo carmine (with furosemide) may help localize the site of the orifice upon dye excretion with the urine, usually within 10 min of injection.

Once identified, the ureteral orifice is intubated with a hydrophilic stiff guidewire. Certain surgeons advocate replacement of this wire with an Amplatz super stiff guide, to reduce the risk of unintentional withdrawal of the guide. A double-lumen catheter is inserted on the guidewire, and a retrograde uretero-pyelogram is performed, with the images kept for subsequent reference during the procedure. Identifying a uretero-enteric stenosis or any obstruction at this stage is essential, to avoid traumatic injury with the endoscopic instruments. After securing the safety guidewire, a flexible ureteroscope is inserted through either direct vision if possible or, alternatively, railroaded on a working guidewire placed in tandem with the security guidewire. Insertion of a UAS can be dangerous and traumatic for the uretero-enteric anastomosis and is thus not advisable. A Foley catheter can be kept in the conduit to drain the irrigation fluid and avoid an overdistended collecting system.

In *neobladders*, injection of contrast material through a flexible cystoscope and fluoroscopy are used to outline the neobladder and afferent limb anatomy. Reflux of contrast material can usually outline the presence of the ureteral orifices [49]. In continent non-orthotopic diversions (e.g., Indiana pouch), insertion of instruments must be done with extreme caution to avoid trauma to the catheterized stoma and inadvertent damage to the delicate sphincteric mechanism.

Once access to the collecting system is achieved, RIRS with the flexible ureteroscope is then completed, with care taken to use the lowest possible irrigation pressure [50], in a urinary system already colonized with bacteria. Dusting of stones is preferred if possible, due to the difficulty and time consumption of multiple withdrawals and insertions of the endoscope, without a UAS.

Hyams et al. reported their experience with retrograde access in patients with urinary diversions. Out of 28 retrograde access attempts, 21 (75%) were successful. The success rate for each type of urinary diversion was 90% for orthotopic neobladders, 73% for ileal conduits, and 33% for Indiana pouches. Patients with ureteral anastomotic stricture has a lower success rate. No complications were reported [51].

Potential complications are pyelonephritis, the risk of which is increased due to the preexisting bacterial colonization. Other possible risks are iatrogenic trauma to the delicate continence mechanisms of the urinary diversion or to the uretero-enteric anastomosis.

Drainage of the collecting system is done with a ureteral single-J stent, and a repeat UPG is performed before retrieval of the stent if there is any doubt regarding the integrity of the anastomosis and urinary system.

6 Flexible Ureteroscopy in Pregnancy

Ureteroscopy for stone management in pregnant patients came a long way in the last two decades since it was contraindicated in the past, due to fears of possible fetal and maternal consequences. Furthermore, the medico-legal aspects and unfamiliarity with obstetrical considerations discouraged many urologists from taking an active treatment approach for stone management in pregnant patients.

However, multiple studies have been published in recent years, shedding light on this subject and helping to change the management paradigm in this patient group.

6.1 Stones in Pregnant Patients

The incidence of stones in pregnancy varies widely between 0.07 and 0.5% of pregnancies in different publications. However, a recent Canadian comprehensive population study estimated the incidence of pregnancies with stones to be 0.2%, with almost 80–90% in the second and third trimesters, and the majority being first-time stone formers [52, 53]. Stone presentation seems to be equal on the left and the right side, although the right side is usually more dilated, owing to the mechanical obstruction of the ureter at the pelvic brim by the enlarging uterus.

Calcium phosphate stones are the most common stone type according to certain studies [54], while others suggest the types of stones in pregnancy do not differ from those in nonpregnant women [55]. Regardless, multiple biochemical risk factors for stone formation exist in pregnant women, including elevated urinary calcium, which likely promotes the frequent encrustations seen in urinary drainage stents in pregnancy. In addition, elevated urine pH and uric acid levels have also been observed during pregnancy.

Despite the above factors, pregnancy itself does not seem to increase the incidence of urolithiasis, even among identified stone formers [56]. This is probably the result of the concomitant increase of urinary inhibitors of stone formation, such as citrate and magnesium, in addition to the higher GFR, contributing to urine dilution.

6.2 Presentation

Stones in pregnancy are frequently symptomatic, due to the physiologic dilatation of the urinary tract, facilitating stone migration into the ureters, with the resultant obstruction and renal colic [57]. Indeed, stones are found in the ureter twice as often as in the renal pelvis during pregnancy [58].

When compared with matched pregnancies without stones, pregnancies with stones had an increased risk (OR 1.62) for adverse birth outcomes, including increased risk of low birth weight, premature birth, preeclampsia, and caesarian section [52].

6.3 Diagnosis and Natural History of Pregnancy Stones

When a pregnant woman presents with flank pain, the differential diagnosis is wide, and a high index of suspicion is required for early diagnosis and management.

US is the most widely recommended diagnostic method [59]. Its two main disadvantages, however, are the operator dependence and the inability to differentiate between the physiologic dilatation and an acute obstruction. Documenting ureteral jets, measuring resistive index [60], and using three-dimensional extended imaging US can help improving the performance of US.

The American Urological Association (AUA) introduced imaging recommendations in 2013, which suggested the use of low-dose CT as a second-line imaging modality in the second and third trimester of pregnancy when ultrasound studies failed to secure a diagnosis [61]. This has also been supported by the American College of Obstetricians and Gynecologists (ACOG) [62]. However, concern still exists regarding the potential carcinogenic effects of radiation to the fetus [63]. Consequently, the decision to use this modality must be justified and discussed with the radiologist, after explaining the pros and cons to the patient [64].

The natural history of stones in pregnant patients is also variable according to different publications. Previous studies have suggested high percentages of stone expulsion in pregnant patients, previously estimated around 65% and as high as 84% in one study [65, 66]. This number has recently been reevaluated and found to be around 48% in one study [67].

In a recent large study, including 2863 pregnancies with stones, 26% of pregnant patients eventually had an intervention, most commonly a stent or ureteroscopy [52].

Obstruction by urinary stones in pregnant patients can be complicated by pyelonephritis and, in some cases, premature rupture of membranes, risking fetal loss in extreme cases. Thus, in any case of suspected stone associated with an infection, urgent decompression, with a nephrostomy tube or a ureteral stent, is the rule.

6.4 Definitive Treatment

Drainage procedures with ureteral stents or nephrostomy tubes are only *temporizing measures*, and these tubes are prone to frequent and recurrent encrustations, necessitating periodic replacement every 4–6 weeks, in addition to infectious complications and bothersome urinary symptoms. Due to the need for recurrent procedures to replace the drainage tubes, there is a need for early definitive treatment in cases where multiple such replacements are predicted.

ESWL and PCNL in pregnancy are formally contraindicated due to the serious adverse effects and dangers, both to the fetus and to the mother.

6.5 The Evolution of fURS in Pregnancy

The concerns precluding the routine use of fURS in pregnancy involve primarily the utilization of imaging, whether preoperative evaluation of stone site and volume, or intraoperative fluoroscopy, and the potential consequences for the fetus. Second, the anesthetic risks for both the fetus and the mother were long considered an obstacle to performing any procedure more elaborate than the insertion of a nephrostomy tube or ureteral stent. Third, retrograde access to the upper ureter and collecting system were difficult to achieve with older rigid endoscopes. As a result of these concerns, management of cases presenting with an obstructive stone mainly consisted of drainage with a nephrostomy tube or a ureteral stent alone.

Imagery and radiation are two of the thorniest issues in pregnancy and urolithiasis, due to the potential dangers of radiation to the fetus. Despite the difficulty in accurately evaluating the radiation exposure and its effects on the fetus, recent studies have shown that the teratogenic risk is minimal with radiation doses <50 mGy. This is especially relevant for the period before the eighth week or after the 23rd week of gestation. Stochastic effects (e.g., carcinogenesis) on the other hand are independent of the dose and can occur without a threshold level, thus presenting the main reason for concern.

Regarding the anesthetic angle, the American College of Obstetricians and Gynecologists' Committee on Obstetric Practice and the American Society of Anesthesiologists published in a joint statement in 2017 that a pregnant woman should never be denied medically necessary surgery or have that surgery delayed regardless of trimester because this can adversely affect the pregnant woman and her fetus [68]. In addition, no currently used anesthetic agents have been shown to have any teratogenic effects in humans when using standard concentrations at any gestational age.

The improvement in flexible endoscopes has made it possible to use miniaturized equipment with excellent deflection capacity, able to negotiate tortuous ureters and explore the entirety of the collecting system.

These factors combined, encouraged urologists to take a more proactive approach for stone management during pregnancy, leading to a growing number of ureteroscopic procedures in the pregnant patient.

6.6 Procedure

Preoperative planning is mandatory. The considerations for performing the procedure and the potential risks must be explained to the patient, and a shared decision is always encouraged.

Every decision to perform a URS procedure must be taken in a multidisciplinary team, involving a urologist, obstetrician, neonatologist. Anesthetist, and possibly the radiologist as well.

In case the diagnosis was made with US imaging only, the possibility of "white" (negative) URS must also be discussed. White et al. published in their study that the rate of negative ureteroscopy among patients who underwent renal ultrasound alone, renal ultrasound and low dose computerized tomography, and renal ultrasound and magnetic resonance urography, was 23%, 4.2%, and 20%, respectively [69].

Antibiotic prophylaxis must be given and adapted to the urinary cultures, due to the elevated risk for urinary colonization in pregnant women.

DVT prophylaxis is also mandatory and must be discussed preoperatively. Formal obstetric consultation including fetal monitoring during the procedure are mandatory.

During the procedure itself, the patient is installed in the lithotomy position with the right side elevated, to reduce the pressure of the gravid uterus on the IVC, decreasing the venous return.

The procedure is begun with a cystoscopy, identification of the ureteral orifice, and insertion of a safety guidewire retrogradely. Insertion of the wire must be performed with the greatest attention to any resistance that might signify a stone or other obstruction. Usually, a hydrophilic coated 0.038-in guidewire is used. If the surgeon prefers, this wire can be exchanged for a non-hydrophilic guide wire, less prone to withdrawal, through a ureteral catheter. Regardless, working with a safety guidewire is imperative in these cases, where any change in fetal monitoring or maternal status might necessitate and immediate abortion of the procedure, with time only to insert a ureteral stent or catheter for drainage.

In our institution, we introduce the safety guidewire through the ureteral orifice, followed by a flexible ureteroscope alongside the safety wire that is advanced gradually and under direct endoscopic vision. An alternative is the "follow the wire" approach, reported in 26 pregnant patients in 2009 [70]. In this approach, a semi-rigid ureteroscope is introduced by advancing the guidewire through the ureteroscope into the ureteric orifice and following it stepwise up to the site of obstruction; then the GW was advanced past the obstruction under vision to the kidney, and the ureteroscope was removed and re-introduced.

Regardless of the technique used, this step, in a normal case, would be performed with fluoroscopic guidance. In pregnancy, however, radiation use must be reduced to the minimum and avoided wherever possible.

Although the radiation limit in the previously mentioned ACOG recommendations was 50 mGy, and fluoroscopic imaging produces much less radiation than this limit, the dose-independent carcinogenic risk still exists and needs to be taken into consideration.

The recommendation to the use of fluoroscopy includes using pulsed and not continuous fluoroscopy, with the lowest possible dose settings, and with coning of the image to include only the kidney. The C-arm X-ray *source* must be placed under the patient the farthest possible from the patient, by either lowering the source or elevating the table. To shield the pelvis from radiation, a lead apron may be placed *beneath* the patient's pelvis. Another alternative, allowing for manipulation of the shielded field, is inversion of the C-arm with the X-ray source above the patient, and the apron on the abdomen, shielding the fetus.

Optimally, a simultaneous renal US can guide the insertion of the guidewire or endoscope and the placement of a ureteral stent at the end of the procedure.

After passage of a safety guidewire, the ureter can then be inspected by a flexible or a semirigid ureteroscope, alongside the safety wire. The ureter is generally dilated and accommodating to the insertion of the endoscope, and the gravid uterus does not prevent the retrograde passage. The flexible ureteroscope allows inspection of the collecting system. During the inspection, stones are either extracted, if possible, or fragmented.

If lithotripsy is to be performed, Ho:YAG laser is the ideal method due to its ability to fragment every stone type, small size of new laser fibers allowing better endoscope manipulation, and the inexistent side effects for the fetus. Ho:YAG is safe to use due to the little tissue penetration depth.

The alternative for lithotripsy besides the use of laser is pneumatic lithotripsy. The drawbacks with its use, however, is the potential retropulsion of the stones into the collecting system and that it must be used with a semirigid ureteroscope. Ultrasonic lithotripters's use is limited due to potential risk for auditory damage to the fetus, and electrohydraulic lithotripsy is also avoided due to safety concerns, mainly effects on fetal hearing and uterine contractions [71].

A ureteral stent is preferably left in place for 5–7 days, with specific instructions for removal of the stent, to avoid unintentional prolonged dwelling time (i.e., forgotten stent) and stent encrustation. The strings of the double-J stent can be left in place and attached to the pubis for easier withdrawal. They also would serve as a reminder for the presence of the stent and need for its withdrawal.

6.7 Results

In a review by Laing et al. of 15 studies with a total of 116 procedures, SFR was achieved in 86% of cases, and only two major complications were identified: one ureteral perforation and one case of premature uterine contraction. In another review by Guisti et al., including 8 studies and 198 cases, SFR ranged from 73 to 100% [72].

Semins et al. performed a systematic review of the literature concerning the safety of ureteroscopy in pregnancy. The overall complication rate was 8.3% with two Clavien 1, six Clavien 2, and one Clavien 3 complications being noted. When compared with the complication rates derived from the AUA/EAU ureteral stone guidelines, no statistical difference in the rate of ureteral injury or UTI was shown [73].

Another study focusing on obstetric complications in 46 patients undergoing ureteroscopic stone removal during pregnancy found two (4.3%) obstetric complications, both premature contractions in the third trimester. One was managed with tocolytics and the other required cesarean section [74].

Today, many of the concerns that precluded the use of fURS in pregnant patients are now deconstructed and better understood with recent experience and evidence-based medicine [75–78]. Thus, primary fURS is certainly an option to be considered in a multidisciplinary fashion for the management of stones in pregnant patients. These procedures should preferably be performed by an experienced endourologist in a high-volume center, with available supporting obstetrics and neonatology units.

References

1. Geraghty RM, Jones P, Somani BK. Worldwide trends of urinary stone disease treatment over the last two decades: a systematic review. J Endourol.

2017;31(6):547–56. https://doi.org/10.1089/end.2016.0895.
2. Timmons JW, Malek RS, Hattery RR, Deweerd JH. Caliceal diverticulum. J Urol. 1975;114(1):6–9. https://doi.org/10.1016/s0022-5347(17)66930-1.
3. Waingankar N, Hayek S, Smith AD, Okeke Z. Calyceal diverticula: a comprehensive review. Rev Urol. 2014;16(1):29–43.
4. Wulfsohn MA. Pyelocaliceal diverticula. J Urol. 1980;123(1):1–8. https://doi.org/10.1016/s0022-5347(17)55748-133.
5. Jones JA, Lingeman JE, Steidle CP. The roles of extracorporeal shock wave lithotripsy and percutaneous nephrostolithotomy in the management of pyelocaliceal diverticula. J Urol. 1991;146(3):724–7. https://doi.org/10.1016/s0022-5347(17)37906-5.
6. Canales B, Monga M. Surgical management of the calyceal diverticulum. Curr Opin Urol. 2003;13(3):255–60. https://doi.org/10.1097/00042307-200305000-00015.
7. Liatsikos EN, Bernardo NO, Dinlenc CZ, Kapoor R, Smith AD. Caliceal diverticular calculi: is there a role for metabolic evaluation? J Urol. 2000;164(1):18–20. https://doi.org/10.1016/s0022-5347(05)67439-3.
8. Lechevallier E, Saussine C, Traxer O. Prise en charge des calculs des diverticules caliciels rénaux. Prog Urol. 2008;18(12):989–91. https://doi.org/10.1016/j.purol.2008.09.019.
9. Tan YK, Cha DY, Gupta M. Management of stones in abnormal situations. Urol Clin N Am. 2013;40(1):79–97. https://doi.org/10.1016/j.ucl.2012.10.001.
10. Shalhav AL, Soble JJ, Nakada SY, Wolf JS, McClennan BL, Clayman, R. V. Long-term outcome of caliceal diverticula following percutaneous endosurgical management. J Urol. 1998;160(5):1635–9. https://doi.org/10.1016/s0022-5347(01)62366-8.
11. Grasso M, Lang G, Loisides P, Bagley D, Taylor F. Endoscopic management of the symptomatic caliceal diverticular calculus. J Urol. 1995;153(6):1878–81. https://doi.org/10.1016/s0022-5347(01)67337-3.
12. Khan SA, Khan FR, Fletcher MS, Richenberg JL. Milk of calcium (MOC) cysts masquerading as renal calculi—a trap for the unwary. Cent Eur J Urol. 2012;65(3):170–3. https://doi.org/10.5173/ceju.2012.03.art16.
13. Kourmpetis V, Sofer M. Toward respiratory-gated retrograde intrarenal surgery: a prospective controlled randomized study. J Endourol. 2018;32(9):812–7. https://doi.org/10.1089/end.2018.0231.
14. Soni SD. Modified "Blue Spritz" technique for ureteroscopic localization and management of caliceal diverticula. Videourology. 2018;32(3):2018.
15. Chong TW, Bui MHT, Fuchs GJ. Calyceal diverticula. Urol Clin N Am. 2000;27(4):647–54. https://doi.org/10.1016/s0094-0143(05)70114-2.
16. Smyth N, Somani B, Rai B, Aboumarzouk OM. Treatment options for calyceal diverticula. Curr Urol Rep. 2019;20(7):1–4. https://doi.org/10.1007/s11934-019-0900-x.
17. Hoznek A, Chopin DK, Abbou C-C. Symptomatic caliceal diverticula treated with extraperitoneal laparoscopic marsupialization fulguration and gelatin resorcinol formaldehyde glue obliteration. J Urol. 1998;160(2):352–5. https://doi.org/10.1016/s0022-5347(01)62893-3.
18. Gupta M, Lee MW. Treatment of stones associated with complex or anomalous renal anatomy. Urol Clin N Am. 2007;34(3):431–41. https://doi.org/10.1016/j.ucl.2007.04.004.
19. Yohannes P, Smith AD. The endourological management of complications associated with horseshoe kidney. J Urol. 2002;168(1):5–8. https://doi.org/10.1016/s0022-5347(05)64819-7.
20. Molimard B, Al-Qahtani S, Traxer O. Flexible ureterorenoscopy with holmium laser in horseshoe kidneys. Urology. 2010;76(6):1334–7. https://doi.org/10.1016/j.urology.2010.02.072.
21. Raj GV, Auge BK, Assimos D, Preminger GM. Metabolic abnormalities associated with renal calculi in patients with horseshoe kidneys. J Endourol. 2004;18(2):157–61. https://doi.org/10.1089/089277904322959798.
22. Bingham G, Leslie SW. Pelvic kidney. Treasure Island: StatPearls; 2020.
23. Weizer AZ, Assimos DG, Preminger GM. Ureteroscopic management of renal calculi in anomalous kidneys. Urology. 2005;65(2):265–9. https://doi.org/10.1016/j.urology.2004.09.055.
24. Harraz AM, Kamal AI, Shokeir AA. Urolithiasis in renal transplant donors and recipients: an update. Int J Surg. 2016;36:693–7. https://doi.org/10.1016/j.ijsu.2016.11.032.
25. Challacombe B, Dasgupta P, Tiptaft R, Glass J, Koffman G, Goldsmith D, Khan MS. Multimodal management of urolithiasis in renal transplantation. BJU Int. 2005;96(3):385–9. https://doi.org/10.1111/j.1464-410X.2005.05636.x.
26. Hyams E, Marien T, Bruhn A, Quirouet A, Andonian S, Shah O, Matlaga B. Ureteroscopy for transplant lithiasis. J Endourol. 2012;26(7):819–22. https://doi.org/10.1089/end.2011.0495.
27. Del Pizzo JJ, Jacobs SC, Sklar GN. Ureteroscopic evaluation in renal transplant recipients. J Endourol. 1998;12(2):135–8. https://doi.org/10.1089/end.1998.12.135.
28. Sevinc C, Balaban M, Ozkaptan O, Karadeniz T. Flexible ureterorenoscopy and laser lithotripsy for the treatment of allograft kidney lithiasis. Transplant Proc. 2015;47(6):1766–71. https://doi.org/10.1016/j.transproceed.2015.06.020.
29. Reeves T, Agarwal V, Somani BK. Donor and post-transplant ureteroscopy for stone disease in patients with renal transplant: evidence from a systematic review. Curr Opin Urol. 2019;29(5):548–55. https://doi.org/10.1097/MOU.0000000000000618.
30. Mosayyebi A, Manes C, Carugo D, Somani BK. Advances in ureteral stent design and materials. Curr Urol Rep. 2018;19(5):1–9. https://doi.org/10.1007/s11934-018-0779-y.
31. Bouzidi H, Traxer O, Doré B, Amiel J, Hadjadj H, Conort P, Daudon M. Caractéristiques des incrusta-

tions des endoprothèses urétérales chez les patients lithiasiques. Prog Urol. 2008;18(4):230–7. https://doi.org/10.1016/j.purol.2008.02.004.
32. Rouprêt M, Daudon M, Hupertan V, Gattegno B, Thibault P, Traxer O. Can ureteral stent encrustation analysis predict urinary stone composition? Urology. 2005;66(2):246–51. https://doi.org/10.1016/j.urology.2005.03.054.
33. Acosta-Miranda AM, Milner J, Turk TMT. The FECal double-J: a simplified approach in the management of encrusted and retained ureteral stents. J Endourol. 2009;23(3):409–15. https://doi.org/10.1089/end.2008.0214.
34. Tunney M, Gorman S. Evaluation of a poly(vinyl pyrollidone)-coated biomaterial for urological use. Biomaterials. 2002;23(23):4601–8. https://doi.org/10.1016/s0142-9612(02)00206-5.
35. Thomas A, Cloutier J, Villa L, Letendre J, Ploumidis A, Traxer O. Prospective analysis of a complete retrograde ureteroscopic technique with holmium laser stent cutting for management of encrusted ureteral stents. J Endourol. 2017;31(5):476–81. https://doi.org/10.1089/end.2016.0816.
36. Ishii H, Couzins M, Aboumarzouk O, Somani BK. Outcomes of systematic review of ureteroscopy for stone disease in the obese and morbidly obese population. J Endourol. 2016;30(2):135–45. https://doi.org/10.1089/end.2015.0547.
37. Stevens J, Cai J, Pamuk W, J. L. The effect of age on the association between body-mass index and mortality. N Engl J Med. 1998;338(1):1–7. https://doi.org/10.1056/nejm199801013380101.
38. Duffey BG, Pedro RN, Monga M. Lithogenic risk factors in the morbidly obese population. J Urol. 2008;179(4):1401–6. https://doi.org/10.1016/j.juro.2007.11.072.
39. Spatola L, Ferraro PM, Gambaro G, Badalamenti S, Dauriz M. Metabolic syndrome and uric acid nephrolithiasis: insulin resistance in focus. Metabolism. 2018;83:225–33. https://doi.org/10.1016/j.metabol.2018.02.008.
40. Juan HC, Lin HY, Juan YS. Abdominal fat distribution on computed tomography predicts ureteric calculus fragmentation by shock wave lithotripsy. Eur Radiol. 2012;22(8):1624–30. https://doi.org/10.1007/s00330-012-2413-6.
41. Cloutier J, Villa L, Traxer O, Daudon M. Kidney stone analysis: "Give me your stone, I will tell you who you are!". World J Urol. 2015;33(2):157–69. https://doi.org/10.1007/s00345-014-1444-9.
42. Calvert RC, Burgess NA. Urolithiasis and obesity: metabolic and technical considerations. Curr Opin Urol. 2005;15(2):113–7. https://doi.org/10.1097/01.mou.0000160626.36236.22.
43. Mancini JG, Raymundo EM, Ferrandino MN. Factors affecting patient radiation exposure during percutaneous nephrolithotomy. J Urol. 2010;184(6):2373–7. https://doi.org/10.1016/j.juro.2010.08.033.
44. Chew BH, Zavaglia B, Miller NL. A multicenter comparison of the safety and effectiveness of ureteroscopic laser lithotripsy in obese and normal weight patients. J Endourol. 2013;27(6):710–4. https://doi.org/10.1089/end.2012.0605.
45. Andreoni C, Afane J, Olweny E, Clayman RV. Flexible ureteroscopic lithotripsy: first-line therapy for proximal ureteral and renal calculi in the morbidly obese and superobese patient. J Endourol. 2001;15(5):493–8. https://doi.org/10.1089/089277901750299285.
46. Davis NF, Burke JP, McDermott T, Flynn R, Manecksha RP, Thornhill JA. Bricker versus Wallace anastomosis: a meta-analysis of ureteroenteric stricture rates after ileal conduit urinary diversion. Can Urol Assoc J. 2015;9(5–6):284. https://doi.org/10.5489/cuaj.2692.
47. Okhunov Z, Duty B, Smith AD, Okeke Z. Management of urolithiasis in patients after urinary diversions. BJU Int. 2011;108(3):330–6. https://doi.org/10.1111/j.1464-410x.2011.10194.x.
48. Ramachandra MN, Somani BK. Challenges of retrograde ureteroscopy in patients with urinary diversion: outcomes and lessons learnt from a systematic review of literature. Urol Int. 2018;101(3):249–55. https://doi.org/10.1159/000488325.
49. Nelson CP, Wolf JS, Montie JE, Faerber GJ. Retrograde ureteroscopy in patients with orthotopic ileal neobladder urinary diversion. J Urol. 2003;170(1):107–10. https://doi.org/10.1097/01.ju.0000070962.91546.bd.
50. Doizi S, Traxer O. Flexible ureteroscopy: technique, tips and tricks. Urolithiasis. 2017;46(1):47–58. https://doi.org/10.1007/s00240-017-1030-x.
51. Hyams ES, Winer AG, Shah O. Retrograde ureteral and renal access in patients with urinary diversion. Urology. 2009;74(1):47–50. https://doi.org/10.1016/j.urology.2009.02.050.
52. Ordon M, Dirk J, Slater J, Kroft J, Dixon S, Welk B. Incidence, treatment and implications of kidney stones during pregnancy: a matched population-based cohort study. J Endourol. 2019;34(2):215–21. https://doi.org/10.1089/end.2019.0557.
53. Swartz MA, Lydon-Rochelle MT, Porter MP. Admission for nephrolithiasis in pregnancy and risk of adverse birth outcomes. Obstet Gynecol. 2007;109(5):1099–104. https://doi.org/10.1097/01.AOG.0000259941.90919.c0.
54. Ross AE, Handa S, Lingeman JE, Matlaga BR. Kidney stones during pregnancy: an investigation into stone composition. Urol Res. 2008;36(2):99–102. https://doi.org/10.1007/s00240-008-0138-4.
55. Coe FL, Parks JH, Lindheimer MD. Nephrolithiasis during pregnancy. N Engl J Med. 1978;298(6):324–6. https://doi.org/10.1056/nejm197802092980608.
56. Maikranz P, Lindheimer M, Coe F. 8 Nephrolithiasis in pregnancy. Baillieres Clin Obstet Gynaecol. 1994;8(2):375–86. https://doi.org/10.1016/s0950-3552(05)80326-8.
57. Kroovant RL. Stones in pregnancy. In: Coe FLFM, Pak CYC, Parks JH, Preminger GM, editors. Kidney stones: medical and surgical management. Philadelphia: Lippincott-Raven; 1996. p. 1059–64.

58. White J, Ory J, Lantz Powers AG, Ordon M, Kroft J, Cox A. Urological issues in pregnancy: a review for urologists. Can Urol Assoc J. 2020;14(10):352. https://doi.org/10.5489/cuaj.6526.
59. Moş C, Holt G, Hălbac M. The sensitivity of transabdominal ultrasound in the diagnosis of ureterolithiasis. Med Ultrason. 2010;12(3):188–97.
60. Shokeir AA, Mahran MR, Abdulmaaboud M. Renal colic in pregnant women: role of renal resistive index. Urology. 2000;55(3):344–7. https://doi.org/10.1016/s0090-4295(99)00475-6.
61. Fulgham PF, Assimos DG, Pearle MS, Preminger GM. Clinical effectiveness protocols for imaging in the management of ureteral calculous disease: AUA technology assessment. J Urol. 2013;189(4):1203–13. https://doi.org/10.1016/j.juro.2012.10.031.
62. Committee Opinion No. 723. Committee Opinion No. 723: Guidelines for diagnostic imaging during pregnancy and lactation. Obstet Gynecol. 2017;130(4):e210–6. https://doi.org/10.1097/aog.0000000000002355.
63. Pearce MS, Salotti JA, Berrington de González A. Radiation exposure from CT scans in childhood and subsequent risk of leukaemia and brain tumours: a retrospective cohort study. Lancet. 2012;380(9840):499–505. https://doi.org/10.1016/s0140-6736(12)60815-0.
64. White WM, Zite NB, Gash J, Waters WB, Thompson W, Klein FA. Low-dose computed tomography for the evaluation of flank pain in the pregnant population. J Endourol. 2007;21(11):1255–60. https://doi.org/10.1089/end.2007.0017.
65. Parulkar BG, Hopkins TB, Wollin MR, Howard PJ, Lal A. Renal colic during pregnancy: a CASE for conservative treatment. J Urol. 1998;159(2):365–8. https://doi.org/10.1016/s0022-5347(01)63918-1.
66. Stothers L, Lee LM. Renal colic in pregnancy. J Urol. 1992;148(5):1383–7. https://doi.org/10.1016/s0022-5347(17)36917-3.
67. Burgess KL, Gettman MT, Rangel LJ, Krambeck AE. Diagnosis of urolithiasis and rate of spontaneous passage during pregnancy. J Urol. 2011;186(6):2280–4. https://doi.org/10.1016/j.juro.2011.07.103.
68. American College of Obstetricians and Gynecologists. Nonobstetric surgery during pregnancy. ACOG Committee Opinion No. 775. Obstet Gynecol. 2019;133:e285–6.
69. White WM, Johnson EB, Zite NB, Beddies J, Krambeck AE, Hyams E, Marien T, Shah O, Matlaga B, Pais VM Jr. Predictive value of current imaging modalities for the detection of urolithiasis during pregnancy: a multicenter, longitudinal study. J Urol. 2013;189(3):931–4. https://doi.org/10.1016/j.juro.2012.09.076.
70. Tawfiek ER. Ureteroscopy during pregnancy with follow-the-wire technique. Afr J Urol. 2009;15(4):245–9. https://doi.org/10.1007/s12301-009-0044-1.
71. Watterson JD, Girvan AR, Beiko DT, et al. Ureteroscopy and holmium: YAG laser lithotripsy: an emerging definitive management strategy for symptomatic ureteral calculi in pregnancy. Urology. 2002;60:383–7.
72. Giusti G, Proietti S, Graziotti P. Sky is no limit for ureteroscopy: extending the indications and special circumstances. World J Urol. 2014;33(2):257–73. https://doi.org/10.1007/s00345-014-1345-y.
73. Semins MJ, Matlaga BR. Kidney stones during pregnancy. Nat Rev Urol. 2014;11(3):163–8. https://doi.org/10.1038/nrurol.2014.17.
74. Johnson EB, Krambeck AE, White WM, Hyams E, Beddies J, Marien T, Shah O, Matlaga B, Pais VM Jr. Obstetric complications of ureteroscopy during pregnancy. J Urol. 2012;188:151–4.
75. Bjazevic J, Razvi H. Stones in pregnancy and pediatrics. Asian J Urol. 2018;5(4):223–34. https://doi.org/10.1016/j.ajur.2018.05.006.
76. Laing KA, Lam TBL, McClinton S, Cohen NP, Traxer O, Somani BK. Outcomes of ureteroscopy for stone disease in pregnancy: results from a systematic review of the literature. Urol Int. 2012;89(4):380–6. https://doi.org/10.1159/000343732.
77. Ishii H, Aboumarzouk OM, Somani BK. Current status of ureteroscopy for stone disease in pregnancy. Urolithiasis. 2013;42(1):1–7. https://doi.org/10.1007/s00240-013-0635-y.
78. Duvdevani M, Sfoungaristos S, Razvi H. Stones in special situations. World J Urol. 2017;35(9):1381–93. https://doi.org/10.1007/s00345-017-2011-y.

Complications of Flexible Ureteroscopy

Etienne Xavier Keller, Vincent De Coninck, B. M. Zeeshan Hameed, Olivier Traxer, and Bhaskar K. Somani

Abstract

Ureteroscopy is generally considered a minimally invasive surgery mostly associated with minor complications, but possibly leading to devastating and potentially lethal damages to the patient. Complications of ureteroscopy include fever, urinary tract infection, abscess, urosepsis, hematuria, hemorrhage, vascular lesions, fistulae, fornix rupture, post-obstructive diuresis, ureteral wall injury, perforation, avulsion and intussusception, vesicoureteral reflux and hydronephrosis, urethral injury, preterm labor, ureteral stent migration, forgotten ureteral stents, pain and renal colic, ureteral stent discomfort, hospital readmission and reintervention, as well as locked instruments from instrument malfunction or damages.

Risk factors associated with complications of ureteroscopy typically include high patient age, patient comorbidities including renal abnormalities and solitary kidney function, pregnancy, history of urinary tract infection, infectious stone disease, inadequate antibiotic coverage, high and complex stone burden, bilateral surgery, long operative time, high irrigation flow rate and pressure, use of laser, pneumatic or electrohydraulic lithotripters, ureteral dilation, forced instrument insertion and manipulation, larger instrument size, fluoroless interventions, longer stent dwelling time, postinterventional stenting, and in broader manner improper use of instruments and techniques.

The present chapter shall help urologists to prevent, recognize, and treat complications of

Etienne Xavier Keller and Vincent De Coninck contributed equally with all other contributors.

E. X. Keller
Department of Urology, University Hospital Zurich, University of Zurich, Zurich, Switzerland

V. De Coninck
Department of Urology, AZ Klina, Brasschaat, Belgium

B. M. Z. Hameed
Department of Urology, Kasturba Medical College, Manipal Academy of Higher Education, Manipal, Karnataka, India

Innovation Center, Kasturba Medical College, Manipal Academy of Higher Education, Manipal, Karnataka, India

O. Traxer
Service d'Urologie, Sorbonne Université, AP-HP, Hôpital Tenon, Paris, France

GRC n°20, Groupe de Recherche Clinique sur la Lithiase Urinaire, Sorbonne Université, Hôpital Tenon, Paris, France

B. K. Somani (✉)
Department of Urology, Kasturba Medical College, Manipal Academy of Higher Education, Manipal, Karnataka, India

Department of Urology, University Hospital Southampton NHS Trust, University of Southampton, Southampton, UK
e-mail: b.k.somani@soton.ac.uk

G. Zeng et al. (eds.), *Flexible Ureteroscopy*, https://doi.org/10.1007/978-981-19-2936-6_16

ureteroscopy. It also encourages the use of standardized classification systems for reporting of complications, which are warranted to compare results among different studies, to conduct meta-analyses, and to objectively inform health-care workers and properly counsel patients about the hazards of ureteroscopy.

Keywords

Ureteroscopy · Complications · Infection · Sepsis · Bleeding · Hemorrhage · Hematoma · Injury · Damage · Mortality

1 Introduction

Ureteroscopy is a routine urological procedure allowing for diagnosis and treatment of upper urinary tract diseases. It has been subject to a continuous development and has become the worldwide most frequent modality of interventional therapy for kidney stones [1, 2]. Ureteroscopy is considered a minimally invasive surgery, since it generally does not require disruption of anatomical boundaries. Intuitively, this may lead the unexperienced urologist to believe that complications associated with ureteroscopy are rare and of minor grade. Contrarily, improper patient management and disregard of operation techniques and recommendations may cause complications with devastating morbidity or even mortality. The present chapter offers a comprehensive overview of all complications associated with ureteroscopy, including causes, risk factors, preventive measures, and treatment modalities for each complication. By integrating the suggested recommendations in their approach, urologists will be able to undoubtedly enhance patient outcomes.

2 Classification Systems

Two classification systems are available for complications of ureteroscopy: the modified Clavien classification system (MCCS) and the modified Satava classification system (Table 1) [3, 4]. The MCCS for ureteroscopy was introduced in 2012 by Mandal et al., and stratifies perioperative complications (up to 3 months after surgery) into five grades: grade 1 and 2 are considered "minor" complications, while grade 3 and 4 are considered major complications requiring invasive intervention with possible organ dysfunction [3, 5]. Grade 5 corresponds to a lethal complication. The modified Satava classification system was introduced in 2014 by Tepeler et al., and stratifies complications into three grades: grade 1 complications have no consequences for the patient, grade 2 complications require endoscopic surgery, and grade 3 complications require open or laparoscopic surgery [4, 6]. Accordingly, the modified Satava classification system relates to the need of reinterventions, and is rather insensitive to potentially severe complications that would not require surgery.

These two classification systems are objective, reproducible, and standardized systems for quality assessment after ureteroscopy outcomes. They allow for a comparison of results among different studies, which may ultimately allow for a compelling review and meta-analysis. These systems are applicable to any type of study, even if retrospective in its nature. In the present chapter, an effort has been made to explore the applications of these systems, throughout the text, for the sake of the attentive reader.

Table 1 Comparison of classification system for complications of ureteroscopy

Modified Clavien classification system [3]		Modified Satava classification system [4]	
Grade I	Any deviation from the normal postoperative course. Allowed therapeutic regimens are drugs as antiemetics, antipyretics, analgesics, diuretics, electrolytes, and physiotherapy	Grade 1	Incidents without consequences
Grade II	Requiring pharmacological treatment with drugs other than such allowed for grade I complications Blood transfusions and total parenteral nutrition are also included	Grade 2	Incidents treated with endoscopic surgery
Grade III	Requiring surgical, endoscopic, or radiological intervention	Grade 2a	Incidents treated intraoperatively with endoscopic surgery
Grade IIIa	Intervention not under general anesthesia	Grade 2b	Incidents requiring endoscopic retreatment
Grade IIIb	Intervention under general anesthesia	Grade 3	Incidents requiring open or laparoscopic surgery
Grade IV	Life-threatening complication requiring IC/ICU management		
Grade IVa	Single-organ dysfunction		
Grade IVb	Multiorgan dysfunction		
Grade V	Death of a patient		

3 Overall Risk Factors Related to Complications from Ureteroscopy

Several larger studies have evaluated predictors of complications from ureteroscopy in a broader manner. Based on a Japanese inpatient administrative claims database, Sugihara et al. evaluated 12,372 patients undergoing ureteroscopic lithotripsy, of which a subset of 296 patients with severe complications (MCCS grade ≥ IV) (2.4%) was analyzed. On multivariable analysis, female gender, higher age (≥80 years old), higher Charlson Comorbidity Index (≥2), general anesthesia (compared to spinal or epidural), longer operative duration (≥90 min), higher hospital volume (≥39 ureteroscopies per year), and emergency admission (compared to elective) were significant predictors of severe complications [7]. In a similar analysis based 11,885 adult patients from the CROES database, Daels et al. found higher age as well as comorbidities such as diabetes mellitus, obesity, cardiovascular disease, and use of anticoagulants as significant predictors of complications from ureteroscopy [8]. Based on a retrospective study on 1571 ureteroscopies, Bas et al. found the presence of congenital renal abnormalities (e.g., bifid pelvis, complete ureteral duplication, calyceal diverticulum, horseshoe kidney, pelvic ectopia, malrotation) as the sole significant and independent predictor of complications on multivariable analysis, despite having additionally found stone burden as a predictor on univariable analysis [9].

In a smaller-sized retrospective premillennial (1997–1999) analysis, Schuster et al. found kidney stone location (compared to ureteral stones), longer operative time, and lower surgeon expertise as predictors of complications [10]. In a prospective observational study on 120 patients, Mandal et al. found larger stones (>10 mm), midureteral stones (versus distal ureteral stones), impacted stones, and surgeon experience (resident versus consultant) as predictors of complications following ureteroscopy for ureteral stones [3].

3.1 Operative Time

Arguably, the causative link between operative time and complications is multifactorial. Complications may arise from prolonged exposition to risk factors during surgery (e.g., high intrarenal pressure), but longer operative time may inversely arise from an early complication of surgery (e.g., ureteral perforation during instrument insertion).

Altogether, operative time is the most commonly reported risk factor associated with complications from ureteroscopy [3, 9–16]. In a recent retrospective study on 736 patients, Whitehurst et al. found higher stone burden, use of UAS, and postoperative ureteral stenting to be associated with longer operative time [14]. In that study, longer operative time was also associated with higher complications grade (MCCS grade ≥ III), infectious complications, lower stone-free rate, and lower day-case procedures rate. A recent systematic review concluded that stone complexity, patient risk factors, surgeon experience, bilateral surgery, and instrumentation are strong predictors of longer operative time and associated complications [17]. Of interest, in the study by Sugihara et al. the risk of complications was similarly higher for interventions ranging 60–89 min and 90–119 min operative time (OR 1.46 and 1.58, respectively), compared to interventions <60 min. This risk was markedly higher starting from 120 min operative time (OR 2.24 for 120–149 min) [7]. Accordingly, a maximal operative time of 90–120 min seems to be a generally accepted recommendation for ureteroscopy, beyond which a staged procedure or a different approach should be considered [17].

4 Infectious Complications

4.1 Fever and Urinary Tract Infection

Fever after ureteroscopy (MCCS grade I, Satava grade 1) has been reported with an incidence varying from 0.2 to 15% [3, 9, 11, 16, 18–29]. Interestingly, urinary tract infection (UTI) following ureteroscopy (MCCS grade II, Satava grade 1) has also been reported with an incidence varying from 0.2 to 15% [3, 9–11, 21–28, 30–32]. This overlap is not surprising, since fever has been frequently used as a surrogate sign of UTI in many publications. Notably, fever was still in use as a sign of severe urinary tract infection, namely, urosepsis, until recently [33].

Risk factors for fever and UTI include female gender, high ASA score, preoperative bacteriuria, hydronephrosis, presence of urinary stents, high stone burden, longer operative time, proximal ureteral stones, struvite stones, cardiovascular disease and Crohn's disease [15, 16, 31, 34].

4.2 Urosepsis

Urosepsis is one of the most severe complications of ureteroscopy (MCCS grade IVa–IVb, Satava grade 1–3). Urosepsis incidence ranges between 0.1 and 4.3% [3, 9, 10, 16, 18, 21, 24, 25, 27–29, 35–38].

Urosepsis and SIRS are typically caused by the activity of UTI pathogens within the urinary system, resulting in a systemic release of inflammatory cytokines by the immune system, inducing a cascade of events typically leading to fever, tachycardia, tachypnea, white blood cell release, and eventual life-threatening organ dysfunctions. The most common pathogens include *Escherichia coli*, Proteus, Pseudomonas species, Serratia, and group B Streptococci, as well as Candida species [39–42].

Risk factors include recent UTI, infectious stones, large stone burden, high irrigation flow rate, high irrigation pressure, prolonged stent dwelling time, chronic drains, immunocompromised status, elderly age, female gender, and anatomic abnormalities of the collecting system [16, 38, 39, 43–46]. In a contemporary prospective observational study based on 463 patients undergoing flexible ureteroscopy, Ozgor et al. paradoxically found lower patient age as an independent and significant predictor for infectious complications, next to longer operation time and renal abnormalities [15]. The authors could not find any explanation to this result.

Diagnosis relies on the recognition of symptoms associated with sepsis. Until recently, sepsis was defined as the presence of at least two out of four systemic inflammatory response syndrome (SIRS) criteria, with a confirmed or suspected infection [47, 48] (Table 2). In 2016, an updated

Table 2 Comparison of sepsis criteria (adapted with permission from Table 5.3 of Keller E.X. et al. (2022) Stones. In: Hubosky S.G., Grasso III M., Traxer O., Bagley D.H. (eds) Advanced Ureteroscopy. Springer, Cham. https://doi.org/10.1007/978-3-030-82351-1_5)

	Systemic inflammatory response syndrome (SIRS)	Sequential organ failure assessment (SOFA)	Quick sequential organ failure assessment (qSOFA)
Score range	0–4 criteria	0–24 points (0–4 points per variable)	0–3 points (1 point per variable)
Definitions	SIRS: Two or more criteria Sepsis: + confirmed or suspected infection Severe sepsis: + organ failure	Sepsis: Life-threatening organ dysfunction in response to infection Organ dysfunction: Acute change in total SOFA score ≥2 points consequent to infection	Bedside criteria to identify adult patients with suspected infection who are likely to have poor outcomes if ≥2 points
Vital parameters	Temperature >38 °C or <36 °C	Glasgow Coma Scale	Altered mentation
	Heart rate >90/min	Mean arterial pressure, +/− concomitant administration of vasopressors	Systolic blood pressure ≤ 100 mmHg
	Respiratory rate >20/min	Urine output/24 h	Respiratory rate ≥22/min
Laboratory tests	$PaCO_2$ <32 mmHg	PaO_2/FiO_2 ratio	
	White blood cell count >12,000/mm^3, <4000/mm^3 or >10% immature band forms	Platelet count	
		Bilirubin	
		Serum creatinine	
References	Bone et al. [47]	Singer et al. [33]	Singer et al. [33]

definition of sepsis has been proposed in a consensus article, abandoning the use of SIRS criteria [33]. This new proposal presupposes the presence of a life-threatening organ dysfunction and follows a Sequential Organ Failure Assessment (SOFA) scoring. This updated definition was shown to have a superior predictive validity over SIRS criteria for mortality [49]. A major limitation to the SOFA scoring is the complexity of parameter retrieval, which may lead to delayed identification of sepsis. Therefore, a "quick SOFA" scoring (qSOFA) has been proposed. Other biomarkers of systemic response to infection such as procalcitonin or bone morphogenetic protein endothelial cell precursor-derived regulator (BMPER) are currently been explored as additional criteria to help in management of urosepsis. Procalcitonin accurately predicts the presence of bacteremia and bacterial load and may be a helpful biomarker to monitor microbial activity [50]. The combination of procalcitonin with BMPER has recently been shown to reach an area under the curve of 0.90 for the prediction of urosepsis [46].

In the setting of urolithiasis-associated sepsis, the SOFA score has been shown to achieve the best performance for predicting in-hospital mortality or prolonged intensive care unit (ICU) stay, followed by SIRS criteria, and lastly by the qSOFA score (adjusted area under the receiver operating characteristic curve 0.94, 0.72, and 0.71, respectively) [51].

4.3 Perirenal Abscess

Perirenal abscess after ureteroscopy (MCCS grade II–IV, Satava grade 1–3) has been reported in one study with an incidence of 0.06% [9]. Perirenal abscess may be related to urinoma and subcapsular, perirenal or retroperitoneal hematoma, since the common underlying pathophysiological mechanism seems to be associated with high intrarenal pressure and iatrogenic trauma of the pelvicalyceal system. Perirenal abscess typically becomes symptomatic after 7–14 days after ureteroscopy. Patients may present with lumbar pain, fever or urosepsis. Diagnosis is made by sonography, computed tomography or magnetic resonance imaging.

4.4 Prevention of Infectious Complications

Preoperative urine culture and antibiotic treatment in case of significant bacterial growth is a commonly recognized recommendation. Intraoperative sight of purulent urine is an alarming sign and shall mostly impel surgeons to interrupt the intervention [52]. In a recent prospective observational study by Pietropaolo et al. this strategy could prevent further complications in 96% of all analyzed 76 patients undergoing ureteroscopy after prior sepsis and emergency drainage due to ureteric stones [53]. These results are in line with prior results from a smaller retrospective study considering adequate antibiotic coverage, with infectious complications similar between patients with or without previous drainage of obstructive pyelonephritis [54]. Contrarily, a matched-pair comparison of 69 patients with or without prior urosepsis found a higher overall complication rate (20% vs. 7%), longer hospital length of stay (2.5 days vs. 0.6 days), and longer courses of postoperative antibiotics (1.7 days vs. 0.4 days) following intervention in favor of patients with prior urosepsis [55]. However, in that study, severe complications such as urosepsis following ureteroscopy were similar between both groups (1.4% in both groups).

In the absence of significant preoperative bacterial growth, an antibiotic prophylaxis may decrease the incidence of pyuria after ureteroscopy, while it does not significantly reduce the rate of postoperative fever and UTI [32, 34, 56–58]. Accordingly, both the EAU and AUA guidelines recommend a single preoperative dose of prophylactic antibiotics [59, 60]. Prolonged postoperative antibiotic therapy does not seem to decrease infectious complications. Routine urinary stone culture is not generally recommended, but may be more informative than preoperative urine culture in cases with suspected infection [61].

There is compelling evidence in literature supporting the association of high intrarenal pressure with infectious complications (see above). Whether reduced intrarenal pressure during ureteroscopy may prevent fever and infectious complications is a topic of ongoing debate. Particularly, the routine use of an ureteral access sheath (UAS) to decrease intrarenal pressure is a debatable strategy [62]. A prospective analysis from the Clinical Research Office of the Endourological Society (CROES) favors the use of UAS to prevent fever an infectious complication. In that study, a significantly higher risk of urosepsis was found in the absence of a UAS (0.94% without UAS, versus 0.47% with UAS, respectively) [63]. These data must be interpreted with caution, since the use of a UAS depended on surgeon's preference in that study, therefore potentially having led to a selection bias.

Reusable ureteroscopes have been linked to nosocomial infection caused by instrument contamination [64]. More studies are necessary to evaluate the possible influence of reusable versus disposable instruments and ureteroscopes on infectious complications from ureteroscopy [65].

4.5 Treatment of Infectious Complications

Fever may be treated conservatively with antipyretics, provided that the absence of signs indicating UTI or urosepsis. Depending on the clinical course, an additional antibiotic therapy may be indicated. Optimally, a fully microbial sampling (urinary culture and blood culture) shall be performed before starting antibiotic therapy.

Treatment of urosepsis consists of early recognition (SIRS criteria and/or SOFA score), immediate resuscitation if needed, diagnostic workup to identify the source of infection, appropriate drainage of the urinary tract and culture-based antibiotic therapy.

Perirenal abscess mostly can be treated conservatively with prolonged antibiotic therapy. Depending on the clinical presentation and clinical course, abscess and urinary drainage may be indicated [9]. Seldom, patients must be treated with a nephrectomy [66].

In rare cases, infectious complication may have a lethal course, especially in cases of delayed initiation of supportive care, antibiotic therapy and appropriate drainage or decompression of the urinary tract [52, 67, 68].

5 Hematologic and Vascular Complications

5.1 Bleeding and Hematuria

Transient hematuria resolving spontaneously within 48 h (MCCS grade I, Satava grade 1) shall be differentiated from persistent hematuria lasting more than 48 h (MCCS grade I–IV, Satava 1–3) [3]. Transient hematuria may occur in 0.2% up to 19.9% patients after ureteroscopy, while persistent hematuria is being reported with an incidence of only 0.1–5.7% [3, 9, 11, 21, 22, 24–28, 30, 35, 37, 69, 70]. Urinary clot retention has a reported incidence up to 1.6% [3, 20, 28].

Causes of bleeding and hematuria associated with ureteroscopy are iatrogenic organ injury from excessive irrigation pressure, mechanical stress of tissues, or by ancillary devices such as laser ultrasonic or electrohydraulic lithotripters, as well as tissue vaporization. Active aspiration over the working channel of the ureteroscope is another less well-known cause of bleeding, either due to traumatic tissue damages at the tip of the ureteroscope, or because of intrarenal pressure drop with consequence mucosal tissue bleeding. Organ injuries are discussed later in this book chapter.

Anticoagulants, antiplatelet drugs and bleeding diatheses have been reported as risk factors associated with bleeding complications in a recent meta-analysis [71]. In a study by Westerman et al. continuation or bridging of anticoagulants also increased the risk of perioperative bleeding, whereas continuous antiplatelet therapy was not associated with bleeding complications [72, 73].

5.2 Prevention of Bleeding Complications

Iatrogenic trauma may be prevented by gentle usage of appropriate instruments. Miniaturized, smaller size ureteroscopes and instruments have been associated with lower postoperative hematuria rate [74]. Since intrarenal pressure cannot currently be adequately monitored by any ureteroscope or dedicated ancillary device to date, it may be advisable to limit irrigation pressure to levels that would prevent organ injuries. It is conceivable that pressure-sensor may be integrated to ureteroscopes in near future [75]. For laser vaporization purposes such as endoscopic management of upper tract urothelial carcinoma, bleeding may be prevented by using a "noncontact technique" with low pulse energy, low pulse frequency and long pulse duration when using Holmium:YAG, or alternatively by using a continuously emitting laser such as the Thulium:YAG laser [76–82]. Recently, the Thulium fiber laser has emerged as a promising source of energy with low bleeding proprieties [83–87].

Concerning anticoagulants, antiplatelet drugs and bleeding diatheses, a patient-centered approach should be taken to limit the risks of bleeding complications [71].

5.3 Treatment of Bleeding Complications

Mucosal bleeding usually subsides spontaneously within a few minutes of low-pressure irrigation with the ureteroscope. In case of prolonged mucosal bleeding causing impaired visibility, the intervention shall be postponed and the placement of a ureteral stent is recommended to ensure proper urinary drainage.

Blood transfusion has been reported in up to 0.7% of patients after ureteroscopy [3, 7, 21, 25]. Angiographic techniques and emergency open surgery for bleeding complications are exceptionally necessary to treat live-threatening bleeding complications [27]. The later interventions may typically occur in face of distinct clinical situations, as discussed hereafter.

5.3.1 Subcapsular, Perirenal and Retroperitoneal Hematoma Formation

Subcapsular, perirenal, and retroperitoneal hematoma (MCCS grade I–IV, Satava grade 1–3) may occur with an incidence up to 2.2% [3, 9, 23, 28, 35, 52, 88–96]. Risk factors include larger stones, longer operation time, higher irrigation system pressure, higher grade of ipsilateral hydronephrosis, lower body mass index, thinner kidney cortex thickness, and a history of chronic kidney disease [88, 97]. Additionally, insufficiently treated UTI has been proposed as a risk factor for renal hematoma, due to tissue fragility caused by neutrophil infiltration of renal parenchyma [94, 97]. Iatrogenic organ perforation during ureteral stent placement has also been reported as a cause of hematoma and may be associated with the use of traumatic guidewires [98, 99]. Patients may present with lumbar pain, macroscopic hematuria, fever, or hypovolemic shock. Diagnosis is usually made by angiographic computed tomography.

Treatment mostly relies on conservative management, but blood transfusion, drainage, selective embolization or repair of the ruptured pelvicalyceal system may be necessary based on individual case appreciation. Nephrectomy is rarely necessary, but may present as a last-instance therapy for life-threatening bleeding complications [9, 35, 52].

5.3.2 Endoureterotomy or Endopyelotomy

Endoureterotomy or endopyelotomy for treatment of ureteral strictures or ureteropelvic junction stenosis are particularly prone to bleeding complications (MCCS grade I–IV, Satava grade 1–3). Blood transfusion rates up to 10% have been reported in historical series using cold knife or electrocautery incision [100]. Nowadays, preferred incision techniques include visual laser incision or Acucise balloon dilation, with blood transfusion rates up to 8% [101, 102].

Preventive measures include consideration of anatomical boundaries to avoid injury of crossing vessels. Aberrant anatomical vessels or incisions performed at wrong locations may result in life-threatening bleeding complications [102–104]. Immediate placement of a dilated ureteral balloon may have a tamponade effect limiting the bleeding. Definitive treatment mostly relies on vascular embolization, endovascular repair, or open repair.

5.3.3 Renal Pseudoaneurysm

Renal pseudoaneurysm is a rare complication (MCCS grade III–IV, Satava grade 2–3) caused by injury of a renal artery with bleeding containment within surrounding connective tissue and hematoma. Life-threatening hemorrhage may suddenly occur when arterial pressure surpasses the tamponade effect of the surrounding tissue. It has been reported after endopyelotomy, as well as after laser or electrohydraulic lithotripsy, independently of UAS use [105–111]. It may frequently remain unrecognized because of an asymptomatic course, eventually evolving to unexplained anemia, abdominal pain, fever, or hematuria. Diagnosis relies on angiographic computed tomography. Treatment consists of embolization or surgical intervention [105–111].

5.3.4 Arteriovenous Fistula

Intrarenal arteriovenous fistula (MCCS grade III–IV, Satava grade 2–3) has been reported by few authors after laser or electrohydraulic lithotripsy. Arguably, these iatrogenic fistulae are caused by damages to renal arteries and veins during lithotripsy, leading to a connection between a high-pressure artery and a low-pressure vein. Up to date, all reports in literature presented with hematuria and were treated by selective embolization [52, 112–114].

5.3.5 Ureteroiliac Fistula

Ureteroiliac fistula is rare complication (MCCS grade IV, Satava grade 3) with only two documented cases related to ureteroscopy in literature to date [115, 116]. In both cases, acute hemorrhage occurred during the intervention, namely, at dilation of a ureteral stenosis [115], as well as a consequence of unexpected patient position change while passing the ureteroscope over the iliac vessel crossing [116]. The latter case was successfully treated by emergency open vascular repair.

5.4 Deep-Vein Thrombosis

Deep-vein thrombosis (MCCS grade II–IV, Satava grade 1–3) related to ureteroscopy is exceptional [117]. Nevertheless, prolonged operative time in lithotomy position may arguably present as a risk factor. Consequently, it may be advisable to follow general international guidelines on thromboprophylaxis recommending prophylaxis with low-molecular-weight heparin or antiembolism stockings in high-risk patients until complete mobilization of the patient [118].

5.5 Cerebrovascular Accident and Transient Ischemic Attack

Cerebrovascular accident and transient ischemic attack (MCCS grade II–IV, Satava grade 1–3) have only been rarely reported in association with ureteroscopy [21, 25, 27]. It remains unsolved whether risk factors directly related to ureteroscopy are associated with these severe vascular complications. In case of stroke-like symptoms, according diagnostic and therapeutic measures should be rapidly considered to minimize the detrimental neurological effects.

6 Organ Injuries

6.1 Kidney Injury

Vascular injuries leading to bleeding complications have already been discussed above. Organ injuries with secondary organ function disorders will be detailed here.

6.1.1 Fornix Rupture

Fornix rupture (MCCS grade I–IV, Satava grade 1–3) has been attributed to high intrarenal pressure and appears as a natural pressure relief valve mechanism [119]. It typically becomes symptomatic with renal colic pain in face of obstructive uropathy [120]. Based on animal studies, fornix rupture may occur at intrarenal pressure levels ranging from 60 to 80 cmH_2O [121–123].

During ureteroscopy, fornix rupture may impair visibility because of tissue bleeding. Also, fornix rupture may cause a substantive irrigation fluid extravasation or postoperative urinoma and hematoma, which in turn may lead to infectious complications. As simple as it may appear to understand, fornix rupture may be prevented by maintaining low intrapelvic pressure during ureteroscopy [124]. This may be easily achieved by limiting irrigation inflow pressure, and accordingly avoiding devices that may cause undesirable high-pressure levels [125]. If needed, higher irrigation flow may subsequently be achieved by using a UAS [62].

6.1.2 Transient Serum Creatinine Elevation

Transient serum creatinine elevation (MCCS grade I, Satava grade 1) is frequently overserved in clinical routine after ureteroscopy, but has been seldom reported in literature. According to prospective observational studies, incidence ranges between 1.4 and 1.6% [3, 24]. Causes, risk factors and consequences of this assumingly benign complication needs to be evaluated in future studies. Other markers of acute kidney injury such as the kidney injury molecule-1 (KIM-1) may be used in conjunction with evaluations on creatinine elevation [126].

6.1.3 Post-Obstructive Diuresis

Post-obstructive diuresis (MCCS grade IV, Satava grade 1) is defined as diuresis >4 L/day following relief of a prolonged urinary obstruction. This medical condition may cause severe fluid and electrolyte disbalances [127]. Ibrahim et al. reported on an incidence of 1.4% in a series of 148 patients undergoing ureteroscopy for urolithiasis [24]. In that study, post-obstructive diuresis exclusively occurred in patients with an obstructed solitary kidney. Predictors of this potentially lethal complication include high serum creatinine, high serum bicarbonate, and urinary retention on admission. Despite the risks associated with post-obstructive diuresis, urgent drainage of the obstructed urinary path is necessary to reduce the risk of severe chronic renal failure [128].

6.2 Ureteral Injury

6.2.1 Difficult Ureteral Access

The ureter acts a helpful natural pathway for retrograde access to the kidney during ureteroscopy [36]. The inherent downside of this pathway is that the ureter also acts as a natural bottleneck to ureteroscopy. Particularly, three narrow portions of the ureter may hinder primary insertion: the ureteral orifice, the iliac vessels crossing, and the pyeloureteral junction.

Cross-sectional size of most flexible ureteroscopes is ≤9 F [75], which remarkably goes in hand with cross-sectional size of native human ureters (≤9 F in 96% of all patients, based on a CT-analysis) [129]. Nevertheless, primary insertion of a ureteroscope along the upper urinary tract is not possible in 1–37% of patients without prior dilation [130, 131]. Insertion failure is defined as the surgeon's decision to resign ureteroscope insertion due to high resistance to the retrograde progression of the ureteroscope along the urinary tract (MCCS grade I–III, Satava grade 2a–2b). A narrow ureteral orifice or intramural part of the ureter is the main cause of access failure. This can be resolved by placing a ureteral stent for 1 week allowing passive ureteral dilation. Prestenting is preferred since active ureteral dilation using a serial, coaxial, or balloon dilator have a 5% associated risk of ureteral perforation [132]. Ureteroscope and UAS insertion failures becomes negligible after prestenting, thereby decreasing the risk of severe injury by up to sevenfold [62, 133, 134]. Disadvantages of prestenting are the need for a secondary intervention (MCCS grade III, Satava grade 2b) and stent-related morbidity that result in reduced quality of life in up to 80% of patients [135]. As a last resort, minimal dilation up to the size of the ureteroscope can be performed, since performing ureteroscopy with resistance has a significant risk (22%) of ureteral stricture development [136, 137].

Predictors of successful primary ureteroscope insertion are a smaller sized instrument, previous history of ipsilateral ureteral stenting or ureteroscopy, as well as more than one-half of proximal ureteral opacification on computed tomography urography [130, 131, 134].

6.2.2 Classification of Ureteral Wall Injuries

Considering the observation of frequently occurring ureteral wall injuries associated with UAS use, Traxer et al. proposed an endoscopic classification of ureteral wall injuries in 2013 (Table 3)

Table 3 Comparison of endoscopic classification of ureteral wall injury

Traxer classification [133]		Post-ureteroscopic lesion scale (PULS) [138]	
Grade 0 (low)	No lesion, only mucosal petechiae	Grade 0	No lesion
Grade 1 (low)	Ureteral mucosal erosion without smooth muscle injury	Grade 1	Superficial mucosal lesion and/or significant mucosal edema/hematoma
Grade 2 (high)	Ureteral wall injury, including mucosa and smooth muscle, with adventitial preservation (periureteral fat not seen)	Grade 2	Submucosal lesion
Grade 3 (high)	Ureteral wall injury, including mucosa and smooth muscle, with adventitial perforation (periureteral fat seen)	Grade 3	Perforation with less than 50% (partial) transection
Grade 4	Total ureteral avulsion	Grade 4	More than 50% but less than 100% (partial) transection
		Grade 5	Complete transection

[133]. In the same year, Schoentaler et al. proposed a similar grading system, namely, the post-ureteroscopic lesion scale (PULS) (Table 3) [138].

6.2.3 Ureteral Wall Injuries

Incidences of mucosal erosions and false passages (MCCS grade I–III, Satava grade 1–2) during ureteroscopy ranges from 0.13 to 46.5% [11, 22, 24, 27, 28, 30, 35, 37, 69, 70, 133, 139–141]. Incidence of ureteral perforations (MCCS grade III, Satava grade 2) ranges from 0.3 to 7.4% [3, 9–11, 21, 22, 24, 25, 30, 35, 37, 69, 70, 139, 142]. The associated fluid extravasation has an incidence of up to 4% [11, 26, 30].

Traxer et al. reported ureteral injuries in up to 46.5% patients undergoing ureteroscopy with a 12/14 F UAS [133]. In that study, severe ureteral injury involving the smooth muscle layers was noticed in 13.3% of cases. In another study on 148 prestented patients undergoing ureteroscopy with 14/16 F UAS, superficial ureteral mucosa lesions were found in 39.9% of patients, deeper mucosal ureteral lesions in 17.6% and circumferential perforation in 4.7% [140]. A later study on 101 patients with no prestenting and 9.5/11.5 F or 12/14 F UAS, PULS grade 1 and 2 lesions were found in 38.6% and 2.9% of the patients, respectively [141]. In that study, injuries were exclusively found in the proximal or distal ureter. The distal ureter is possibly more prone to false passage, because of its oblique insertion in the bladder causing a medioposterior ureteral wall stress when instruments and ancillary devices are inserted retrogradely. This hypothesis has yet to be confirmed [25].

Causes of ureteral mucosa erosion, false passage and perforation are usually insertion of a guidewire, ureteral access sheath or ureteroscope, as well as lithotripsy, stone extraction, and ureteral dilation. Risk factors include larger ureteroscopes and UAS, absence of prestenting, male gender, increasing age, and longer operative time [10, 74, 143]. Smaller sized UAS were found to be associated with lower rate of severe ureteral lesions, with no UAS having the lowest rate of ureteral lesions [143]. In a recent prospective analysis by Monga et al., male gender, large stone burden, longer time of sheath insertion, and a more difficult subjective rating for sheath placement were associated with higher grade ureteral wall injuries [144].

Preventive measures include consideration of all the abovementioned causes and risk factors. Instruments shall always be adapted to the patient's anatomy, and not vice versa. In case of resistance, the intervention shall be postponed, as discussed above. Other less well explored preventive measures are associated to technique of ureteroscopy, which presupposes trivial rules such that ancillary devices shall always be manipulated with great care under direct vision. Impacted stones within the ureter should always be targeted in their center, since energy application to their periphery entails a high risk of accidental damages to the ureteral wall.

Of interest, preoperative Tamsulosin has been found to lower the risk of ureteral wall injuries associated with ureteroscopy [145]. A recent meta-analysis on this subject confirmed a significantly lower need for ureteral dilation, higher stone-free status, shorter operative time, and shorter hospital stay in favor of the Tamsulosin treatment group [146].

Treatment is dictated by the severity of ureteral wall injuries. Mucosal erosion may trigger the need for postoperative stenting, without otherwise compromising the operative course. In case of more severe ureteral lesions with massive fluid extravasation, consequent urinary drainage shall be warranted, eventually leading to percutaneous nephrostomy tube placement [11, 24, 35, 69].

6.2.4 Extraureteral Stone Migration

Ureteral wall injury may be further complicated by submucosal or extraureteral stone migration (MCCS grade I–III, Satava grade 2). Incidence reported in a large case series (n = 8150) was 0.15%, when using a semirigid ureteroscopies for ureteral stones [69]. Although debatable, submucosal fragments shall be retrieved in order to prevent chronic inflammation and subsequent stricture formation. Contrarily, extraureteral stones may be left untreated, provided that signs for infectious stones are excluded.

6.2.5 Ureteral Avulsion

Ureteral avulsion is relatively rare, devastating complication of ureteroscopy (MCCS grade IIIb, Satava grade 3) occurring with an incidence of 0.04–0.9% [3, 21, 22, 25, 28, 35, 37, 69, 70, 139, 147, 148]. Due to its thinner muscular wall, the proximal ureter is most prone to ureteral avulsion [25].

Most reported ureteral avulsions are the result of excessive longitudinal stress forces on the ureter during urinary stone retrieval [3, 21, 22, 25, 28, 35, 37, 69, 70, 139]. This may typically occur when a stone is entrapped within a basket and too large to be passed through the ureteral lumen. Another risk factor is endopyelotomy, where the incised and fragilized ureteropelvic junction becomes particularly vulnerable and prone to ureteral avulsion [100]. Ureteral avulsion has also been associated to the use of UAS, although it remains unclear whether UAS was a direct cause of avulsion in that study [149].

Another, possibly less well-known and devastating mechanism of ureteral injury is the "scabbard" ureteral avulsion. It involves a proximal and distal discontinuity of the ureter with a resultant scabbard, since the ureter is withdrawn like a sheath on the ureteroscope [149–151]. The tapered design of a semirigid ureteroscopes has been reported as a risk factor, since the larger proximal shaft may become wedged in the intramural distal ureter [151]. Ureteral avulsion may also occur in any unusual, unexpected situation such as instrument failure or breakage, which will be discussed later in the according paragraph.

Ureteral avulsion is best prevented by avoiding forced extraction of large stones or stone fragments. Unfortunately, no tensile force sensors are available in ureteroscopes to date. Hence, signs of ureteral wall damage should always be observed under direct visual control during ureteroscope retrieval. Adequate choice of baskets may also prevent unexpected entrapment of stones and fragments. Particularly, tipless baskets at least 4 mm larger than the targeted stone may disengage more easily when opened and gently pushed retrogradely next to the entrapped stone [152]. Entrapped stones are best managed by insertion of a laser fiber parallelly to the basket in the working channel, in order to perform in situ laser lithotripsy with subsequent stone fragment size reduction. Another option is to cut the wires of the basket or to dismantle the handle of the basket.

Treatment of ureteral avulsion involves either immediate or postponed repair. The latter option may be beneficial in order to discuss various ureteral reconstruction methods with the patient. In such cases, immediate nephrostomy tube insertion is recommended until postponed repair. Ureteral reconstruction methods include ureteral reimplantation to the bladder (with a psoas hitch or a Boari flap), ureteroureterostomy, transureteroureterostomy, ureterocalicostomy, ileal interposition graft, and autotransplantation [151, 153].

6.2.6 Ureteral Intussusception

Ureteral intussusception (MCCS grade IIIb, Satava grade 3) may occur spontaneously due to the presence of a ureteral tumor or stone, or may be secondary to iatrogenic injury [154]. Iatrogenic injury is typically associated to percutaneous endopyelotomy and ureteral stent exchange. Only one case of ureteral intussusception has been directly related to ureteroscopy in literature to date [155].

6.2.7 Vesicoureteral Reflux

Transitory vesicoureteral reflux (MCCS grade I, Satava grade 1) has a low incidence of 0.1% after ureteroscopy [35]. Comparatively, reflux may occur in 10–20% of patients after dilatation of the ureterovesical junction [156, 157]. Vesicoureteral reflux after ureteroscopy mostly resolves without any additional therapy. Persistent vesicoureteral reflux may be treated conservatively, or by submucosal collagen injection, depending on the clinical situation [35, 156].

6.2.8 Ureteral Stricture

Historical case series using older 11.5 F rigid ureteroscopes or 13 F flexible ureteroscopes reported about ureteral stricture (MCCS grade IIIb, Satava grade 2–3) rates up to 5% [142]. More recent reports revealed a decreasing risk of ureteral stricture with improving instruments and techniques, such that current incidence ranges between 0.4 and 3%, mostly depending on length of follow-up [9, 19, 21, 22, 25, 28, 35, 139, 158]. Risk factors are not well defined, but multiple causes have been attributed to ureteral stricture formation after ureteroscopy: mechanical trauma (perforation), thermal injury (laser energy), chronic inflammation (stones or foreign bodies), chronic infection (tuberculosis and schistosomiasis), as well as ischemic injuries (impacted stones) [159–161]. According to an evaluation on 71 patients undergoing ureteroscopy with a UAS, only patient (1.4%) was found to have a subsequent ureteral stricture (at the ureteropelvic junction) after a mean follow-up of 11 months [162]. A more recent analysis focusing on 56 patients with high-grade ureteral lesions after ureteroscopy with a UAS, stricture rate was 1.8% at a median 30 months follow-up [163].

Flank pain, kidney function impairment, and particularly persisting hydronephrosis are the most frequently reported signs indicating ureteral stricture. Incidence of persisting hydronephrosis ranges from 15.1 to 32.1%, according to studies with a maximal follow-up of 6 months [164–167]. In the aforementioned more recent analysis on a subgroup of 56 patients with documented high-grade ureteral injury at the time of ureteroscopy, only 5.6% were found with persisting hydronephrosis at a median follow-up of 30 months [163]. In another study, the incidence rate of silent obstruction was 1.9% [168]. In that study, a cost-analysis revealed that routine postoperative imaging after ureteroscopy may be a cost-effective strategy to prevent loss of kidney function caused by prolonged silent obstruction and its attendant morbidity. Risk factors associated with persisting hydronephrosis after ureteroscopy are prior ipsilateral ureteroscopy, impacted stones, increasing number of stones, increasing stone diameter, increasing preoperative grade of hydronephrosis, longer operative time, as well as documented perioperative ureteral injury [164–167].

Preventive measures cannot be adequately formulated, since validated risk factors still have to established yet. Any type of ureteral injury may arguably result in ureteral stricture. Therefore, iatrogenic ureteral injury should always be prevented, as discussed above. Particularly, some authors proposed miniaturized ureteroscopes to prevention injuries to the ureteral wall [22, 142, 169]. Impacted stones shall be entirely removed, since the associated chronic inflammation may cause stone granuloma which in turn have been associated with stricture formation [170–172]. This also forms the rationale for authors recommending to postpone lithotripsy when an endopyelotomy has been performed in the presence of urinary stone [173].

Management of ureteral stricture and silent persisting hydronephrosis is based on regular follow-up controls and shall be tailored to each patient separately. No clear recommendations are available to date. Kidney function monitoring and imaging methods such as dynamic scintigraphy and computed tomography urography may help identifying patients at risk of kidney function deterioration.

Definitive treatment may consist of stricture dilation, incision, resection, buccal ureteroplasty, ureteral reimplantation or renal autotransplantation [19, 22, 139, 174, 175]. In the absence of ischemia, balloon dilation may be effective for short stricture in up to 89% of the cases [176]. Success rate up to 80% have been reported for endoureterotomy of benign ureteral strictures [177]. In case of endourological treatment failure, open or laparoscopic surgical repair may be required.

6.3 Bladder Injury

6.3.1 Urinary Retention

Incidence of urinary retention following ureteroscopy (MCCS grade III, Satava grade 1) ranges from 0.1 to 1.4% [10, 19, 23, 24, 27]. It mainly occurs in elderly male patients. Risk factors include bladder outlet obstruction and neurogenic bladder dysfunction. Treatment consists of temporary placement of a Foley catheter, eventually accompanied by disease-specific additional measures.

6.4 Urethra Injury

6.4.1 Urethral Injury

To the best of our knowledge, only one study to date evaluated urethral injury associated with ureteroscopy (MCCS grade I–IIIb, Satava grade 1–3), with only one patient out of a retrospective case series with 1235 patients undergoing semi-rigid ureteroscopy [139]. Future studies shall clarify causes and long-term risk of such damages occurring during ureteroscopy.

6.5 Other Organ Dysfunctions

6.5.1 Bowel

Postoperative ileus (lasting more than 1 day) (MCCS grade I–II, Satava grade 1) has been reported in 22 out of 5133 cases (0.4%) by Elashry [22]. Predictive factors of this rare complication are unknown.

7 Instrument-Related Complications

7.1 Instrument Malfunction and Damage

Incidence of instrument malfunction (MCCS grade I–IV, Satava grade 1–3) ranges from 0.1 to 5.3% [9, 10, 19, 24, 30, 35, 69]. The cause and type of malfunction dictates the severity of associated complications. Mostly, problems arising from ancillary devices malfunction, dilation balloon breakage, loss of manipulation range, or loss of view have a limited impact on the patient and will mainly entail risks of higher medical cost burden.

Flexible ureteroscopes are particularly prone to minor malfunctions such as loss of deflection range, obstruction of working channel, or damages to the image transport medium cause loss of vision [178]. A less well known and possibly disastrous damage to flexible ureteroscopes is the dismantling of the bending rubber covering the deflectable distal part a flexible ureteroscope, which may cause instrument retainment, as discussed later [179].

These instrument malfunctions may either arise from forced manipulation during surgery, or from high-level disinfection and sterilization processes [180]. Of note, it is still debated whether the use of UAS may prevent, or contrarily cause instrument damages during flexible ureteroscopy [181–183].

Prevention of instrument malfunctions include adequate use, disinfection, sterilization and storage according to manufacturers' instructions. Damages to reusable may be prevented by tailoring the type of instruments and ancillary devices to each patient separately. In case of instrument malfunction, every effort should be put to safely remove the faulty instrument and replace it, such that a minor malfunction may not escalate into a major complication.

7.2 Locked Instruments

Few reports on locked instruments (MCCS grade IIIb, Satava grade 2–3) have been published to date, exclusively concerning flexible ureteroscopes. A common risk factor seems to be forced manipulation when a flexible ureteroscope is pulled through a stenotic infundibulum in maximal deflection [184, 185]. In such cases manual straightening of the deflectable mechanism may be achieved by passing a coaxial dilator alongside the ureteroscope [184]. In case of failure, one may try to remove the ureteroscope without damaging the urinary tract by cutting the handle of the flexible ureteroscope or by cutting the distal part through a percutaneous access.

Another probably underreported event is the buildup of stone fragments along and distally to ureteroscope during lithotripsy, which may cause ureteroscope entrapment within the ureter. This complication eventually led to open instrument extraction in a recent case report [186].

Again, such devastating complication are best prevented by proper and gently manipulation of instruments, where instruments shall be adapted to the anatomy and not vice versa.

7.3 Damages from Lithotripters

Damages associated with the use of lithotripters are mainly relating to ureteral wall injuries, followed by kidney and vascular injuries (MCCS grade I–IV, Satava grade 1–3) as discussed above. Of interest, complications arising from ureteroscopy seem not to differ whether lithotripsy is performed by the means of laser or pneumatic energy [3, 187].

8 Implant-Related Complications

8.1 Ureteral Stent Migration

Design of ureteral stents is such that it shall prevent migration within the urinary tract, with the double-J endings as a prime example preventing ante- and retrograde stent migration. Still, ureteral stent migration (MCCS grade III, Satava grade 2–3) has an incidence ranging from 0.1 to 26.3% [3, 9, 19, 24, 27, 28, 35, 36, 69, 188]. Migration mostly is retrograde. Causes are incorrect stent placement, inadequate stent length, as well as ureteral peristalsis. Accordingly, preventive measures include appropriate stent length evaluation, proximal curl placement in the pelvis instead of the upper calyx, as well as verification of the presence of a distal curl within the bladder [189]. Early diagnosis and prompt treatment with stent repositioning or stent removal may prevent an avoidable secondary procedure.

8.2 Intravascular Ureteral Stent Migration

Intravascular ureteral stent migration (MCCS grade III–IV, Satava grade 2–3) is a rare complication that has been reported in several cases to date [190–209]. In all cases, the cause was inadvertent ureteral wall perforation with stent insertion either directly into the inferior vena cava, through iliac vein toward the inferior vena cava, through the gonadal vein toward the inferior vena cava, or through the iliac artery to the aorta. In two cases, the ureteral stent migrated up to the pulmonary artery [190, 195]. The most commonly reported risk factor was the absence of intraoperative fluoroscopy during stent insertion. Another recognized risk factor may be Boari-flap reconstruction [206, 209]. Patients may present with persisting postoperative gross hematuria, thromboembolism, dyspnea, and obstructive uropathy, or may remain asymptomatic. Treatment is commonly based on endovascular surgery, or more seldom open surgical removal.

8.3 Forgotten Ureteral Stent

All ureteral stents have a maximal dwell time, beyond which stent material deterioration, encrustation, fragmentation, and obstruction (MCCS grade I–IV, Satava grade 1–3) may occur [210]. In such cases, potentially severe secondary complications such as UTI, urosepsis, fistulizing perinephric abscess, complete loss of ureteral function, and even death may occur [211–213]. Large bladder stone formation at the distal stent loop has also been reported as a frequent complication from forgotten ureteral stents [214, 215].

The largest prospective observational study to date included 68 cases with a mean ureteral stent dwell time of 17 months [216]. In that study, most patients presented with UTI (60%) or kidney function deterioration (25%). Particularly long dwell times of 8–25 years have been reported in literature [215, 217, 218]. Most cases may safely be managed by complex stent extraction interventions, including combined antegrade and retrograde endoscopy, as well as open surgery in selected cases [219, 220]. Extracorporeal shockwave lithotripsy may be an adequate option for well-selected patients [221]. The combination of flexible ureteroscopy and laser stent cutting seems to be an adequate approach which may allow for a majority of cases to be managed endoscopically [222].

Preventive measures include consideration of maximal dwell time recommended by manufacturers, rising adequate patient awareness about any implanted stent, use of stent extraction strings, as well as tracking of patients by the means of stent registries [223]. Particularly, multiple authors suggest the use of mobile phone applications to warrant all these preventive measures [221, 224–226]. Of note, ureteral stent extraction strings seem not to be associated with a higher risk of infection [227, 228].

8.4 Ureteral Access Sheaths

The risks and benefits of UAS have already been discussed in detail earlier in this chapter. It should be recalled that ureteral wall injury is the main risk associated with the use of UAS, while its benefits may stem from lowering intrarenal pressure and therefore lowering infectious as well as bleeding complications [62]. A recent meta-analysis by Huang et al. exemplifies these associations, since the use of UAS was associated with a higher risk of postoperative complications, while its use was not associated with higher intraoperative complications rate, nor longer hospitalization duration [229]. Another study found a higher risk of hospital readmission associated to the use of UAS [230]. Therefore, UAS should not be routinely inserted when performing flexible ureteroscopy, but shall rather be based on a patient-specific basis [62].

9 Pregnancy-Related Complications

9.1 Preterm Labor

Suspected obstructive uropathy represents a conundrum during pregnancy, since therapeutic imaging modalities are limited by the potentially deleterious effect of X-rays on the fetus, and because both renal colic and active intervention may induce preterm labor (MCCS grade III–V, Satava grade 3) [231–233]. This is aggravated by the fact that, due to gestational hypercalciuria and hyperuricosuria, ureteral stents are prone to encrustation and shall therefore be regularly exchanged to prevent secondary complications from stent failures [234]. Finally, the risk of preterm labor seems to increase when the time to intervention is delayed in patients with acute renal colic [235]. Consequently, several authors have proposed emergency ureteroscopy as an adequate diagnostic and therapeutic method, considering urolithiasis is causative in many cases. Early intervention with ureteroscopic stone clearance would therefore achieve a quadruple role: prevent preterm labor by relief of renal colic, prevent kidney function deterioration by relief of an eventual ureteral obstruction, treat the cause in case urolithiasis, and subside the need for longer ureteral stent dwelling time. In case of emergency URS, lithotripsy shall only be performed by the means of laser energy and not with any of pneumatic, electrohydraulic, ultrasonic lithotripters, since these energy sources may induce premature labor or eventually bear a direct hazard for the fetus [232].

Incidence of preterm labor in patients undergoing emergency ureteroscopy ranges from 4.4 to 8.7% [236, 237]. In another meta-analysis including 108 patients, only one case of preterm labor occurred and was managed by tocolytics, such that the authors deeded ureteroscopy during pregnancy safe, with complication rates comparable to nonpregnant patients [238]. A multidisciplinary approach is recommended in case of suspected obstructive uropathy during pregnancy [233, 239]. Both fetal monitoring and obstetrical services available, especially in the third trimester when the risk of preterm labor is increased. Future studies shall clarify benefits and harms associations with delayed intervention versus ureteral stent insertion versus emergency ureteroscopy.

10 Mortality

Lethal ureteroscopy (MCCS grade V) is an extremely unfortunate and rare event, with only 72 patients reported in literature to date [3, 7, 9, 21, 52, 240, 241]. According to a recent systematic review, the most frequent cause of death is urosepsis (57%), followed by cardiac-related (14%), respiratory-related (7%) multiple organ failure (7%), and hemorrhagic (5%) complications, as well as isolated cases with pulmonary thromboembolism intracardiac thromboembolism, disseminated intravascular coagulation, and venous gas embolism [241]. Based on currently available data, three times more reports of death were found in female, compared to males, while more than 60% of all deaths occurred in the elderly. Possible patient-related risk-factors include comorbidities, such as hypertension, ischemic heart disease, diabetes mellitus, recurrent UTIs, neurogenic bladder, and liver disease. Risk factors specific to urosepsis and hemorrhagic complications following ureteroscopy have been discussed above in the according paragraph. Some authors have reported on inadequate management of preventable causes of death, such as insufficient or incorrect antibiotic coverage, prolonged operative time despite bleeding or unrecognized perirenal hematoma [10, 21, 27]. Considering the one death case associated to gas embolism, the authors hypothesized air bubbles generated during laser lithotripsy, air from repeated ureteroscope extraction and insertion, air bubbles from irrigation, or peripheral venous catheter-related air embolism as possible causes of gas embolism [242].

11 Patient-Reported Outcomes

11.1 Pain and Renal Colic

Incidence of pain following ureteroscopy (MCCS grade I–IIIb, Satava grade 1–2b) ranges from 1.1 to 10.2% [10, 19, 22, 25, 26, 30]. It is usually located in the ipsilateral flank, lower abdomen or grain, and is mainly caused by distension of the upper urinary tract, which stimulates nociceptive mechanoreceptors in the ureter and kidney [243]. Risk factors include female gender, larger stone burden, ureteral dilatation and ureteral access sheath time [244, 245]. Of interest, balloon dilation was found to cause more severe pain, compared to dilation with UAS [245]. No study to date has linked side of surgery, stone location, preoperative stenting, size of ureteral access sheath, or postoperative stenting with pain following ureteroscopy. Mostly, conservative measures such as analgesics are sufficient for adequate pain treatment. Nonsteroidal anti-inflammatory drugs seem most adequate against renal colic, based on data from emergency management of renal colic [246]. Recently, corticosteroids have been proposed to reduce postoperative pain after ureteroscopy [247]. In that retrospective matched-pairs analysis, rate of renal colic, rate of parenteral analgesic therapy as well as analgesic consumption were found significantly lower on the day of surgery. This effect was not present anymore from postoperative day 1, and rate of postoperative ureteral stenting as well as unplanned medical visits was similar between treatment groups. In up to 2.2% of patients following stent-free ureteroscopy, ureteral stenting is required for persisting pain that is resistant to conventional analgesics [3, 27, 35].

11.2 Ureteral Stent Discomfort

Ureteral stent discomfort (MCCS grade I, Satava grade 1) has been reported with widely differing incidence rates, ranging from 1.1 to 88% [21, 248, 249]. Several symptom scores have been developed to address quality of life of patients with stone disease, including the Ureteral stent symptom questionnaire (USSQ), Wisconsin Stone Quality of Life Questionnaire (WISQOL), Cambridge Renal Stone PROM (CReSP), and Urinary Stones and Intervention Quality of Life (USIQoL) [250–253]. These questionnaires commonly explore symptoms such as urinary symptoms, body pain, general health, work performance, sexual matters, social domains, emotional domains, stone-related domains, vitality domains, impacts of dietary changes, gastrointestinal symptoms, and psychosocial health.

Increasing evidence on the burden of stent-related symptoms and the safety stent-free ureteroscopy feed the debate about the rationale for routine stenting following ureteroscopy [19, 254–259]. It therefore seems justified to find a balance between a low rate of stent-related discomfort and prevention of more severe complications such as UTI, urosepsis, kidney function failure, hemorrhage, and secondary interventions, as discussed in the subchapters above.

Based on all risk factors discussed in this book chapter, ureteral stenting after ureteroscopy may be considered for patients with previous history of UTI, infectious stones, high ASA score, immunocompromised status, solitary kidney, larger stone size, longer operation time, intraoperative bleeding complications, impacted stones, after endoureterotomy or endopyelotomy, and higher-grade ureteral lesions. Of note, use of ureteral stent extraction strings does not seem to alter stent-related symptoms, nor is it associated with higher infectious complications [227, 260]. Also, use of a ureteral access sheath does not imply the routine use of postoperative stenting, but rather depends on evaluation of ureteral wall lesions on ureteroscope retrieval at the end of the procedure [9, 166].

12 Readmission and Secondary Intervention

12.1 Hospital Readmission

Readmission (MCCS grade I–IV, Satava grade 1–3) rate ranges from 2.17 to 5.8% [230, 261–266]. The main cause for readmission is fever or signs of urosepsis, followed by ureteral stent related symptoms. Risk factors include younger age, female sex, diabetes mellitus, hypertension, chronic obstructive pulmonary disease, lower body mass index, ASA score ≥ 3, higher stone burden, bilateral procedure, use of a UAS, history of psychiatric diagnosis, lower income, and uninsured status. Of interest, the use of postoperative ureteral stent has been variably associated with higher, or lower readmission rates.

12.2 Secondary Intervention

12.2.1 Stone Migration and Residual Fragments

Migration of stones or stone fragments located in the ureter to the pelvicalyceal system caused by ureteroscopy (MCCS grade I–IIIb, Satava grade 1–2b) has a reported incidence between 0.1 and 7.4% [3, 22, 24, 27, 28, 30, 35, 37, 69]. Residual fragments >4 mm seems to corroborate an increased risk of stone growth, complications (59%) and reinterventions (38%) [267]. Stone migration may be prevented by low irrigation flow rate, using laser lithotripsy instead of pneumatic lithotripsy, or by using antiretropulsion devices [187, 268, 269]. Residual fragments shall ideally be excluded by inspecting the whole pelvicalyceal system and the urinary tract at the end of the procedure.

12.2.2 Ureteral Obstruction and Steinstrasse

Incidence of ureteral obstruction or steinstrasse following ureteroscopy (MCCS grade I–IIIb, Satava grade 1–2b) ranges from 0.3 to 2.5% [3, 9–11, 21, 23, 25, 36]. Causes include mucosal edema or aggregation of stone fragments or blot clots in the ureter. It is characterized by flank pain that can be relieved with ureteral stenting or nephrostomy in expectation of another ureteroscopy in case of residual fragments.

13 Conclusion

Although considered minimally invasive, ureteroscopy is frequently associated with complications, ranging from spontaneously vanishing minor events, up to devastating and potentially lethal damages to the patient. The prudent urologist should be aware of all possible complications, together with their etiopathogenic causes and associated risk factors. This awareness allows to perform ureteroscopy in optimal conditions, possibly preventing complications and allowing the surgeon early recognition and treatment of threatening conditions. Additionally, the urologist should be aware of all technical characteristics of his instruments and ancillary devices, together with their weaknesses and strengths. Several debated topics such as the real impact and limits of intrarenal pressure and operative time need to be further clarified in future studies. The use of standardized classification systems complications shall always be incorporated when reporting on case series in order to warrant comparison of results among different studies, to conduct meta-analyses, inform surgeons, and properly counsel patients about the hazards of ureteroscopy.

Disclosures Financial Disclosure: Dr. Etienne Xavier Keller is a consultant for Coloplast, Olympus, Debiopharm, and Recordati. Dr. Vincent De Coninck is a consultant for Boston Scientific, BD Bard, and Coloplast. Dr. Olivier Traxer is a—consultant for Coloplast, Rocamed, Olympus, EMS, Boston Scientific, and IPG Medical.

Funding Support None.

References

1. De Coninck V, Keller EX, Somani B, et al. Complications of ureteroscopy: a complete overview. WJU. 2020;38(9):2147–66.
2. Geraghty RM, Jones P, Somani BK. Worldwide trends of urinary stone disease treatment over the last two decades: a systematic review. J Endourol. 2017;31(6):547–56.
3. Mandal S, Goel A, Singh MK, Kathpalia R, Nagathan DS, Sankhwar SN, et al. Clavien classification of semirigid ureteroscopy complications: a prospective study. Urology. 2012;80(5):995–1001.
4. Tepeler A, Resorlu B, Sahin T, Sarikaya S, Bayindir M, Oguz U, et al. Categorization of intraoperative ureteroscopy complications using modified Satava classification system. World J Urol. 2014;32(1):131–6.
5. Dindo D, Demartines N, Clavien PA. Classification of surgical complications: a new proposal with evaluation in a cohort of 6336 patients and results of a survey. Ann Surg. 2004;240(2):205–13.
6. Oguz U, Resorlu B, Ozyuvali E, Bozkurt OF, Senocak C, Unsal A. Categorizing intraoperative complications of retrograde intrarenal surgery. Urol Int. 2014;92(2):164–8.
7. Sugihara T, Yasunaga H, Horiguchi H, Nishimatsu H, Kume H, Ohe K, et al. A nomogram predicting severe adverse events after ureteroscopic lithotripsy: 12,372 patients in a Japanese national series. BJU Int. 2013;111(3):459–66.
8. Daels FPJ, Gaizauskas A, Rioja J, Varshney AK, Erkan E, Ozgok Y, et al. Age-related prevalence of diabetes mellitus, cardiovascular disease and anticoagulation therapy use in a urolithiasis population and their effect on outcomes: the Clinical Research Office of the Endourological Society Ureteroscopy Global Study. World J Urol. 2014;33(6):859–64.
9. Bas O, Tuygun C, Dede O, Sari S, Cakici MC, Ozturk U, et al. Factors affecting complication rates of retrograde flexible ureterorenoscopy: analysis of 1571 procedures—a single-center experience. World J Urol. 2017;35(5):819–26.
10. Schuster TG, Hollenbeck BK, Faerber GJ, Wolf JS Jr. Complications of ureteroscopy: analysis of predictive factors. J Urol. 2001;166(2):538–40.
11. El-Nahas AR, El-Tabey NA, Eraky I, Shoma AM, El-Hefnawy AS, El-Assmy AM, et al. Semirigid ureteroscopy for ureteral stones: a multivariate analysis of unfavorable results. J Urol. 2009;181(3):1158–62.
12. Komori M, Izaki H, Daizumoto K, Tsuda M, Kusuhara Y, Mori H, et al. Complications of flexible ureteroscopic treatment for renal and ureteral calculi during the learning curve. Urol Int. 2015;95(1):26–32.
13. Knipper S, Tiburtius C, Gross AJ, Netsch C. Is prolonged operation time a predictor for the occurrence of complications in ureteroscopy? Urol Int. 2015;95(1):33–7.
14. Whitehurst L, Pietropaolo A, Geraghty R, Kyriakides R, Somani BK. Factors affecting operative time during ureteroscopy and stone treatment and its effect on outcomes: retrospective results over 6.5 years. Ther Adv Urol. 2020;12:1756287220934403.
15. Ozgor F, Sahan M, Cubuk A, Ortac M, Ayranci A, Sarilar O. Factors affecting infectious complications following flexible ureterorenoscopy. Urolithiasis. 2018;47(5):481–6.
16. Fan S, Gong B, Hao Z, Zhang L, Zhou J, Zhang Y, et al. Risk factors of infectious complications following flexible ureteroscope with a holmium laser: a retrospective study. Int J Clin Exp Med. 2015;8(7):11252–9.
17. Lane J, Whitehurst L, Hameed BMZ, Tokas T, Somani BK. Correlation of operative time with outcomes of ureteroscopy and stone treatment: a systematic review of literature. Curr Urol Rep. 2020;21(4):1.
18. Berardinelli F, De Francesco P, Marchioni M, Cera N, Proietti S, Hennessey D, et al. Infective complications after retrograde intrarenal surgery: a new standardized classification system. Int Urol Nephrol. 2016;48(11):1757–62.
19. Cheung MC, Lee F, Leung YL, Wong BB, Chu SM, Tam PC. Outpatient ureteroscopy: predictive factors for postoperative events. Urology. 2001;58(6):914–8.
20. Cohen J, Cohen S, Grasso M. Ureteropyeloscopic treatment of large, complex intrarenal and proximal ureteral calculi. BJU Int. 2013;111(3 Pt B):E127–31.
21. de la Rosette J, Denstedt J, Geavlete P, Keeley F, Matsuda T, Pearle M, et al. The clinical research office of the endourological society ureteroscopy global study: indications, complications, and outcomes in 11,885 patients. J Endourol. 2014;28(2):131–9.
22. Elashry OM, Elgamasy AK, Sabaa MA, Abo-Elenien M, Omar MA, Eltatawy HH, et al. Ureteroscopic management of lower ureteric calculi: a 15-year single-centre experience. BJU Int. 2008;102(8):1010–7.

23. Hyams ES, Munver R, Bird VG, Uberoi J, Shah O. Flexible ureterorenoscopy and holmium laser lithotripsy for the management of renal stone burdens that measure 2 to 3 cm: a multi-institutional experience. J Endourol. 2010;24(10):1583–8.
24. Ibrahim AK. Reporting ureteroscopy complications using the modified Clavien classification system. Urol Ann. 2015;7(1):53–7.
25. Perez Castro E, Osther PJ, Jinga V, Razvi H, Stravodimos KG, Parikh K, et al. Differences in ureteroscopic stone treatment and outcomes for distal, mid-, proximal, or multiple ureteral locations: the Clinical Research Office of the Endourological Society ureteroscopy global study. Eur Urol. 2014;66(1):102–9.
26. Salem HK. A prospective randomized study comparing shock wave lithotripsy and semirigid ureteroscopy for the management of proximal ureteral calculi. Urology. 2009;74(6):1216–21.
27. Somani BK, Giusti G, Sun Y, Osther PJ, Frank M, De Sio M, et al. Complications associated with ureterorenoscopy (URS) related to treatment of urolithiasis: the Clinical Research Office of Endourological Society URS Global study. World J Urol. 2017;35(4):675–81.
28. Ogreden E, Oguz U, Demirelli E, Benli E, Sancak EB, Gulpinar MT, et al. Categorization of ureteroscopy complications and investigation of associated factors by using the modified Clavien classification system. Turk J Med Sci. 2016;46(3):686–94.
29. Southern JB, Higgins AM, Young AJ, Kost KA, Schreiter BR, Clifton M, et al. Risk factors for postoperative fever and systemic inflammatory response syndrome after ureteroscopy for stone disease. J Endourol. 2019;33(7):516–22.
30. Mursi K, Elsheemy MS, Morsi HA, Ali Ghaleb AK, Abdel-Razzak OM. Semi-rigid ureteroscopy for ureteric and renal pelvic calculi: predictive factors for complications and success. Arab J Urol. 2013;11(2):136–41.
31. Sohn DW, Kim SW, Hong CG, Yoon BI, Ha US, Cho YH. Risk factors of infectious complication after ureteroscopic procedures of the upper urinary tract. J Infect Chemother. 2013;19(6):1102–8.
32. Chew BH, Flannigan R, Kurtz M, Gershman B, Arsovska O, Paterson RF, et al. A single dose of intraoperative antibiotics is sufficient to prevent urinary tract infection during ureteroscopy. J Endourol. 2016;30(1):63–8.
33. Singer M, Deutschman CS, Seymour CW, Shankar-Hari M, Annane D, Bauer M, et al. The third international consensus definitions for sepsis and septic shock (sepsis-3). JAMA. 2016;315(8):801–10.
34. Hsieh CH, Yang SS, Lin CD, Chang SJ. Are prophylactic antibiotics necessary in patients with preoperative sterile urine undergoing ureterorenoscopic lithotripsy? BJU Int. 2014;113(2):275–80.
35. Geavlete P, Georgescu D, Nita G, Mirciulescu V, Cauni V. Complications of 2735 retrograde semi-rigid ureteroscopy procedures: a single-center experience. J Endourol. 2006;20(3):179–85.
36. Giusti G, Proietti S, Villa L, Cloutier J, Rosso M, Gadda GM, et al. Current standard technique for modern flexible ureteroscopy: tips and tricks. Eur Urol. 2016;70(1):188–94.
37. Taie K, Jasemi M, Khazaeli D, Fatholahi A. Prevalence and management of complications of ureteroscopy: a seven-year experience with introduction of a new maneuver to prevent ureteral avulsion. Urol J. 2012;9(1):356–60.
38. Bloom J, Fox C, Fullerton S, Matthews G, Phillips J. Sepsis after elective ureteroscopy. Can J Urol. 2017;24(5):9017–23.
39. Zhong W, Leto G, Wang L, Zeng G. Systemic inflammatory response syndrome after flexible ureteroscopic lithotripsy: a study of risk factors. J Endourol. 2015;29(1):25–8.
40. Scotland KB, Lange D. Prevention and management of urosepsis triggered by ureteroscopy. Res Rep Urol. 2018;10:43–9.
41. Gautam G, Singh AK, Kumar R, Hemal AK, Kothari A. Beware! Fungal urosepsis may follow endoscopic intervention for prolonged indwelling ureteral stent. J Endourol. 2006;20(7):522–4.
42. Blackmur JP, Maitra NU, Marri RR, Housami F, Malki M, McIlhenny C. Analysis of factors' association with risk of postoperative urosepsis in patients undergoing ureteroscopy for treatment of stone disease. J Endourol. 2016;30(9):963–9.
43. Nevo A, Mano R, Baniel J, Lifshitz DA. Ureteric stent dwelling time: a risk factor for post-ureteroscopy sepsis. BJU Int. 2017;120(1):117–22.
44. Mitsuzuka K, Nakano O, Takahashi N, Satoh M. Identification of factors associated with postoperative febrile urinary tract infection after ureteroscopy for urinary stones. Urolithiasis. 2016;44(3):257–62.
45. Nevo A, Mano R, Schreter E, Lifshitz DA. Clinical implications of stent culture in patients with indwelling ureteral stents prior to ureteroscopy. J Urol. 2017;198(1):116–21.
46. Xu CG, Guo YL. Diagnostic and prognostic values of BMPER in patients with urosepsis following ureteroscopic lithotripsy. Biomed Res Int. 2019;2019:1–9.
47. Bone RC, Balk RA, Cerra FB, Dellinger RP, Fein AM, Knaus WA, et al. Definitions for sepsis and organ failure and guidelines for the use of innovative therapies in sepsis. The ACCP/SCCM Consensus Conference Committee. American College of Chest Physicians/Society of Critical Care Medicine. Chest. 1992;101(6):1644–55.
48. Levy MM, Fink MP, Marshall JC, Abraham E, Angus D, Cook D, et al. 2001 SCCM/ESICM/ACCP/ATS/SIS International Sepsis Definitions Conference. Crit Care Med. 2003;31(4):1250–6.
49. Seymour CW, Liu VX, Iwashyna TJ, Brunkhorst FM, Rea TD, Scherag A, et al. Assessment of clinical criteria for sepsis: for the Third International

Consensus Definitions for Sepsis and Septic Shock (Sepsis-3). JAMA. 2016;315(8):762–74.
50. van Nieuwkoop C, Bonten TN, van't Wout JW, Kuijper EJ, Groeneveld GH, Becker MJ, et al. Procalcitonin reflects bacteremia and bacterial load in urosepsis syndrome: a prospective observational study. Crit Care. 2010;14(6):R206.
51. Shi B, Shi F, Xu K, Shi L, Tang H, Wang N, et al. The prognostic performance of Sepsis-3 and SIRS criteria for patients with urolithiasis-associated sepsis transferred to ICU following surgical interventions. Exp Ther Med. 2019;18(5):4165–72.
52. Cindolo L, Castellan P, Primiceri G, Hoznek A, Cracco CM, Scoffone CM, et al. Life-threatening complications after ureteroscopy for urinary stones: survey and systematic literature review. Minerva Urol Nefrol. 2017;69(5):421–31.
53. Pietropaolo A, Hendry J, Kyriakides R, Geraghty R, Jones P, Aboumarzouk O, et al. Outcomes of elective ureteroscopy for ureteric stones in patients with prior urosepsis and emergency drainage: prospective study over 5 year. from a Tertiary Endourology Centre. Eur Urol Focus. 2020;6(1):151–6.
54. Kanno T, Matsuda A, Sakamoto H, Higashi Y, Yamada H. Safety and efficacy of ureteroscopy after obstructive pyelonephritis treatment. Int J Urol. 2013;20(9):917–22.
55. Youssef RF, Neisius A, Goldsmith ZG, Ghaffar M, Tsivian M, Shin RH, et al. Clinical outcomes after ureteroscopic lithotripsy in patients who initially presented with urosepsis: matched pair comparison with elective ureteroscopy. J Endourol. 2014;28(12):1439–43.
56. Martov A, Gravas S, Etemadian M, Unsal A, Barusso G, D'Addessi A, et al. Postoperative infection rates in patients with a negative baseline urine culture undergoing ureteroscopic stone removal: a matched case-control analysis on antibiotic prophylaxis from the CROES URS global study. J Endourol. 2015;29(2):171–80.
57. Qiao LD, Chen S, Lin YH, Li JX, Hu WG, Hou JP, et al. Evaluation of perioperative prophylaxis with fosfomycin tromethamine in ureteroscopic stone removal: an investigator-driven prospective, multicenter, randomized, controlled study. Int Urol Nephrol. 2018;50(3):427–32.
58. Knopf HJ, Graff HJ, Schulze H. Perioperative antibiotic prophylaxis in ureteroscopic stone removal. Eur Urol. 2003;44(1):115–8.
59. Skolarikos A, Thomas K. EAU guidelines on urolithiasis, last update March 2020. 2020. https://uroweb.org/guideline/urolithiasis. Accessed 18 Mar 2020.
60. Assimos D, Krambeck A, Miller NL, Monga M, Murad MH, Nelson CP, et al. Surgical management of stones: American Urological Association/Endourological Society Guideline. Part I. J Urol. 2016;196(4):1153–60.
61. Eswara JR, Shariftabrizi A, Sacco D. Positive stone culture is associated with a higher rate of sepsis after endourological procedures. Urolithiasis. 2013;41(5):411–4.
62. De Coninck V, Keller EX, Rodriguez-Monsalve M, Audouin M, Doizi S, Traxer O. Systematic review of ureteral access sheaths: facts and myths. BJU Int. 2018;122(6):959–69.
63. Traxer O, Wendt-Nordahl G, Sodha H, Rassweiler J, Meretyk S, Tefekli A, et al. Differences in renal stone treatment and outcomes for patients treated either with or without the support of a ureteral access sheath: The Clinical Research Office of the Endourological Society Ureteroscopy Global Study. World J Urol. 2015;33(12):2137–44.
64. Chang CL, Su LH, Lu CM, Tai FT, Huang YC, Chang KK. Outbreak of ertapenem-resistant *Enterobacter cloacae* urinary tract infections due to a contaminated ureteroscope. J Hosp Infect. 2013;85(2):118–24.
65. Ofstead CL, Heymann OL, Quick MR, Johnson EA, Eiland JE, Wetzler HP. The effectiveness of sterilization for flexible ureteroscopes: a real-world study. Am J Infect Control. 2017;45(8):888–95.
66. Podoynicyn AAP, Romanov DVR, EA O, SBU U, VVD D, VVB B. Bilateral acute purulent destructive pyelonephritis after retrograde ureteroscopy and lithotripsy. Urologiia. 2019;5:114–8.
67. Ferrer R, Martin-Loeches I, Phillips G, Osborn TM, Townsend S, Dellinger RP, et al. Empiric antibiotic treatment reduces mortality in severe sepsis and septic shock from the first hour: results from a guideline-based performance improvement program. Crit Care Med. 2014;42(8):1749–55.
68. Whitehurst L, Jones P, Somani BK. Mortality from kidney stone disease (KSD) as reported in the literature over the last two decades: a systematic review. World J Urol. 2018;37(5):759–76.
69. Georgescu D, Multescu R, Geavlete B, Geavlete P. Intraoperative complications after 8150 semirigid ureteroscopies for ureteral lithiasis: risk analysis and management. Chirurgia (Bucur). 2014;109(3):369–74.
70. Tanriverdi O, Silay MS, Kadihasanoglu M, Aydin M, Kendirci M, Miroglu C. Revisiting the predictive factors for intra-operative complications of rigid ureteroscopy: a 15-year experience. Urol J. 2012;9(2):457–64.
71. Sharaf A, Amer T, Somani BK, Aboumarzouk OM. Ureteroscopy in patients with bleeding diatheses, anticoagulated, and on anti-platelet agents: a systematic review and meta-analysis of the literature. J Endourol. 2017;31(12):1217–25.
72. Westerman ME, Sharma V, Scales J, Gearman DJ, Ingimarsson JP, Krambeck AE. The effect of antiplatelet agents on bleeding-related complications after ureteroscopy. J Endourol. 2016;30(10):1073–8.
73. Westerman ME, Scales JA, Sharma V, Gearman DJ, Ingimarsson JP, Krambeck AE. The effect of anticoagulation on bleeding-related complications following ureteroscopy. Urology. 2017;100:45–52.

74. Atis G, Arikan O, Gurbuz C, Yildirim A, Erol B, Pelit S, et al. Comparison of different ureteroscope sizes in treating ureteral calculi in adult patients. Urology. 2013;82(6):1231–5.
75. Keller EX, De Coninck V, Traxer O. Next-generation fiberoptic and digital ureteroscopes. Urol Clin N Am. 2019;46(2):147–63.
76. Defidio L, De Dominicis M, Di Gianfrancesco L, Fuchs G, Patel A. First collaborative experience with thulium laser ablation of localized upper urinary tract urothelial tumors using retrograde intra-renal surgery. Arch Ital Urol Androl. 2011;83(3):147–53.
77. Bozzini G, Gastaldi C, Besana U, Calori A, Casellato S, Parma P, et al. Thulium-laser retrograde intra renal ablation (T-RIRA) of upper urinary tract transitional cell carcinoma: an ESUT study. Minerva Urol Nephrol. 2020;73(1):114–21.
78. Defidio L, Antonucci M, De Dominicis M, Fuchs G, Patel A. Thulium–Holmium:YAG duo laser in conservative upper tract urothelial cancer treatment: 13 years experience from a tertiary national referral center. J Endourol. 2019;33(11):902–8.
79. Musi G, Mistretta FA, Marenghi C, Russo A, Catellani M, Nazzani S, et al. Thulium laser treatment of upper urinary tract carcinoma: a multi-institutional analysis of surgical and oncological outcomes. J Endourol. 2018;32(3):257–63.
80. Emiliani E, Herrmann TR, Breda A. Thulium laser for the treatment of upper urinary tract carcinoma (UTUC)? Are we there, yet? World J Urol. 2015;33(4):595–7.
81. Yoshida T, Taguchi M, Inoue T, Kinoshita H, Matsuda T. Thulium laser ablation facilitates retrograde intra-renal surgery for upper urinary tract urothelial carcinoma. Int J Urol. 2018;25(4):379–80.
82. Proietti S, Rodríguez-Socarrás ME, Eisner BH, Lucianò R, Basulto Martinez MJ, Yeow Y, et al. Thulium:YAG versus Holmium:YAG laser effect on upper urinary tract soft tissue: evidence from an ex vivo experimental study. J Endourol. 2020;35(4):544–51.
83. Taratkin M, Netsch C, Enikeev D, Gross AJ, Herrmann TRW, Korolev D, et al. The impact of the laser fiber-tissue distance on histological parameters in a porcine kidney model. World J Urol. 2020;39(5):1607–12.
84. Becker B, Enikeev D, Glybochko P, Rapoport L, Taratkin M, Gross AJ, et al. Effect of optical fiber diameter and laser emission mode (cw vs pulse) on tissue damage profile using 1.94 microm Tm:fiber lasers in a porcine kidney model. World J Urol. 2020;38(6):1563–8.
85. Pal D, Paul A, Shekhar NK, Chowdhury SD, Sen R, Chatterjee K, et al. COM stone dusting and soft tissue ablation with Q-switched thulium fiber laser. IEEE J Sel Top Quant. 2019;25(1):1–8.
86. Arkhipova V, Enikeev M, Laukhtina E, Kurkov A, Andreeva V, Yaroslavsky I, et al. Ex vivo and animal study of the blue diode laser, Tm fiber laser, and their combination for laparoscopic partial nephrectomy. Lasers Surg Med. 2020;52(5):437–48.
87. Keller EX, Traxer O. Upper tract urothelial carcinoma: ureteroscopic management. In: Autorino R, Liatsikos E, Porpiglia F, editors. New technologies and techniques in minimally invasive surgery: an ESUT collection. Torino: Edizioni Minerva Medica; 2019. p. 277–85.
88. Bai J, Li C, Wang S, Liu J, Ye Z, Yu X, et al. Subcapsular renal haematoma after holmium:yttrium–aluminum–garnet laser ureterolithotripsy. BJU Int. 2012;109(8):1230–4.
89. Chiu PK, Chan CK, Ma WK, To KC, Cheung FK, Yiu MK. Subcapsular hematoma after ureteroscopy and laser lithotripsy. J Endourol. 2013;27(9):1115–9.
90. Paiva MM, da Silva RD, Jaworski P, Kim FJ, Molina WR. Subcapsular hematoma after ureteroscopy and laser lithotripsy. Can J Urol. 2016;23(4):8385–7.
91. Tao W, Cai CJ, Sun CY, Xue BX, Shan YX. Subcapsular renal hematoma after ureteroscopy with holmium:yttrium–aluminum–garnet laser lithotripsy. Lasers Med Sci. 2015;30(5):1527–32.
92. Vaidyanathan S, Samsudin A, Singh G, Hughes PL, Soni BM, Selmi F. Large subcapsular hematoma following ureteroscopic laser lithotripsy of renal calculi in a spina bifida patient: lessons we learn. Int Med Case Rep J. 2016;9:253–9.
93. Riley JM, Stearman L, Troxel S. Retrograde ureteroscopy for renal stones larger than 2.5 cm. J Endourol. 2009;23(9):1395–8.
94. Xu L, Li G. Life-threatening subcapsular renal hematoma after flexible ureteroscopic laser lithotripsy: treatment with superselective renal arterial embolization. Urolithiasis. 2013;41(5):449–51.
95. Meng HZ, Chen SW, Chen GM, Tan FQ, Wang CJ, Shen BH. Renal subcapsular hemorrhage complicating ureterolithotripsy: an unknown complication of a known day-to-day procedure. Urol Int. 2013;91(3):335–9.
96. Yahsi S, Tonyali S, Ceylan C, Yildiz KY, Ozdal L. Intraparenchymal hematoma as a late complication of retrograde intrarenal surgery. Int Braz J Urol. 2017;43(2):367–70.
97. Kao M-H, Wang C-C. Risk factors for developing a perirenal hematoma after flexible ureteroscopic lithotripsy. Urol Sci. 2016;27(3):166–70.
98. Altay B, Erkurt B, Kiremit MC, Guzelburc V. A rare complication of ureteral double-J stenting after flexible ureteroscopy: renal parenchymal perforation. Turk J Urol. 2015;41(2):96–8.
99. Karaköse A, Yüksel MB. An extremely rare complication of double-J stenting: renal parenchymal perforation with no hematoma. Curr Urol. 2011;5(3):165–8.
100. Gerber GS, Lyon ES. Endopyelotomy: patient selection, results, and complications. Urology. 1994;43(1):2–10.
101. el-Nahas AR. Retrograde endopyelotomy: a comparison between laser and Acucise balloon cutting catheter. Curr Urol Rep. 2007;8(2):122–7.

102. Walz J, Lecamus C, Lechevallier E, Barriol D, Bretheau D, Albert P, et al. Complications of acucise (R) balloon endopyelotomy. Prog Urol. 2003;13(1):39–45.
103. Kim FJ, Herrell SD, Jahoda AE, Albala DM. Complications of acucise endopyelotomy. J Endourol. 1998;12(5):433–6.
104. Lopes RI, Torricelli FC, Gomes CM, Carnevale F, Bruschini H, Srougi M. Endovascular repair of a nearly fatal iliac artery injury after endoureterotomy. Scand J Urol. 2013;47(5):437–9.
105. Jubber I, Patel PR, Hori S, Al-Hayek S. Renal pseudoaneurysm: a rare and potentially fatal complication following ureteroscopy and laser fragmentation of stones. Ann R Coll Surg Engl. 2018;100(3):e51–e2.
106. Aston W, Whiting R, Bultitude M, Challacombe B, Glass J, Dasgupta P. Pseudoaneurysm formation after flexible ureterorenoscopy and electrohydraulic lithotripsy. Int J Clin Pract. 2004;58(3):310–1.
107. Angelsen A, Talseth T, Mjones JG, Hedlund H. Hypertension and pseudoaneurism on the renal artery following retrograde endopyelotomy (Acucise). Scand J Urol Nephrol. 2000;34(1):79–80.
108. Durner L, El Howairis MEF, Buchholz N. Renal pseudoaneurysm after flexible ureterorenoscopy—an unusual complication. Urol Int. 2017;99(4):484–6.
109. Ngo TC, Lee JJ, Gonzalgo ML. Renal pseudoaneurysm: an overview. Nat Rev Urol. 2010;7(11):619–25.
110. Watanabe M, Padua HM, Nguyen HT, Alomari AI. Renal pseudoaneurysm following laser lithotripsy: endovascular treatment of a rare complication. J Pediatr Urol. 2010;6(4):420–2.
111. Pelzman DL, Semins MJ. Endoscopic diagnosis of renal pseudoaneurysm following ureteroscopy. Can J Urol. 2019;26(6):10061–3.
112. Rudnick DM, Dretler SP. Intrarenal pseudoaneurysm following ureterorenoscopy and electrohydraulic lithotripsy. J Urol. 1998;159(4):1290–1.
113. Tiplitsky SI, Milhoua PM, Patel MB, Minsky L, Hoenig DM. Case report: intrarenal arteriovenous fistula after ureteroscopic stone extraction with holmium laser lithotripsy. J Endourol. 2007;21(5):530–2.
114. Abogunrin FA. Renal arteriovenous fistula: a rare complication of electro-hydraulic lithotripsy. S Afr J Surg Suid-Afrikaanse tydskrif vir chirurgie. 2012;50(4):134–5.
115. Eres Saez FJ, Sarmentero Ortiz E, Todoli J, Colomer Gonzalez FJ, de Pena R, Zaragoza OJ. Ureteroiliac fistula as a complication of ureterorenoscopy. Arch Esp Urol. 1989;42(3):275–7.
116. Alapont Alacreu JM, Rico E, Pontones Moreno JL, Oliver Amorós F, Palmero Martí JL, Boronat Tormo F, et al. Complicaciones de la uretero-renoscopia. Actas Urol Esp. 2003;27(9):692–9.
117. Grasso M, Bagley D. Small diameter, actively deflectable, flexible ureteropyeloscopy. J Urol. 1998;160(5):1648–53. discussion 53–4
118. Violette PD, Cartwright R, Briel M, Tikkinen KA, Guyatt GH. Guideline of guidelines: thromboprophylaxis for urological surgery. BJU Int. 2016;118(3):351–8.
119. Hinman F. Peripelyic extravasation during intravenous urography, evidence for an additional route for backflow after ureteral obstruction. J Urol. 1961;85(3):385–95.
120. Chapman JP, Gonzalez J, Diokno AC. Significance of urinary extravasation during renal colic. Urology. 1987;30(6):541–5.
121. Thomsen HS, Larsen S, Talner LB. Pyelorenal backflow during retrograde pyelography in normal and ischemic porcine kidneys. A radiologic and pathoanatomic study. Eur Urol. 1982;8(5):291–7.
122. Thomsen HS, Talner LB, Higgins CB. Intrarenal backflow during retrograde pyelography with graded intrapelvic pressure. A radiologic study. Investig Radiol. 1982;17(6):593–603.
123. Tokas T, Herrmann TRW, Skolarikos A, Nagele U, Training, Research in Urological S, et al. Pressure matters: intrarenal pressures during normal and pathological conditions, and impact of increased values to renal physiology. World J Urol. 2018;37(1):125–31.
124. Thomsen HS, Dorph S, Olsen S. Pyelorenal backflow in rabbits following clamping of the renal vein and artery: radiologic and microscopic investigation. Acta Radiol Diagn (Stockh). 1982;23(2):143–8.
125. Proietti S, Dragos L, Somani BK, Buttice S, Talso M, Emiliani E, et al. In vitro comparison of maximum pressure developed by irrigation systems in a kidney model. J Endourol. 2017;31(5):522–7.
126. Fahmy N, Sener A, Sabbisetti V, Nott L, Lang RM, Welk BK, et al. Urinary expression of novel tissue markers of kidney injury after ureteroscopy, shockwave lithotripsy, and in normal healthy controls. J Endourol. 2013;27(12):1455–62.
127. Peterson LJ, Yarger WE, Schocken DD, Glenn JF. Post-obstructive diuresis: a varied syndrome. J Urol. 1975;113(2):190–4.
128. Hamdi A, Hajage D, Van Glabeke E, Belenfant X, Vincent F, Gonzalez F, et al. Severe post-renal acute kidney injury, post-obstructive diuresis and renal recovery. BJU Int. 2012;110(11 Pt C):E1027–34.
129. Zelenko N, Coll D, Rosenfeld AT, Smith RC. Normal ureter size on unenhanced helical CT. AJR Am J Roentgenol. 2004;182(4):1039–41.
130. Hudson RG, Conlin MJ, Bagley DH. Ureteric access with flexible ureteroscopes: effect of the size of the ureteroscope. BJU Int. 2005;95(7):1043–4.
131. Hubosky SG, Healy KA, Grasso M, Bagley DH. Accessing the difficult ureter and the importance of ureteroscope miniaturization: history is repeating itself. Urology. 2014;84(4):740–2.
132. Kuntz NJ, Neisius A, Tsivian M, Ghaffar M, Patel N, Ferrandino MN, et al. Balloon dilation of the ureter: a contemporary review of outcomes and complications. J Urol. 2015;194(2):413–7.
133. Traxer O, Thomas A. Prospective evaluation and classification of ureteral wall injuries resulting from insertion of a ureteral access sheath during retrograde intrarenal surgery. J Urol. 2013;189(2):580–4.

134. Viers BR, Viers LD, Hull NC, Hanson TJ, Mehta RA, Bergstralh EJ, et al. The difficult ureter: clinical and radiographic characteristics associated with upper urinary tract access at the time of ureteroscopic stone treatment. Urology. 2015;86(5):878–84.
135. Joshi HB, Stainthorpe A, MacDonagh RP, Keeley FX Jr, Timoney AG, Barry MJ. Indwelling ureteral stents: evaluation of symptoms, quality of life and utility. J Urol. 2003;169(3):1065–9. discussion 9
136. Ansari MS. Re: Complications of ureteroscopy: analysis of predictive factors. J Urol. 2002;167(4):1801–2.
137. Ambani SN, Faerber GJ, Roberts WW, Hollingsworth JM, Wolf JS Jr. Ureteral stents for impassable ureteroscopy. J Endourol. 2013;27(5):549–53.
138. Schoenthaler M, Buchholz N, Farin E, Ather H, Bach C, Bach T, et al. The Post-Ureteroscopic Lesion Scale (PULS): a multicenter video-based evaluation of inter-rater reliability. World J Urol. 2014;32(4):1033–40.
139. Fuganti PE, Pires S, Branco R, Porto J. Predictive factors for intraoperative complications in semirigid ureteroscopy: analysis of 1235 ballistic ureterolithotripsies. Urology. 2008;72(4):770–4.
140. Miernik A, Wilhelm K, Ardelt PU, Adams F, Kuehhas FE, Schoenthaler M. Standardized flexible ureteroscopic technique to improve stone-free rates. Urology. 2012;80(6):1198–202.
141. Guzelburc V, Guven S, Boz MY, Erkurt B, Soytas M, Altay B, et al. Intraoperative evaluation of ureteral access sheath-related injuries using post-ureteroscopic lesion scale. J Laparoendosc Adv Surg Tech Part A. 2016;26(1):23–6.
142. Kramolowsky EV. Ureteral perforation during ureterorenoscopy: treatment and management. J Urol. 1987;138(1):36–8.
143. Lildal SK, Andreassen KH, Jung H, Pedersen MR, Osther PJS. Evaluation of ureteral lesions in ureterorenoscopy: impact of access sheath use. Scand J Urol. 2018;52(2):157–61.
144. Loftus CJ, Ganesan V, Traxer O, Schold JD, Noble M, Sivalingam S, et al. Ureteral wall injury with ureteral access sheaths: a randomized prospective trial. J Endourol. 2020;34(9):932–6.
145. Rashahmadi N, Sofimajidpour H, Saedi A, Moradi G. The effect of tamsulosin on the quality and complications of ureteroscopy: a double blind clinical trial. Med Sci. 2018;22(91):272–8.
146. Alsaikhan B, Koziarz A, Lee JY, Pace KT. Preoperative alpha-blockers for ureteroscopy for ureteral stones: a systematic review and meta-analysis of randomized controlled trials. J Endourol. 2020;34(1):33–41.
147. Alobaid K, Faty M, El-Nahas A, Al-Terki A, Khan Z. Renal fungus ball in a patient with retroperitoneal fibrosis: unique complication in a rare disease. Mycoses. 2018;61(6):410–6.
148. Sawazaki H, Yoshikawa T, Takahashi T, Taki Y, Takeuchi H. Ureteral avulsion: a rare complication of ureteroscopy. Hinyokika Kiyo. 2007;53(9):641–4.
149. Tanimoto R, Cleary RC, Bagley DH, Hubosky SG. Ureteral avulsion associated with ureteroscopy: insights from the MAUDE database. J Endourol. 2016;30(3):257–61.
150. Ordon M, Schuler TD, Honey RJ. Ureteral avulsion during contemporary ureteroscopic stone management: "the scabbard avulsion". J Endourol. 2011;25(8):1259–62.
151. Gaizauskas A, Markevicius M, Gaizauskas S, Zelvys A. Possible complications of ureteroscopy in modern endourological era: two-point or "scabbard" avulsion. Case Rep Urol. 2014;2014:308093.
152. Chotikawanich E, Korman E, Monga M. Complications of stone baskets: 14-year review of the manufacturer and user facility device experience database. J Urol. 2011;185(1):179–83.
153. Giusti G, Proietti S, Peschechera R, Taverna G, Graziotti P. Total ureteral replacement by means of Boari vesical flap and psoas hitching: a case report. Minerva Urol Nefrol. 2014;66(1):97–9.
154. Sewell J, Blecher G, Tsai K, Bishop C. Calculus-related ureteral intussusception: a case report and literature review. Int J Surg Case Rep. 2015;12:63–6.
155. Bernhard PH, Reddy PK. Retrograde ureteral intussusception: a rare complication. J Endourol. 1996;10(4):349–51.
156. Garvin TJ, Clayman RV. Balloon dilation of the distal ureter to 24 F: an effective method for ureteroscopic stone retrieval. J Urol. 1991;146(3):742–5.
157. Richter S, Shalev M, Lobik L, Buchumensky V, Nissenkorn I. Early postureteroscopy vesicoureteral reflux—a temporary and infrequent complication: prospective study. J Endourol. 1999;13(5):365–6.
158. El-Abd AS, Suliman MG, Abo Farha MO, Ramadan AR, El-Tatawy HH, El-Gamal OM, et al. The development of ureteric strictures after ureteroscopic treatment for ureteric calculi: a long-term study at two academic centres. Arab J Urol. 2019;12(2):168–72.
159. Roberts WW, Cadeddu JA, Micali S, Kavoussi LR, Moore RG. Ureteral stricture formation after removal of impacted calculi. J Urol. 1998;159(3):723–6.
160. Sharfi AR, Rayis AB. The continuing challenge of bilharzial ureteric stricture. Scand J Urol Nephrol. 1989;23(2):123–6.
161. Sener TE, Cloutier J, Audouin M, Villa L, Traxer O. A guidewire introducer as a ureteral foreign body: a case report. Can Urol Assoc J. 2015;9(5–6):E384–6.
162. Delvecchio FC, Auge BK, Brizuela RM, Weizer AZ, Silverstein AD, Lallas CD, et al. Assessment of stricture formation with the ureteral access sheath. Urology. 2003;61(3):518–22. discussion 22
163. Stern KL, Loftus CJ, Doizi S, Traxer O, Monga M. A prospective study analyzing the association between high-grade ureteral access sheath injuries and the formation of ureteral strictures. Urology. 2019;128:38–41.
164. Gokce MI, Telli O, Ozkidik M, Akinci A, Hajiyev P, Soygur T, et al. Evaluation of postoperative hydronephrosis following ureteroscopy in pediatric population: incidence and predictors. Urology. 2016;93:164–9.

165. Gokce MI, Esen B, Gulpinar B, Huseynov A, Ozkidik M, Suer E. Evaluation of postoperative hydronephrosis following semirigid ureteroscopy: incidence and predictors. Turk J Urol. 2017;43(2):171–5.
166. Barbour ML, Raman JD. Incidence and predictors for ipsilateral hydronephrosis following ureteroscopic lithotripsy. Urology. 2015;86(3):465–71.
167. Kim SW, Ahn JH, Yim SU, Cho YH, Shin BS, Chung HS, et al. Clinical factors associated with postoperative hydronephrosis after ureteroscopic lithotripsy. Investig Clin Urol. 2016;57(5):343–50.
168. Sutherland TN, Pearle MS, Lotan Y. How much is a kidney worth? Cost-effectiveness of routine imaging after ureteroscopy to prevent silent obstruction. J Urol. 2013;189(6):2136–41.
169. Harmon WJ, Sershon PD, Blute ML, Patterson DE, Segura JW. Ureteroscopy: current practice and long-term complications. J Urol. 1997;157(1):28–32.
170. Dretler SP, Young RH. Stone granuloma: a cause of ureteral stricture. J Urol. 1993;150(6):1800–2.
171. Doddamani D, Kumar R, Hemal AK. Stone granuloma—not to be forgotten as a delayed complication of ureteroscopy. Urol Int. 2002;68(2):129–31.
172. Narcisi F, Castellani D, Di Marco G, Fileni A, Galatioto GP, Mancinotti A, et al. Uncommon complication of endoscopic ureterolithotripsy: the stone granuloma. Int J Urol. 2006;13(3):289–90.
173. Giddens JL, Grotas AB, Grasso M. Stone granuloma causes ureteropelvic junction obstruction after percutaneous nephrolithotomy and antegrade endopyelotomy. J Urol. 2000;164(1):118–9.
174. Zhao LC, Weinberg AC, Lee Z, Ferretti MJ, Koo HP, Metro MJ, et al. Robotic ureteral reconstruction using buccal mucosa grafts: a multi-institutional experience. Eur Urol. 2017;73(3):419–26.
175. Tran G, Ramaswamy K, Chi T, Meng M, Freise C, Stoller ML. Laparoscopic nephrectomy with autotransplantation: safety, efficacy and long-term durability. J Urol. 2015;194(3):738–43.
176. Richter F, Irwin RJ, Watson RA, Lang EK. Endourologic management of benign ureteral strictures with and without compromised vascular supply. Urology. 2000;55(5):652–7.
177. Wolf JS Jr, Elashry OM, Clayman RV. Long-term results of endoureterotomy for benign ureteral and ureteroenteric strictures. J Urol. 1997;158(3 Pt 1):759–64.
178. Afane JS, Olweny EO, Bercowsky E, Sundaram CP, Dunn MD, Shalhav AL, et al. Flexible ureteroscopes: a single center evaluation of the durability and function of the new endoscopes smaller than 9 Fr. J Urol. 2000;164(4):1164–8.
179. Huynh M, Telfer S, Pautler S, Denstedt J, Razvi H. Retained digital flexible ureteroscopes. J Endourol Case Rep. 2017;3(1):24–7.
180. Abraham JB, Abdelshehid CS, Lee HJ, Box GN, Deane LA, Le T, et al. Rapid communication: effects of Steris 1 sterilization and Cidex orthophthalaldehyde high-level disinfection on durability of new-generation flexible ureteroscopes. J Endourol. 2007;21(9):985–92.
181. Multescu R, Geavlete B, Georgescu D, Geavlete P. Improved durability of flex-Xc digital flexible ureteroscope: how long can you expect it to last? Urology. 2014;84(1):32–5.
182. Traxer O, Dubosq F, Jamali K, Gattegno B, Thibault P. New-generation flexible ureterorenoscopes are more durable than previous ones. Urology. 2006;68(2):276–9.
183. Pietrow PK, Auge BK, Delvecchio FC, Silverstein AD, Weizer AZ, Albala DM, et al. Techniques to maximize flexible ureteroscope longevity. Urology. 2002;60(5):784–8.
184. Hubosky SG, Raval AJ, Bagley DH. Locked deflection during flexible ureteroscopy: incidence and elucidation of the mechanism of an underreported complication. J Endourol. 2015;29(8):907–12.
185. Anderson JK, Lavers A, Hulbert JC, Monga M. The fractured flexible ureteroscope with locked deflection. J Urol. 2004;171(1):335.
186. Wallace B, Nham E, Watterson J, Mahoney J, Skinner T. "Between a Rock and a Hard Place": a case report of stone fragment impaction causing a retained ureteroscope requiring open surgical intervention. J Endourol Case Rep. 2020;6(1):7–9.
187. Maghsoudi R, Amjadi M, Norizadeh D, Hassanzadeh H. Treatment of ureteral stones: a prospective randomized controlled trial on comparison of Ho:YAG laser and pneumatic lithotripsy. Indian J Urol. 2008;24(3):352–4.
188. Ray RP, Mahapatra RS, Mondal PP, Pal DK. Long-term complications of JJ stent and its management: a 5 years review. Urol Ann. 2015;7(1):41–5.
189. Slaton JW, Kropp KA. Proximal ureteral stent migration: an avoidable complication? J Urol. 1996;155(1):58–61.
190. Michalopoulos AS, Tzoufi MJ, Theodorakis G, Mentzelopoulos SD. Acute postoperative pulmonary thromboembolism as a result of intravascular migration of a pigtail ureteral stent. Anesth Analg. 2002;95(5):1185–8. table of contents
191. Sabnis RB, Ganpule AP, Ganpule SA. Migration of double J stent into the inferior vena cava and the right atrium. Indian J Urol. 2013;29(4):353–4.
192. Farshi AR, Roshandel MR. Intracardiac migration of ureteral double-J stent: a case report and review. Can Urol Assoc J. 2015;9(9–10):E661–4.
193. Ioannou CV, Velegrakis J, Kostas T, Georgakarakos E, Touloupakis E, Anezinis P, et al. Caval migration of a ureteral J-stent after simultaneous ureter and iliac vein perforation during its placement for obstructive pyelonephritis. Int Angiol. 2009;28(5):421–4.
194. Hajji M, Bennani MS, Bekkali S, Jroundi L. Intracaval migration of ureteral stent. J Belg Soc Radiol. 2015;99(1):28–30.
195. Arab D, Zadeh AA, Eskandarian R, Asaadi M, Ghods K. An extremely rare complication of ureteral pigtail stent placement: a case report. Nephro-urol Mon. 2016;8(3):e36527.
196. Falahatkar S, Hemmati H, Gholamjani MK. Intracaval migration: an uncommon complica-

tion of ureteral double-J stent placement. J Endourol. 2012;26(2):119–21.

197. Tang Z, Li D, Xiao L, Wan Y, Luo K, Huang L, et al. Re: Intracaval migration: an uncommon complication of ureteral double-J stent placement. (From: Falahatkar S, Hemmati H, Gholamjani Moghaddam K. J Endourol 2012;26:119–121). J Endourol. 2012;26(8):1100–1. author reply 2
198. Hastaoglu IO, Tokoz H, Kavlak E, Bilgen F. Double J ureteral stent displaced through the right ventricle. Interact Cardiovasc Thorac Surg. 2014;18(6):853–4.
199. Ozveren B, Sahin A. Re: Intracaval migration: an uncommon complication of ureteral double-J stent placement. (From: Falahatkar S, Hemmati H, Gholamjani Moghaddam K. J Endourol 2012;26:119–121). J Endourol. 2013;27(8):1069–71.
200. Marques V, Parada B, Rolo F, Figueiredo A. Intracaval misplacement of a double-J ureteral stent. BMJ Case Rep. 2018;2018:bcr2017221713.
201. Garrido Abad P, Fernandez Arjona M, Fernandez Gonzalez I, Santos Arrontes D, Pereira SI. Proximal migration of a Double J catheter: case report and review of the literature. Arch Esp Urol. 2008;61(3):428–31.
202. Li D, Xiao L, Tang Z, Qi L, Luo K, Huang L, et al. Management of intravenous migration of urologic catheter. Urology. 2013;82(1):248–52.
203. Hu C, Zhu A, Zhu X, Liang T, Lu X. Endovascular removal of a misplaced ureteral stent in the vena cava: a complication of ultrasound-guided percutaneous nephrolithotomy. Clin Case Rep. 2020;9(1):77–9.
204. Chathuranga Ambegoda ALAM, Sagara Ruwan Kumara MG, Sandamalee K, Abeygunasekera AM. Cystoscopic extraction of an inadvertently placed ureteral stent in inferior vena cava. Asian J Urol. 2020;7(4):373–5.
205. Wang D, Sun H, Yang C, Ding D, Qian W, Yu D. Management of a ureteral stent displaced into the abdominal aorta: a case report. Urology. 2020;144:e10–e4.
206. Kochhar G, Rudrawadi S, Rajan K, Laddha PJ. Black pearl in urology: inadvertent anastomosis of gonadal vein to ureter leading to malpostioning of stent into the inferior vena cava. Turk J Urol. 2019;45(−1):178–80.
207. Jiang C, Fu S, Chen J, Chen Y, Chen D, Mishra P, et al. Migration of a double J stent into the inferior vena cava. Medicine. 2019;98(20):e15668.
208. Hoekx L, Tilborghs S, Vaganée D, De Wachter S. Intravascular double J stent migration: a case report, review, and management algorithm. Urol Ann. 2019;11(1):93.
209. Mao X-W, Xu G, Xiao J-Q, Wu H-F. Ureteral double J stent displaced into vena cava and management with laparoscopy: a case report and review of the literature. World J Clin Cases. 2018;6(16):1160–3.
210. Fiuk J, Bao Y, Calleary JG, Schwartz BF, Denstedt JD. The use of internal stents in chronic ureteral obstruction. J Urol. 2015;193(4):1092–100.
211. Lee SW, Kim JH. Renocolic fistula secondary to a perinephric abscess: a late complication of a forgotten double J stent. J Korean Med Sci. 2009;24(5):960–2.
212. Singh V, Srinivastava A, Kapoor R, Kumar A. Can the complicated forgotten indwelling ureteric stents be lethal? Int Urol Nephrol. 2005;37(3):541–6.
213. Kumar S, Dutt UK, Navriya SC, Mammen KJ. Ileal ureteral substitution after "panureteral damage: a devastating complication of forgotten double-J stent". J Endourol Case Rep. 2020;6(3):217–9.
214. Coulier B, Lefebvre G. Forgotten ureteral double-J stent complicated by severe encrustation in the bladder. J Belg Soc Radiol. 2016;100(1):77.
215. Al-Hajjaj M, Kazan MN. Neglected double J stent for 8 years with giant bladder calculi formation: a case report. Urol Case Rep. 2020;32:101195.
216. Abdelaziz AY, Fouda WB, Mosharafa AA, Abelrasoul MA, Fayyad A, Fawzi K. Forgotten ureteral stents: risk factors, complications and management. Afr J Urol. 2018;24(1):28–33.
217. Kandemir A, Sönmez M. Treatment of fragmented and severely encrusted ureteral double-J stent forgotten for 11 years through multimodal endourological methods. Urol Ann. 2019;11(3):310.
218. Kim DS, Lee SH. Huge encrusted ureteral stent forgotten for over 25 years: a case report. World J Clin Cases. 2020;8(23):6043–7.
219. Sen V, Bozkurt HI, Yonguc T, Aydogdu O, Yarimoglu S, Degirmenci T, et al. Forgotten and fragmented ureteral J stent with stone formation: combined endoscopic management. Int Braz J Urol. 2015;41(3):602–3.
220. Lam JS, Gupta M. Tips and tricks for the management of retained ureteral stents. J Endourol. 2002;16(10):733–41.
221. Hameed BMZ, Shah MJ, Naik N, Amaresh M, Hegde P, Beary RH, et al. Are technology-driven mobile phone applications (Apps) the new currency for digital stent registries and patient communication: prospective outcomes using urostentz app. Adv Urol. 2021;2021:1–7.
222. Thomas A, Cloutier J, Villa L, Letendre J, Ploumidis A, Traxer O. Prospective analysis of a complete retrograde ureteroscopic technique with holmium laser stent cutting for management of encrusted ureteral stents. J Endourol. 2017;31(5):476–81.
223. Larkin S, Preston D. Where are the stents? A computerized tracking system to eliminate the forgotten ureteral stent. Urol Pract. 2015;2(3):106–8.
224. Ziemba JB, Ludwig WW, Ruiz L, Carvalhal E, Matlaga BR. Preventing the forgotten ureteral stent by using a mobile point-of-care application. J Endourol. 2017;31(7):719–24.
225. Molina WR, Pessoa R, Donalisio da Silva R, Kenny MC, Gustafson D, Nogueira L, et al. A new patient safety smartphone application for prevention of "forgotten" ureteral stents: results from a clinical pilot study in 194 patients. Patient Saf Surg. 2017;11(1):1.

226. Ulker V, Atalay HA, Cakmak O, Yucel C, Celik O, Kozacioglu Z. Smartphone-based stent tracking application for prevention of forgotten ureteral double-J stents: a prospective study. Int Braz J Urol. 2019;45(2):376–83.
227. Barnes KT, Bing MT, Tracy CR. Do ureteric stent extraction strings affect stent-related quality of life or complications after ureteroscopy for urolithiasis: a prospective randomised control trial. BJU Int. 2014;113(4):605–9.
228. Frohlich M, Fehr J, Sulser T, Eberli D, Mortezavi A. Extraction strings for ureteric stents: is there an increased risk for urinary tract infections? Surg Infect (Larchmt). 2017;18(8):936–40.
229. Huang J, Zhao Z, AlSmadi JK, Liang X, Zhong F, Zeng T, et al. Use of the ureteral access sheath during ureteroscopy: a systematic review and meta-analysis. PLoS One. 2018;13(2):e0193600.
230. Du K, Wang RS, Vetter J, Paradis AG, Figenshau RS, Venkatesh R, et al. Unplanned 30-day encounters after ureterorenoscopy for urolithiasis. J Endourol. 2018;32(12):1100–7.
231. Parulkar BG, Hopkins TB, Wollin MR, Howard PJ Jr, Lal A. Renal colic during pregnancy: a case for conservative treatment. J Urol. 1998;159(2):365–8.
232. Srirangam SJ, Hickerton B, Van Cleynenbreugel B. Management of urinary calculi in pregnancy: a review. J Endourol. 2008;22(5):867–75.
233. Matlaga B, Semins M. Management of urolithiasis in pregnancy. Int J Women's Health. 2013;5:599.
234. Smith CL, Kristensen C, Davis M, Abraham PA. An evaluation of the physicochemical risk for renal stone disease during pregnancy. Clin Nephrol. 2001;55(3):205–11.
235. Zhang S, Liu G, Duo Y, Wang J, Li J, Li C. Application of ureteroscope in emergency treatment with persistent renal colic patients during pregnancy. PLoS One. 2016;11(1):e0146597.
236. Buttice S, Lagana AS, Vitale SG, Netsch C, Tanidir Y, Cantiello F, et al. Ureteroscopy in pregnant women with complicated colic pain: is there any risk of premature labor? Arch Ital Urol Androl. 2017;89(4):287–92.
237. Johnson EB, Krambeck AE, White WM, Hyams E, Beddies J, Marien T, et al. Obstetric complications of ureteroscopy during pregnancy. J Urol. 2012;188(1):151–4.
238. Semins MJ, Trock BJ, Matlaga BR. The safety of ureteroscopy during pregnancy: a systematic review and meta-analysis. J Urol. 2009;181(1):139–43.
239. Somani BK, Dellis A, Liatsikos E, Skolarikos A. Review on diagnosis and management of urolithiasis in pregnancy: an ESUT practical guide for urologists. World J Urol. 2017;35(11):1637–49.
240. Cindolo L, Castellan P, Scoffone CM, Cracco CM, Celia A, Paccaduscio A, et al. Mortality and flexible ureteroscopy: analysis of six cases. World J Urol. 2016;34(3):305–10.
241. Bhanot R, Pietropaolo A, Tokas T, Kallidonis P, Skolarikos A, Keller EX, et al. Predictors and strategies to avoid mortality following ureteroscopy for stone disease: a systematic review from European Association of Urologists Sections of Urolithiasis (EULIS) and Uro-technology (ESUT). Eur Urol Focus. 2021. https://doi.org/10.1016/j.euf.2021.02.014.
242. Chang CP, Liou CC, Yang YL, Sun MS. Fatal gas embolism during ureteroscopic holmium: yttrium–aluminium–garnet laser lithotripsy under spinal anesthesia—a case report. Minim Invasive Ther Allied Technol. 2008;17(4):259–61.
243. Pedersen KV, Drewes AM, Frimodt-Moller PC, Osther PJ. Visceral pain originating from the upper urinary tract. Urol Res. 2010;38(5):345–55.
244. Oguz U, Sahin T, Senocak C, Ozyuvali E, Bozkurt OF, Resorlu B, et al. Factors associated with postoperative pain after retrograde intrarenal surgery for kidney stones. Turk J Urol. 2017;43(3):303–8.
245. Kourambas J, Byrne RR, Preminger GM. Does a ureteral access sheath facilitate ureteroscopy? J Urol. 2001;165(3):789–93.
246. Pathan SA, Mitra B, Straney LD, Afzal MS, Anjum S, Shukla D, et al. Delivering safe and effective analgesia for management of renal colic in the emergency department: a double-blind, multigroup, randomised controlled trial. Lancet. 2016;387(10032):1999–2007.
247. Hamidi N, Ozturk E, Yikilmaz TN, Atmaca AF, Basar H. The effect of corticosteroid on postoperative early pain, renal colic and total analgesic consumption after uncomplicated and unstented ureteroscopy: a matched-pair analysis. World J Urol. 2018;36(6):979–84.
248. Al-Kandari AM, Al-Shaiji TF, Shaaban H, Ibrahim HM, Elshebiny YH, Shokeir AA. Effects of proximal and distal ends of double-J ureteral stent position on postprocedural symptoms and quality of life: a randomized clinical trial. J Endourol. 2007;21(7):698–702.
249. Giannarini G, Keeley FX Jr, Valent F, Manassero F, Mogorovich A, Autorino R, et al. Predictors of morbidity in patients with indwelling ureteric stents: results of a prospective study using the validated Ureteric Stent Symptoms Questionnaire. BJU Int. 2011;107(4):648–54.
250. Joshi HB, Newns N, Stainthorpe A, MacDonagh RP, Keeley FX Jr, Timoney AG. Ureteral stent symptom questionnaire: development and validation of a multidimensional quality of life measure. J Urol. 2003;169(3):1060–4.
251. Penniston KL, Antonelli JA, Viprakasit DP, Averch TD, Sivalingam S, Sur RL, et al. Validation and reliability of the Wisconsin stone quality of life questionnaire. J Urol. 2017;197(5):1280–8.
252. Ragab M, Baldin N, Collie J, Tran MGB, Al-Hayek S, Parsy KS, et al. Qualitative exploration of the renal stone patients' experience and development of the renal stone-specific patient-reported outcome measure. BJU Int. 2020;125(1):123–32.
253. Joshi HB, Johnson H, Pietropaolo A, Raja A, Joyce AD, Somani B, et al. Urinary Stones and Intervention

Quality of Life (USIQoL): development and validation of a new core universal patient-reported outcome measure for urinary calculi. Eur Urol Focus. 2021;8(1):283–90.
254. Seklehner S, Sievert KD, Lee R, Engelhardt PF, Riedl C, Kunit T. A cost analysis of stenting in uncomplicated semirigid ureteroscopic stone removal. Int Urol Nephrol. 2017;49(5):753–61.
255. Jeong H, Kwak C, Lee SE. Ureteric stenting after ureteroscopy for ureteric stones: a prospective randomized study assessing symptoms and complications. BJU Int. 2004;93(7):1032–4.
256. Makarov DV, Trock BJ, Allaf ME, Matlaga BR. The effect of ureteral stent placement on post-ureteroscopy complications: a meta-analysis. Urology. 2008;71(5):796–800.
257. Clayman RV. Ureteric stenting after ureteroscopy for ureteric stones: a prospective randomized study assessing symptoms and complications. J Urol. 2005;173(6):2022.
258. Borboroglu PG, Amling CL, Schenkman NS, Monga M, Ward JF, Piper NY, et al. Ureteral stenting after ureteroscopy for distal ureteral calculi: a multi-institutional prospective randomized controlled study assessing pain, outcomes and complications. J Urol. 2001;166(5):1651–7.
259. Denstedt JD, Wollin TA, Sofer M, Nott L, Weir M, RJ DAH. A prospective randomized controlled trial comparing nonstented versus stented ureteroscopic lithotripsy. J Urol. 2001;165(5):1419–22.
260. Fröhlich M, Fehr J, Sulser T, Eberli D, Mortezavi A. Extraction strings for ureteric stents: is there an increased risk for urinary tract infections? Surg Infect. 2017;18(8):936–40.
261. Bloom J, Matthews G, Phillips J. Factors influencing readmission after elective ureteroscopy. J Urol. 2016;195(5):1487–91.
262. Kumar M, Pandey S, Aggarwal A, Sharma D, Garg G, Agarwal S, et al. Unplanned 30-day readmission rates in patients undergoing endo-urological surgeries for upper urinary tract calculi. Investig Clin Urol. 2018;59(5):321–7.
263. Mittakanti HR, Conti SL, Pao AC, Chertow GM, Liao JC, Leppert JT, et al. Unplanned emergency department visits and hospital admissions following ureteroscopy: do ureteral stents make a difference? Urology. 2018;117:44–9.
264. Kim TJ, Lee IJ, Lee JK, Lee HM, Jeong CW, Hong SK, et al. Analysis of factors affecting re-admission after retrograde intrarenal surgery for renal stone. World J Urol. 2018;37(6):1205–10.
265. Michel KF, Patel HD, Ziemba JB. Emergency department and hospital revisits after ambulatory surgery for kidney stones: an analysis of the Healthcare Cost and Utilization Project. Urolithiasis. 2021;49(5):433–41.
266. Carlos EC, Peters CE, Wollin DA, Winship BB, Davis LG, Li J, et al. Psychiatric diagnoses and other factors associated with emergency department return within 30 days of ureteroscopy. J Urol. 2019;201(3):556–62.
267. Chew BH, Brotherhood HL, Sur RL, Wang AQ, Knudsen BE, Yong C, et al. Natural history, complications and re-intervention rates of asymptomatic residual stone fragments after ureteroscopy: a report from the EDGE Research Consortium. J Urol. 2016;195(4 Pt 1):982–6.
268. Hendlin K, Weiland D, Monga M. Impact of irrigation systems on stone migration. J Endourol. 2008;22(3):453–8.
269. Kroczak T, Ghiculete D, Sowerby R, Ordon M, Lee JY, Pace KT, et al. Dual usage of a stone basket: stone capture and retropulsion prevention. Can Urol Assoc J. 2018;12(8):280–3.

Postoperative Care and Quality of Life After Flexible Ureteroscopy

Iliya Saltirov, Kremena Petkova, Ognyan Gatsev, Petar Petrov, Stefan Hristoforov, and Daniela Petrova

Abstract

Recent advancements in endoscopic technologies, disposables, and intracorporeal lithotripsy devices expanded the indications for flexible ureteroscopy (fURS) in the treatment of ureteral and renal stones, and increased its efficacy and safety. Postoperative care and follow-up are important stages of the surgical treatment and aim timely diagnosis and treatment of complications to reduce procedure-related morbidity. Apart from the surgical intervention, patients' quality of life is affected by the postoperative pain, presence of postoperative drainage (stent or nephrostomy), intra- and postoperative complications, absence from work, and economic burden, which may have an adverse impact on the reconvalescence period following minimally invasive management of stones. Therefore, understanding patients' needs and preferences is essential to optimize stone treatment and recurrence prevention, and reduce the impact of stone disease and intervention on patients' health and quality of life.

I. Saltirov (✉) · K. Petkova · O. Gatsev · P. Petrov
S. Hristoforov · D. Petrova
Department of Urology and Nephrology, Military Medical Academy, Sofia, Bulgaria
e-mail: saltirov@vma.bg; dan_petrova@abv.bg

Keywords

Flexible ureterorenoscopy · Endourology · Postoperative care · Quality of life · Urolithiasis

1 Postoperative Care Following fURS

1.1 Introduction

With the technical advancements during the last years, flexible ureteroscopy (fURS) has become a recommended minimally invasive treatment modality for renal stones, together with shockwave lithotripsy (SWL) and percutaneous nephrolithotomy (PCNL). Technological improvements such as miniaturization of the flexible endoscopes with better flexibility and visualization, the "chip on the tip" technology and an adequate working channel, accommodating both enough irrigation and working instruments, expanded the indications for fURS [1]. The combination of contemporary flexible endoscopes, high power laser systems (Holmium:YAG and Thulium fiber laser) and different disposables, made ureteroscopy an efficient and safe procedure for the treatment of ureteral and renal stones, irrespective of stone composition [2]. Contemporary indications for fURS are competing with those for SWL and

G. Zeng et al. (eds.), *Flexible Ureteroscopy*, https://doi.org/10.1007/978-981-19-2936-6_17

miniaturized PCNL (Mini-PNL)—mid-sized stones in the kidney up to 15–20 mm. Selected larger stones, stones in patients contraindicated for PCNL, or failure of the other treatment modalities, are also amenable to treatment with fURS. In these cases, fURS offers better stone-free rates compared to SWL and increased safety profile compared to PCNL [3].

fURS is a highly effective minimally invasive treatment option for stones in the upper urinary tract. Postoperative care and follow-up of patients aim at early diagnosis and treatment of complications and include the following:

- Observation of patients' overall medical condition in the early postoperative period.
- Evaluation of specific symptoms, which may be a manifestation of complications, occurring during the operation, or, in the early postoperative period.
- Monitoring for changes in the laboratory findings or postoperative imaging, which may be a manifestation of postureteroscopy complications.

1.2 Postoperative Care of Patients with Infectious Complications Following fURS

1.2.1 Risk Factors and Diagnosis

Postoperative fever and urinary tract infection (UTI) are common complications following fURS. Identification and treatment of risk factors for postoperative fever and infection are crucial to prevent these complications or to treat them successfully. Preoperative urine culture is mandatory before fURS. In patients with negative preoperative urine culture a single-dose antibiotic prophylaxis according to local resistance patterns is recommended before treatment [4–6]. Presence of preoperative UTI is a risk factor for septic complications following fURS, should be treated preoperatively with culture specific antibiotics [7, 8]. Patients with obstruction and infection are managed with drainage of the kidney and culture specific antibiotics, and definitive management of the stone is postponed, after the infection has been treated.

A positive intraoperative pelvic urine culture and stone culture are both risk factors for septic complications following fURS and should be collected, especially in female patients and patients with struvite stones and positive preoperative urine culture [9, 10]. Furthermore, the results of pelvic urine and stone cultures taken intraoperatively, would help guide antibiotic treatment in cases with postoperative infectious complications.

Reusable flexible ureteroscopes, increased intrarenal pressure intraoperatively, and longer operation duration are other risk factors for infectious complications following ureteroscopy [11–16]. Therefore, the team responsible for the postoperative care of the patient should be aware of the intraoperative details in order to monitor the patient for potential complications.

Other risk factors for infectious complications following fURS, which should be taken into consideration during the procedure and the postoperative care, are female gender, longer stent or nephrostomy dwelling time, presence of obstruction, struvite stones, higher stone burden, diabetes, and immunocompromised and elderly patients [9, 17, 18].

Patients with postoperative infectious complications following fURS should be monitored for the following symptoms: pain in the treatment area, fever, tachycardia, tachypnea, hypotonia, oligoanuria.

Patients usually experience some degree of pain in the treatment area in the early postoperative period. Severe pain may be an indicator of complication and should be investigated further. Renal colic pain may be due to obstruction from residual stone fragments, clots, postoperative ureteral oedema or mucosal proliferations from impacted stones. Presence of postoperative obstruction of the kidney is an important risk factor for infectious complications following fURS and can be easily identified on ultrasound in the postoperative period. In cases, when the ultrasound study cannot diagnose the level and cause of obstruction, a computed tomography (CT) may be indicated for the early diagnosis and treatment of complications.

The presence of fever, tachycardia, tachypnea, hypotonia, oligoanuria in the postoperative period are alarming symptoms, which require further investigation. The occurrence of Systemic Inflammatory Response Syndrome (SIRS) symptoms may be an indicator for a potential septic complication, which requires timely diagnosis and management. SIRS is defined as a clinical response to a nonspecific insult of either infectious or noninfectious origin [19]. SIRS is characterized by the presence of two or more of the following symptoms:

- Fever of more than 38 °C or body temperature less than 36 °C.
- Heart rate of more than 90 beats per minute.
- Respiratory rate of more than 20 breaths per minute or arterial carbon dioxide tension ($PaCO_2$) of less than 32 mm Hg.
- Abnormal white blood cell count (>12,000/μL or <4000/μL or >10% immature [band] forms) [19].

Till 2016, the definition of sepsis was systemic response to infection, defined as the presence of SIRS in addition to a documented or presumed infection [20]. However, the SIRS criteria do not indicate a life-threatening response and are present in many patients, who do not have an infection [21]. Therefore, sepsis was defined as a life-threatening organ dysfunction caused by a dysregulated host response to infection [22]. Despite the change in the definition, monitoring of the patient for symptoms, suggesting SIRS in the postoperative period, aids the early diagnosis and treatment of infectious complications following URS.

It is imperative to obtain urine and blood cultures in patients with signs of postoperative infection. Although the results would not be available immediately, it will help guide antibiotic treatment in the event of sepsis. Complete blood count and serum biochemistry should be obtained to check for leukocytosis, increased values of C-reactive protein (CRP) and serum urea and creatinine levels, which may indicate presence of infection and deterioration of renal function. Procalcitonin level is an important indicator of urosepsis, which may help with the early diagnosis and treatment [23].

1.2.2 Treatment

Successful treatment of postoperative infectious complications following fURS, relies on the early diagnosis and include resuscitation, supportive care, monitoring, broad-spectrum antimicrobial agents, and drainage. In cases with obstruction, drainage of the kidney with ureteral stent or nephrostomy tube should be done as soon as possible. Antibiotic therapy should start immediately with a culture specific antibiotic, in cases when preoperative urine culture is available, or, with broad-spectrum antibiotics, until postoperative urine and blood culture sensitivities are obtained. Supportive therapy with electrolyte and intravenous fluids is indicated to maintain adequate organ perfusion. Patients with signs of urosepsis should be transferred in intensive care units for monitoring and resuscitation.

1.2.3 Summary

With the rising number of fURS procedures for treatment of ureteral and renal stones worldwide, the risk of postoperative infectious complications is increasing. Despite the minimally invasive nature of fURS, postoperative urinary tract infection is one of the most common complications that can be even life-threatening.

Prevention and postoperative care of postoperative infectious complications in fURS is based on the following:

- Preoperative urine culture and antibiogram.
- Preoperative treatment of urinary tract infections.
- In cases with obstructed and infected kidneys—drainage of the kidney and culture specific antibiotic treatment, and postponed definitive treatment of the stone.
- In patients with negative preoperative urine culture—antibiotic prophylaxis according to local antibiotic resistance patterns and intraoperative pelvic or stone urine culture in cases with obstruction.
- Maintenance of low intrarenal pressure intraoperatively—no abrupt changes in irrigation fluid pressure; use of ureteral access sheath.
- Reducing operation duration up to 90 min. Patients with large stones should be counseled

preoperatively about the possibility of staged procedure.
- Strict adherence to disinfection and sterilization protocols for reusable flexible endoscopes.
- Postoperative drainage of the kidney in patients with infected stones, longer operation duration, intraoperative complications, or patients at increased risk of postoperative complications.

Postoperative follow-up of patients is essential to detect early symptoms of infectious complications. Early diagnosis and treatment is based on imaging, laboratory and microbiologic studies, and antibiotic and supportive therapy. Patients with signs of urosepsis should be transferred to intensive care units for monitoring and treatment.

1.3 Postoperative Care of Patients with Ureteral Injuries Following fURS

1.3.1 Risk Factors and Diagnosis

Miniaturization of endoscopes, advances in endoscopic imaging, and improvement in intracorporeal lithotripsy devices and disposables decreased the rate of intraoperative iatrogenic injuries of the ureter during ureteroscopy.

Intraoperative iatrogenic injuries of the ureter range from mucosal erosion, false passage and perforation to complete ureteral avulsion. These complications may occur during insertion of guidewires, catheters, ureteral access sheath (UAS) or ureteroscope, lithotripsy and stone extraction, as well as ureteroscope retraction out of the ureter. The risk factors for intraoperative complications include use of large-sized instruments, insertion of guidewires and other disposables without endoscopic and fluoroscopic guidance, use of excessive force, attempts on lithotripsy or stone basketing without good endoscopic visibility, use of larger ureteral access sheaths, stone basketing, surgeon experience, and technique [24–35]. Ureteral avulsion and intussusception are the most devastating complications of ureteroscopy. Ureteral avulsion is rare with reported in literature incidence between 0.05% and 0.9% [28, 31–34].

Iatrogenic ureteral injury is usually recognized during the procedure and treatment decisions are made intraoperatively. However, one should be aware that the ureteral injury might not be recognized intraoperatively. Therefore, patients should be monitored postoperatively in order to diagnose and treat it and avoid further complications.

The symptoms of ureteral perforation and urine extravasation, not recognized during the procedure, include pain in the lumbar area or the abdomen, nausea and/or vomiting, fever, or signs of urosepsis. Imaging studies (CT scan, retrograde or antegrade pyelography) reveal urine and contrast extravasation and retroperitoneal urinoma and/or hematoma with or without hydronephrosis, extravasation of contrast, and/or missing part of the ureter.

Treatment of ureteral perforation includes drainage of the kidney with ureteral stent or nephrostomy tube and antibiotic therapy in patients with signs of infection. Ureteral avulsion or major ureteral injuries are usually recognized intraoperatively and surgically repaired immediately or in a staged manner, following drainage of the kidney with nephrostomy tube. The surgical technique depends on the level and degree of injury and the length of the ureteral defect [25, 36]. Long-term complications include ureteral stricture formation and obstruction.

1.3.2 Summary

Intraoperative iatrogenic injuries of the ureter range from mucosal erosion, false passage and perforation to complete ureteral avulsion. Risk factors include forced manipulation of endoscopes and working instruments, large caliber instruments, basketing of proximal ureteral stones, impacted stones, and ureteral abnormalities. Iatrogenic ureteral injury is usually recognized during the procedure and treatment decisions are made intraoperatively. However, some injuries might not be diagnosed intraoperatively and patients should be monitored postoperatively in order to diagnose and treat it, and avoid further complications.

1.4 Postoperative Care of Patients with Hemorrhagic Complications Following fURS

1.4.1 Risk Factors and Diagnosis

Bleeding complications are relatively rare following URS and range from hematuria and compromised visualization, to subcapsular or perirenal hematoma, and arteriovenous fistula. The risk of bleeding complications following fURS is lower than after SWL and percutaneous nephrolithotomy (PCNL), making URS a recommended procedure for patients with bleeding diathesis or on anticoagulation therapy. However, fURS still carries a risk of bleeding complications, especially in anticoagulated patients.

Risk factors for postureteroscopy bleeding include severe hydronephrosis, thin renal cortex, high stone burden, hypertension, preoperative urinary tract infection, prior SWL or PCNL, increased intrarenal pressure, and longer duration of the procedure [37, 38].

Bleeding complications in the postoperative period are manifested with macroscopic hematuria, kidney pain, fever, hemoglobin drop with or without the need for hemotransfusion, and hemodynamic instability, which lead to the diagnosis [39]. Therefore, patients with suspected significant bleeding should be monitored closely in the postoperative period. Ultrasound study may reveal hydronephrosis due to obstruction from blood clots, subcapsular or perirenal hematoma. CT scan and renal angiography are indicated in patients with severe bleeding in order to diagnose the complication and decide on treatment.

1.4.2 Treatment

Treatment of bleeding complications following fURS is based on symptom severity, type of complication, and hemodynamic stability of the patient. Hemodynamically stable patients are treated with bed rest, antibiotics, adequate analgesia and hemostatic agents, and supportive therapy. Hemodynamic monitoring and laboratory studies are mandatory in the postoperative period. Mild bleeding usually resolves after drainage of the kidney with ureteral stent and supportive therapy. Cases with severe bleeding, needing transfusion, and hemodynamically unstable patients can be managed by angiography and selective embolization of the bleeding source. Surgical exploration is needed in cases when the bleeding cannot be managed by conservative approach or angiography.

Cases with perirenal or subcapsular hematoma, no signs of active bleeding and hemodynamically stable patient, can be treated conservatively till spontaneous resolution of the hematoma. Other treatment options include percutaneous drainage of the hematoma or surgical clot evacuation [39].

1.4.3 Summary

Bleeding complications are relatively rare following fURS and range from hematuria and compromised visualization, to subcapsular or perirenal hematoma. Patient monitoring in the postoperative period is essential in order to prevent life-threatening bleeding. Treatment of bleeding complications following fURS is based on the symptoms severity, type of complication and hemodynamic stability of the patient, and ranges from conservative treatment to surgical exploration and nephrectomy.

1.5 Pain Management Following fURS

Postoperative pain is common following fURS and ranges from mild discomfort to acute renal colic. The most common causes of postoperative pain are presence of ureteral catheter or stent, obstruction of the kidney from stone fragments, clots, and/or mucosal edema and inflammation from impacted stones or from the insertion of the ureteroscope and ureteral access sheath (UAS). Postoperative pain may be a symptom of complications from fURS and should be investigated. Ultrasound in the most commonly used imaging modality in the postoperative period following fURS. It may reveal presence of obstruction or other complication and aid diagnosis and treatment.

Postoperative renal colic is treated with nonsteroidal anti-inflammatory drugs (NSAIDs), metamizole and paracetamol, which have fewer side effects than opioid analgesics [7]. However, the use of NSAIDs should be reduced or used with caution in patients with increased cardiovascular risk and history of gastrointestinal complications [40]. Patients with contraindications for NSAIDs use may be treated with a short course of opioid analgesic in the early postoperative period.

Patients with renal colic and obstruction from stone fragments may be treated with medical expulsive therapy to promote spontaneous passage of stone fragments and pain relief [41]. Alpha-blockers have been used off-label to promote the spontaneous passage of stones due to their effects on smooth muscle contraction. Several meta-analyses have found a benefit of MET with higher and faster expulsion rate, lower analgesic requirements, fewer colic episodes, and fewer hospitalizations within treatment groups [41–43]. A more recent randomized study failed to demonstrate increased stone passage rates with alpha-blocker in 1136 patients, but was criticized for the fact that the need for surgery was used as a surrogate end point rather than radiologic testing and that more than 75% of the stones were smaller than 5 mm [44].

Persistent pain and obstruction, not amenable to conservative treatment, are indicated for drainage with ureteral stent or percutaneous nephrostomy or ureteroscopy to remove obstruction, stone fragments and prevent further complications, such as infection and renal function deterioration.

Postoperative pain may be a symptom of other complications following fURS, such as bleeding or formation of perirenal abscess. Therefore, patients should undergo imaging studies (ultrasound, CT scan), if a complication is suspected, in order to treat it in a timely manner. Treatment should be individualized and patients should be monitored closely to prevent further complications.

1.6 Postoperative Drainage Care Following fURS

Routine postoperative stenting is not indicated following fURS and should be done at surgeons' discretion in patients with increased risk of complications [7, 45].

Postoperative drainage of the kidney with ureteral catheter or stent is recommended in the following cases:

- Longer operation duration.
- Larger stone burden and multiple stone fragments.
- Impacted ureteral stones and significant ureteral edema and inflammation.
- Preoperative urinary tract infection.
- Hematuria.
- Residual stone fragments.
- Residual stone burden and staged procedure.
- Intraoperative complications.

Ureteral stenting is not indicated following uncomplicated procedure and clinically insignificant stone fragments <2 mm, in order to prevent stent-related symptoms in the postoperative period, and the need for auxiliary procedure for stent removal [7, 46]. Postoperative drainage with ureteral catheter for 24–48 h is an alternative to ureteral stenting following fURS. Drainage with ureteral catheter helps monitor urine output of the kidney and the presence of significant hematuria, which may indicate the occurrence of postureteroscopy complications. It is related to postoperative pain and discomfort and prolonged hospital stay, but access of the kidney is preserved in cases when ureteral stenting is necessary because of complications.

Stent dwelling time following fURS depends on the indication for ureteral stenting and the risk of infection and encrustation. In most of the cases stents are removed 1–4 weeks postoperatively. However, the optimal stent duration following fURS is not currently defined and stent dwelling time has not been shown to have an effect on residual fragments and postoperative hydronephrosis and ureteral stricture rate [47–49]. Patients should be aware of the presence of ureteral stent and the need for extraction and this should be noted in the medical papers of the patient to prevent complications of forgotten stents.

Ureteral stents often cause stent-related symptoms such as pain, hematuria, and lower urinary tract symptoms (LUTS). Patients should be informed about the possibility of experiencing stent-related symptoms in the postoperative period. Alpha-blockers and antimuscarinics have been shown to reduce stent associated morbidity and are indicated in the postoperative period in patients with ureteral stents [50–52].

Nephrostomy tubes are rarely needed following ureteroscopy, but are necessary in cases with obstruction or occurrence of complication, which cannot be managed by retrograde ureteral stent. Patients should be informed on the need for nephrostomy tube insertion and how to prevent its dislodgment out of the kidney. The team responsible for the postoperative care of the patient should monitor the urine output from the nephrostomy tube in order to diagnose and treat potential complications such as bleeding and tube obstruction.

1.7 Residual Fragments Following fURS

The goal of minimally invasive treatment of stone disease is to render the patient stone free with the minimum number of procedures, or to create small residual fragments, which can be eliminated spontaneously. The lithotripsy strategy during fURS, either dusting or fragmenting, depends on the available laser machine, stone characteristics, and surgeons' experience. It is recommended to extract fragments >2 mm, when possible, in order to prevent postoperative renal colic and obstruction. At the end of the procedure the collecting system should be inspected for clinically significant residual fragments or intraoperative complications. Postoperative follow-up of patients includes imaging studies (ultrasound, plain radiography, or CT scan) to detect residual fragments or obstruction. CT is the imaging study with highest sensitivity and specificity to detect residual stone fragments, but at a higher cost [7, 53].

The term clinically insignificant residual stone fragments (CIRFs), was introduced to define the presence of asymptomatic residual fragments smaller than 4 mm following minimally invasive treatment of stone disease. However, this definition is still controversial as there is no consensus regarding the size of the residual stone fragments, because multiple studies have shown that, the so called CIRFs, have the potential to cause obstruction, stone recurrence and regrowth [54–57]. In a study of Chew et al. fragments ≥4 mm were more likely to regrow ($p < 0.001$) and were associated with more complications ($p = 0.039$) [56]. Fragments ≥2 mm were more likely to grow with time ($p < 0.001$), but were not associated with complications or higher reintervention rates. Rebuck et al. showed that 20% of patients with residual stone fragments ≤4 mm following ureteroscopy, will experience a stone related event in 1.6 years, while the rest of the patients will, either pass their fragments spontaneously, or remain asymptomatic [57]. More recently, Iremashvili et al. found 42% residual stones rate following ureteroscopy [58]. Stone size larger than 2 mm was related to an increased risk of reintervention, and, out of the repeat procedures, 75% were done for a symptomatic stone episode.

Residual fragments are common after stone surgery and data in the literature shows, that small fragments are associated with a significant incidence of stone related events requiring reintervention. Therefore, patients should be followed-up after fURS for asymptomatic obstruction and regrowth of residual fragments. The surgeon should aim at complete stone clearance in order to prevent further stone-related events, additional costs, and impact on patients' health-related quality of life.

2 Quality of Life (QoL) Following fURS

Quality of life (QoL) **is defined as** the degree to which an individual is healthy, comfortable, and able to participate in or enjoy life events [59]. It is a subjective experience, which is difficult to be measured objectively. Urolithiasis can affect QoL in various aspects such as associated morbidity, need for hospitalization and surgical intervention, need for lifestyle and dietary modifications or medical treatment, loss of work time, and economic burden.

The main goal of the urologist, managing stone disease, is to treat the patient with the minimally invasive modality, which offers highest efficacy with minimal morbidity. However, the patients' perspective on the treatment takes into account not only the efficacy and safety of the procedure, but also the pain, impact on his/her QoL, reconvalescence period, and economic burden related to the procedure. When discussing treatment options with the patient, it is of importance to take into account that his/her QoL was impaired before the procedure by the presence of the stone, which is related to pain, urinary infection, emergency room visits, absence of work, need for medication, and so on. Therefore, measuring QoL is important when counseling stone patients on their treatment options.

A patient reported outcome measurement (PROM) is any report of the status of a patient's health condition that comes directly from the patient, without interpretation of the patient's response by a clinician or anyone else [60]. PROM is an instrument to objectively measure the effect of a disease or medical intervention on the health condition of the patient in order to guide treatment decisions, identify patient subgroups with lower QoL, and minimize the risk of complications. Recently, several PROMs specific to urolithiasis have been developed and validated [61–65].

Urolithiasis is a common condition with a relatively high recurrence rate, which affects QoL both in symptomatic and asymptomatic patients. Penniston et al. investigated the QoL in asymptomatic stone formers using the Wisconsin Stone Quality of Life (WiSQoL) questionnaire [66]. WiSQoL results were lower (worse QoL) among patients with stones versus those without, regardless of whether they knew their actual stone status [66]. Age, gender, and duration of stone disease were not associated with differences in QoL. In another study, the same authors evaluated QoL in stone formers, using the SF-36 Health Survey [67]. Impaired QoL was found in stone formers compared to healthy adults regarding general health and pain. Furthermore, female gender, depression, diabetes, hypertension, and overweight/obesity were related to lower QoL scores for many health domains [67]. Patel et al. evaluated the impact of urolithiasis on QoL using the Patient Reported Outcomes Measurement Information System (PROMIS) is an NIH validated questionnaire [65]. Out of the 103 patients, who completed the survey, 74% were recurrent stone formers. The authors found that stone formers had worse pain and physical function than the general population. The number of stone episodes and chronic medical conditions were associated with lower QoL, whereas medical therapy and prevention of stones improved QoL.

Interestingly, patient and urologist perceptions regarding medical treatment of stone disease were found to be different in a study by Bensalah et al. [68]. While the majority of patients in their study would adhere to a long-term medical therapy, rather than experience recurrent stone episodes or repeated interventions, most of the surveyed urologists perceived the opposite [68]. Therefore, understanding patients' needs and preferences is essential to optimize stone treatment and recurrence prevention, and reduce the impact of stone disease and intervention on patients' health and QoL.

Studying the effects of minimally invasive procedures for stone treatment on QoL is important when counseling patients. Postoperative pain, presence of postoperative drainage (stent or nephrostomy), absence from work, economic burden, and reconvalescence period are all factors influencing QoL following surgical intervention for stones. Several studies have found that surgical treatments are associated with lower QoL compared to medical treatment for stones [65, 69]. Hamamoto et al. compared QoL in 262 patients undergoing URS and SWL using the SF-36 Health Survey [70]. QoL was lower for the URS group on discharge despite the higher stone free rates. The longer hospital stay and increased postoperative pain in the URS group were associated with lower QoL scores. Similarly, Atis et al. showed lower pain and emotional well-being scores ($p = 0.012$ and $p = 0.011$, respectively) in the RIRS group compared to SWL [71]. Di Mauro et al. compared QoL between fURS and miniaturized PCNL in 60 patients with stones ≤25 mm with the WiSQoL questionnaire [72]. Interestingly, the authors found higher anxiety and depression scores in the fURS group (3 [range 0–15] vs. 15 [range 6–24], $p < 0.01$). There were no statistically significant differences in satisfaction scores ($p > 0.05$). However, pain scores were lower for the miniaturized PCNL group ($p < 0.05$). Increased stent dwelling time in the fURS group was significantly associated with lower QoL in their patient population.

Routine ureteral stenting is currently not recommended following an uncomplicated URS [7]. However, ureteral stents are commonly placed following fURS, especially in cases with longer procedure, larger stone burden, residual fragments, or presence of intraoperative complications. Ureteral stents have been shown to be associated with significant morbidity and stent-related symptoms such as pain, hematuria, and storage and voiding symptoms, which affect patients' everyday life and work performance, resulting in a negative economic impact [73–76]. The need for auxiliary procedure to remove the stent adds to the discomfort of the patient and increases the costs of treatment.

Joshi et al. analyzed the prevalence of stent-related symptoms and its impact on QoL with the ureteral stent symptom questionnaire (USSQ) [77]. Lower urinary tract symptoms were present in 78% of the patients, and more than 80% experienced pain affecting their daily activities. 58% of the patients had reduced work performance and negative economic impact [77]. Ureteral stents were associated with lower QoL, regarding mobility, ability to perform usual activities, and presence of pain or discomfort ($p < 0.001$). Similar results were reported by Leibovici et al. in a series of 135 patients with unilateral ureteral stents [75]. In their study ureteral stents were associated with significant stent-related symptoms in almost half of the patient population, and had significant negative impact on patients' QoL.

Recently, Ordonez et al. performed a systematic review and meta-analysis assessing the effects of postoperative ureteral stent placement after uncomplicated ureteroscopy [78]. Their findings suggested that stenting may reduce the number of unplanned return visits to the hospital, the need for opioid analgesics, ureteral stricture, and hospital readmission. However, the authors were uncertain of these findings due to the low quality of evidence. Therefore, the decision whether to place a stent or not should be individualized, weighing the benefits of stent placement versus its morbidity and impact on patients' QoL.

3 Patient Education and Decision-Making

Patient education and informed decision-making are an important part of treatment as patient's and surgeon's perspectives may differ significantly. Although URS is a minimally invasive procedure, it has an associated morbidity and reconvalescence period. Taking time to educate the patient on the procedure, the postoperative period and possible complications helps manage patients' expectations. Patients should be aware of the need for postoperative monitoring for residual fragments or late complications such as ureteral stricture, to prevent silent obstruction and loss of kidney function. The need for ureteral stenting and stent-related morbidity should be explained in details, as some patients have fear of ureteral stents and are worried to have an additional procedure for stent removal. It is imperative to inform the patient on the stent dwelling time and the need for stent removal, and this should be noted in patients' medical records in order to prevent complications from forgotten ureteral stents.

4 Conclusions

Recent improvements in endoscopic technologies, disposables, and intracorporeal lithotripsy devices expanded the indications of fURS in the treatment of ureteral and renal stones, and increased its efficacy and safety. Currently, the indications of fURS in stone disease are competing with those of SWL and PCNL. fURS is increasingly used in specific situations with proximal ureteral stones not amenable to semirigid URS, anatomical abnormalities, or in combination with PCNL to reduce the need for multiple nephrostomy tracts or perform antegrade ureteroscopy. The efficacy and safety of fURS alone or in combination with other minimally invasive treatment modalities reduced the need for secondary procedures and the impact of repeated interventions on patients' QoL.

The increased number of fURS procedures worldwide put an emphasis on endourologic training and education in order to prevent complications and increase stone-free rates. Apart from the surgical technique of fURS, surgeons should be aware of postoperative care and monitoring of patients in order to diagnose and treat complications in a timely manner to prevent significant patient morbidity. Good communication with the patient is essential when making treatment decisions. Surgeons should understand that the clinical outcomes do not always correlate with patient perceptions of their own health. The expected benefits of the procedure should be weighed against the pain, impact on QoL, reconvalescence period, and economic burden related to the intervention, and discussed with the patient. Understanding patients' needs and preferences is essential to optimize stone treatment and recurrence prevention, and reduce the impact of stone disease and intervention on patients' health and QoL.

References

1. Wendt-Nordahl G, Mut T, Krombach P, Michel MS, Knoll T. Do new generation flexible ureterorenoscopes offer a higher treatment success than their predecessors? Urol Res. 2011 Jun;39(3):185–8. https://doi.org/10.1007/s00240-010-0331-0.
2. Traxer O, Keller EX. Thulium fiber laser: the new player for kidney stone treatment? A comparison with holmium:YAG laser. World J Urol. 2020;38(8):1883–94. https://doi.org/10.1007/s00345-019-02654-5.
3. Geraghty R, Abourmarzouk O, Rai B, Biyani CS, Rukin NJ, Somani BK. Evidence for Ureterorenoscopy and laser fragmentation (URSL) for large renal stones in the modern era. Curr Urol Rep. 2015;16(8):54. https://doi.org/10.1007/s11934-015-0529-3.
4. Chew BH, Flannigan R, Kurtz M, Gershman B, Arsovska O, Paterson RF, Eisner BH, Lange D. A single dose of intraoperative antibiotics is sufficient to prevent urinary tract infection during ureteroscopy. J Endourol. 2016;30(1):63–8. https://doi.org/10.1089/end.2015.0511.
5. Wolf JS Jr, Bennett CJ, Dmochowski RR, Hollenbeck BK, Pearle MS, Schaeffer AJ. Urologic surgery antimicrobial prophylaxis Best practice policy panel. Best practice policy statement on urologic surgery antimicrobial prophylaxis. J Urol. 2008;179(4):1379–90. https://doi.org/10.1016/j.juro.2008.01.068.
6. Zisman A, Badaan S, Kastin A, Kravtsov A, Amiel GE, Mullerad M. Tailoring antibiotic prophylaxis for Ureteroscopic procedures based on local resistance profiles may Lead to reduced rates of infections and urosepsis. Urol Int. 2020;104(1–2):106–12. https://doi.org/10.1159/000503905.
7. Turk C, Skolarikos A, Neisius A, et al. EAU guidelines on urolithiasis. In: EAoUG Office, editor. EAU guidelines. Edn published at the 35th EAU Annual Meeting, Amsterdam. Arnhem, the Netherlands: European Association of Urology Guidelines Office; 2020.
8. Lo CW, Yang SS, Hsieh CH, Chang SJ. Effectiveness of prophylactic antibiotics against post-Ureteroscopic lithotripsy infections: systematic review and meta-analysis. Surg Infect. 2015;16(4):415–20. https://doi.org/10.1089/sur.2014.013.
9. Yoshida S, Takazawa R, Uchida Y, Kohno Y, Waseda Y, Tsujii T. The significance of intraoperative renal pelvic urine and stone cultures for patients at a high risk of post-ureteroscopy systemic inflammatory response syndrome. Urolithiasis. 2019;47(6):533–40. https://doi.org/10.1007/s00240-019-01112-6.
10. Eswara JR, Shariftabrizi A, Sacco D. Positive stone culture is associated with a higher rate of sepsis after endourological procedures. Urolithiasis. 2013;41(5):411–4. https://doi.org/10.1007/s00240-013-0581-8.
11. Sun J, Xu J, OuYang J. Risk factors of infectious complications following ureteroscopy: a systematic review and meta-analysis. Urol Int. 2020;104(1–2):113–24. https://doi.org/10.1159/000504326.
12. Ofstead CL, Heymann OL, Quick MR, Johnson EA, Eiland JE, Wetzler HP. The effectiveness of sterilization for flexible ureteroscopes: a real-world study. Am J Infect Control. 2017;45(8):888–95. https://doi.org/10.1016/j.ajic.2017.03.016.
13. Osther PJ, Pedersen KV, Lildal SK, Pless MS, Andreassen KH, Osther SS, Jung HU. Pathophysiological aspects of ureterorenoscopic management of upper urinary tract calculi. Curr Opin Urol. 2016;26(1):63–9. https://doi.org/10.1097/MOU.0000000000000235.
14. Osther PJS. Risks of flexible ureterorenoscopy: pathophysiology and prevention. Urolithiasis. 2018;46(1):59–67. https://doi.org/10.1007/s00240-017-1018-6.
15. Tokas T, Herrmann TRW, Skolarikos A, Nagele U. Training and research in urological surgery and technology (T.R.U.S.T.)-group. Pressure matters: intrarenal pressures during normal and pathological conditions, and impact of increased values to renal physiology. World J Urol. 2019;37(1):125–31. https://doi.org/10.1007/s00345-018-2378-4.

16. Auge BK, Pietrow PK, Lallas CD, Raj GV, Santa-Cruz RW, Preminger GM. Ureteral access sheath provides protection against elevated renal pressures during routine flexible ureteroscopic stone manipulation. J Endourol. 2004;18(1):33–6. https://doi.org/10.1089/089277904322836631.
17. Blackmur JP, Maitra NU, Marri RR, Housami F, Malki M, McIlhenny C. Analysis of Factors' Association with risk of postoperative urosepsis in patients undergoing ureteroscopy for treatment of stone disease. J Endourol. 2016;30(9):963–9. https://doi.org/10.1089/end.2016.0300.
18. Youssef RF, Neisius A, Goldsmith ZG, Ghaffar M, Tsivian M, Shin RH, Cabrera F, Ferrandino MN, Scales CD, Preminger GM, Lipkin ME. Clinical outcomes after ureteroscopic lithotripsy in patients who initially presented with urosepsis: matched pair comparison with elective ureteroscopy. J Endourol. 2014;28(12):1439–43. https://doi.org/10.1089/end.2014.0343.
19. Levy MM, Fink MP, Marshall JC, Abraham E, Angus D, Cook D, Cohen J, Opal SM, Vincent JL, Ramsay G. SCCM/ESICM/ACCP/ATS/SIS. 2001 SCCM/ESICM/ACCP/ATS/SIS international sepsis definitions conference. Crit Care Med. 2003;31(4):1250–6. https://doi.org/10.1097/01.CCM.0000050454.01978.3B.
20. Bone RC, Balk RA, Cerra FB, Dellinger RP, Fein AM, Knaus WA, Schein RM, Sibbald WJ. Definitions for sepsis and organ failure and guidelines for the use of innovative therapies in sepsis. The ACCP/SCCM consensus conference committee. American College of Chest Physicians/Society of Critical Care Medicine. Chest. 1992;101(6):1644–55. https://doi.org/10.1378/chest.101.6.1644.
21. Churpek MM, Zadravecz FJ, Winslow C, Howell MD, Edelson DP. Incidence and prognostic value of the systemic inflammatory response syndrome and organ dysfunctions in Ward patients. Am J Respir Crit Care Med. 2015;192(8):958–64. https://doi.org/10.1164/rccm.201502-0275OC.
22. Singer M, Deutschman CS, Seymour CW, Shankar-Hari M, Annane D, Bauer M, Bellomo R, Bernard GR, Chiche JD, Coopersmith CM, Hotchkiss RS, Levy MM, Marshall JC, Martin GS, Opal SM, Rubenfeld GD, van der Poll T, Vincent JL, Angus DC. The third international consensus definitions for sepsis and septic shock (Sepsis-3). JAMA. 2016;315(8):801–10. https://doi.org/10.1001/jama.2016.0287.
23. Sugimoto K, Adomi S, Koike H, Esa A. Procalcitonin as an indicator of urosepsis. Res Rep Urol. 2013;26(5):77–80. https://doi.org/10.2147/RRU.S42711.
24. Atis G, Arikan O, Gurbuz C, Yildirim A, Erol B, Pelit S, Ulus I, Caskurlu T. Comparison of different ureteroscope sizes in treating ureteral calculi in adult patients. Urology. 2013;82(6):1231–5. https://doi.org/10.1016/j.urology.2013.07.021.
25. De Coninck V, Keller EX, Somani B, Giusti G, Proietti S, Rodriguez-Socarras M, Rodríguez-Monsalve M, Doizi S, Ventimiglia E, Traxer O. Complications of ureteroscopy: a complete overview. World J Urol. 2020;38(9):2147–66. https://doi.org/10.1007/s00345-019-03012-1.
26. De Coninck V, Keller EX, Rodríguez-Monsalve M, Audouin M, Doizi S, Traxer O. Systematic review of ureteral access sheaths: facts and myths. BJU Int. 2018;122(6):959–69. https://doi.org/10.1111/bju.14389.
27. Schuster TG, Hollenbeck BK, Faerber GJ, Wolf JS Jr. Complications of ureteroscopy: analysis of predictive factors. J Urol. 2001;166(2):538–40. https://doi.org/10.1016/s0022-5347(05)65978-2.
28. Geavlete P, Georgescu D, Niţă G, Mirciulescu V, Cauni V. Complications of 2735 retrograde semirigid ureteroscopy procedures: a single-center experience. J Endourol. 2006;20(3):179–85. https://doi.org/10.1089/end.2006.20.179.
29. Somani BK, Giusti G, Sun Y, Osther PJ, Frank M, De Sio M, Turna B, de la Rosette J. Complications associated with ureterorenoscopy (URS) related to treatment of urolithiasis: the clinical research Office of Endourological Society URS global study. World J Urol. 2017;35(4):675–81. https://doi.org/10.1007/s00345-016-1909-0.
30. Baş O, Tuygun C, Dede O, Sarı S, Çakıcı MÇ, Öztürk U, Göktuğ G, İmamoğlu A. Factors affecting complication rates of retrograde flexible ureterorenoscopy: analysis of 1571 procedures-a single-center experience. World J Urol. 2017;35(5):819–26. https://doi.org/10.1007/s00345-016-1930-3.
31. de la Rosette J, Denstedt J, Geavlete P, Keeley F, Matsuda T, Pearle M, Preminger G, Traxer O, CROES URS Study Group. The clinical research office of the endourological society ureteroscopy global study: indications, complications, and outcomes in 11,885 patients. J Endourol. 2014;28(2):131–9. https://doi.org/10.1089/end.2013.0436.
32. Taie K, Jasemi M, Khazaeli D, Fatholahi A. Prevalence and management of complications of ureteroscopy: a seven-year experience with introduction of a new maneuver to prevent ureteral avulsion. Urol J. 2012;9(1):356–60.
33. Öğreden E, Oğuz U, Demirelli E, Benli E, Sancak EB, Gülpinar MT, Akbaş A, Reşorlu B, Ayyildiz A, Yalçin O. Categorization of ureteroscopy complications and investigation of associated factors by using the modified Clavien classification system. Turk J Med Sci. 2016;46(3):686–94. https://doi.org/10.3906/sag-1503-9.
34. Bhaskarapprakash AR, Karri L, Velmurugan P, Venkatramanan S, Natarajan K. Ureteral avulsion during semirigid ureteroscopy: a single-Centre experience. Surg Res Pract. 2020;19(2020):3198689. https://doi.org/10.1155/2020/3198689.
35. de la Rosette JJ, Skrekas T, Segura JW. Handling and prevention of complications in stone basketing. Eur Urol. 2006;50(5):991–8.; ; discussion 998-9. https://doi.org/10.1016/j.eururo.2006.02.033.
36. Georgescu D, Mulţescu R, Geavlete B, Geavlete P. Intraoperative complications after 8150 semirigid

ureteroscopies for ureteral lithiasis: risk analysis and management. Chirurgia (Bucur). 2014;109(3):369–74.
37. Bai J, Li C, Wang S, Liu J, Ye Z, Yu X, Xi Q, Ni M, He D. Subcapsular renal haematoma after holmium:yttrium-aluminum-garnet laser ureterolithotripsy. BJU Int. 2012;109(8):1230–4. https://doi.org/10.1111/j.1464-410X.2011.10490.x.
38. Tiplitsky SI, Milhoua PM, Patel MB, Minsky L, Hoenig DM. Case report: intrarenal arteriovenous fistula after ureteroscopic stone extraction with holmium laser lithotripsy. J Endourol. 2007;21(5):530–2. https://doi.org/10.1089/end.2006.0371.
39. Chiu PK, Chan CK, Ma WK, To KC, Cheung FK, Yiu MK. Subcapsular hematoma after ureteroscopy and laser lithotripsy. J Endourol. 2013;27(9):1115–9. https://doi.org/10.1089/end.2013.0128.
40. Coxib and traditional NSAID Trialists' (CNT) Collaboration, Bhala N, Emberson J, Merhi A, Abramson S, Arber N, Baron JA, Bombardier C, Cannon C, Farkouh ME, GA FG, Goss P, Halls H, Hawk E, Hawkey C, Hennekens C, Hochberg M, Holland LE, Kearney PM, Laine L, Lanas A, Lance P, Laupacis A, Oates J, Patrono C, Schnitzer TJ, Solomon S, Tugwell P, Wilson K, Wittes J, Baigent C. Vascular and upper gastrointestinal effects of non-steroidal anti-inflammatory drugs: meta-analyses of individual participant data from randomised trials. Lancet. 2013;382(9894):769–79. https://doi.org/10.1016/S0140-6736(13)60900-9.
41. Hollingsworth JM, Canales BK, Rogers MA, Sukumar S, Yan P, Kuntz GM, Dahm P. Alpha blockers for treatment of ureteric stones: systematic review and meta-analysis. BMJ. 2016;1(355):i6112. https://doi.org/10.1136/bmj.i6112.
42. Campschroer T, Zhu X, Vernooij RW, Lock MT. Alpha-blockers as medical expulsive therapy for ureteral stones. Cochrane Database Syst Rev. 2018;4(4):CD008509.
43. Seitz C, Liatsikos E, Porpiglia F, Tiselius HG, Zwergel U. Medical therapy to facilitate the passage of stones: what is the evidence? Eur Urol. 2009;56(3):455–71.
44. Pickard R, Starr K, MacLennan G, et al. Medical expulsive therapy in adults with ureteric colic: a multicentre, randomised, placebo-controlled trial. Lancet. 2015;386(9991):341–9.
45. Wang CJ, Huang SW, Chang CH. Indications of stented uncomplicated ureteroscopic lithotripsy: a prospective randomized controlled study. Urol Res. 2009;37(2):83–8. https://doi.org/10.1007/s00240-009-0175-7.
46. Denstedt JD, Wollin TA, Sofer M, Nott L, Weir M, D'A Honey RJ. A prospective randomized controlled trial comparing nonstented versus stented ureteroscopic lithotripsy. J Urol. 2001;165(5):1419–22.
47. Paul CJ, Brooks NA, Ghareeb GM, Tracy CR. Pilot study to determine optimal stent duration following ureteroscopy: three versus seven days. Curr Urol. 2018;11(2):97–102. https://doi.org/10.1159/000447201.
48. Auge BK, Sarvis JA, L'esperance JO, Preminger GM. Practice patterns of ureteral stenting after routine ureteroscopic stone surgery: a survey of practicing urologists. J Endourol. 2007;21(11):1287–91. https://doi.org/10.1089/end.2007.0038.
49. Pengfei S, Yutao L, Jie Y, Wuran W, Yi D, Hao Z, Jia W. The results of ureteral stenting after ureteroscopic lithotripsy for ureteral calculi: a systematic review and meta-analysis. J Urol. 2011;186(5):1904–9. https://doi.org/10.1016/j.juro.2011.06.066.
50. Zhou L, Cai X, Li H, et al. Effects of alpha-blockers, antimuscarinics, or combination therapy in relieving ureteral stent-related symptoms: a meta-analysis. J Endourol. 2015;29(6):650–6.
51. Beddingfield R, Pedro RN, Hinck B, et al. Alfuzosin to relieve ureteral stent discomfort: a prospective, randomized, placebo controlled study. J Urol. 2009;181(1):170–6.
52. Wang CJ, Huang SW, Chang CH. Effects of specific alpha-1A/1D blocker on lower urinary tract symptoms due to double-J stent: a prospectively randomized study. Urol Res. 2009;37(3):147–52.
53. Macejko A, Okotie OT, Zhao LC, Liu J, Perry K, Nadler RB. Computed tomography-determined stone-free rates for ureteroscopy of upper-tract stones. J Endourol. 2009;23(3):379–82. https://doi.org/10.1089/end.2008.0240.
54. Tan YH, Wong M. How significant are clinically insignificant residual fragments following lithotripsy? Curr Opin Urol. 2005;15(2):127–31. https://doi.org/10.1097/01.mou.0000160628.43860.f9.
55. Sarica K, Yuruk E. What should we do with residual fragments. Arch Esp Urol. 2017;70(1):245–50.
56. Chew BH, Brotherhood HL, Sur RL, Wang AQ, Knudsen BE, Yong C, Marien T, Miller NL, Krambeck AE, Charchenko C, Humphreys MR. Natural history, complications and re-intervention rates of asymptomatic residual stone fragments after ureteroscopy: a report from the EDGE research consortium. J Urol. 2016;195(4 Pt 1):982–6. https://doi.org/10.1016/j.juro.2015.11.009.
57. Rebuck DA, Macejko A, Bhalani V, Ramos P, Nadler RB. The natural history of renal stone fragments following ureteroscopy. Urology. 2011;77(3):564–8. https://doi.org/10.1016/j.urology.2010.06.056.
58. Iremashvili V, Li S, Penniston KL, Best SL, Hedican SP, Nakada SY. Role of residual fragments on the risk of repeat surgery after flexible ureteroscopy and laser lithotripsy: single center study. J Urol. 2019;201(2):358–63. https://doi.org/10.1016/j.juro.2018.09.053.
59. Jenkinson C. Quality of life. Encyclopædia Britannica Date Published: May 06, 2020. Available at: https://www.britannica.com/topic/quality-of-life. Accessed: January 15, 2021.
60. US Food and Drug Administration. Patient reported outcome measures: use in medical product development to support labelling claims. In: Guidance for industry. Rockville, MD: US FDA; 2009.

61. Penniston KL, Antonelli JA, Viprakasit DP, Averch TD, Sivalingam S, Sur RL, Pais VM Jr, Chew BH, Bird VG, Nakada SY. Validation and reliability of the Wisconsin stone quality of life questionnaire. J Urol. 2017;197(5):1280–8. https://doi.org/10.1016/j.juro.2016.11.097.
62. Talwar R, Ziemba J. Validated methods of assessing quality of life in stone disease. Curr Urol Rep. 2018;19(4):25. https://doi.org/10.1007/s11934-018-0776-1.
63. Joshi HB, Johnson H, Pietropaolo A, Raja A, Joyce AD, Somani B, Philip J, Biyani CS, Pickles T. Urinary stones and intervention quality of life (USIQoL): development and validation of a new Core universal patient-reported outcome measure for urinary calculi. Eur Urol Focus. 2021;S2405–4569(20):30313–8. https://doi.org/10.1016/j.euf.2020.12.011.
64. Newnham EA, Harwood KE, Page AC. Evaluating the clinical significance of responses by psychiatric inpatients to the mental health subscales of the SF-36. J Affect Disord. 2007;98(1–2):91–7. https://doi.org/10.1016/j.jad.2006.07.001.
65. Patel N, Brown RD, Sarkissian C, De S, Monga M. Quality of life and urolithiasis: the patient - reported outcomes measurement information system (PROMIS). Int Braz J Urol. 2017;43(5):880–6. https://doi.org/10.1590/S1677-5538.
66. Penniston KL, Sninsky BC, Nakada SY. Preliminary evidence of decreased disease-specific health-related quality of life in asymptomatic stone patients. J Endourol. 2016;30(Suppl 1):S42–5. https://doi.org/10.1089/end.2016.0074.
67. Penniston KL, Nakada SY. Health related quality of life differs between male and female stone formers. J Urol. 2007;178(6):2435–40.; ; discussion 2440. https://doi.org/10.1016/j.juro.2007.08.009.
68. Bensalah K, Tuncel A, Raman JD, Bagrodia A, Pearle M, Lotan Y. How physician and patient perceptions differ regarding medical management of stone disease. J Urol. 2009;182(3):998–1004. https://doi.org/10.1016/j.juro.2009.05.025.
69. Bensalah K, Tuncel A, Gupta A, Raman JD, Pearle MS, Lotan Y. Determinants of quality of life for patients with kidney stones. J Urol. 2008;179(6):2238–43.; ; discussion 2243. https://doi.org/10.1016/j.juro.2008.01.116.
70. Hamamoto S, Unno R, Taguchi K, Naiki T, Ando R, Okada A, Inoue T, Okada S, AbdelRazek M, Kohri K, Yasui T. SMART study group. Determinants of health-related quality of life for patients after urinary lithotripsy: ureteroscopic vs. shock wave lithotripsy. Urolithiasis. 2018;46(2):203–10. https://doi.org/10.1007/s00240-017-0972-3.
71. Atis G, Culpan M, Ucar T, Sendogan F, Kazan HO, Yildirim A. The effect of shock wave lithotripsy and retrograde intrarenal surgery on health-related quality of life in 10-20 mm renal stones: a prospective randomized pilot study. Urolithiasis. 2021;49(3):247–53. https://doi.org/10.1007/s00240-020-01219-1.
72. Di Mauro D, La Rosa VL, Cimino S, Di Grazia E. Clinical and psychological outcomes of patients undergoing retrograde intrarenal surgery and miniaturised percutaneous nephrolithotomy for kidney stones. A preliminary study. Arch Ital Urol Androl. 2020;91(4):256–60. https://doi.org/10.4081/aiua.2019.4.256.
73. Damiano R, Autorino R, De Sio M, Cantiello F, Quarto G, Perdonà S, Sacco R, D'Armiento M. Does the size of ureteral stent impact urinary symptoms and quality of life? A prospective randomized study. Eur Urol. 2005;48(4):673–8. https://doi.org/10.1016/j.eururo.2005.06.006.
74. Joshi HB, Stainthorpe A, Keeley FX Jr, MacDonagh R, Timoney AG. Indwelling ureteral stents: evaluation of quality of life to aid outcome analysis. J Endourol. 2001;15(2):151–4. https://doi.org/10.1089/089277901750134421.
75. Leibovici D, Cooper A, Lindner A, Ostrowsky R, Kleinmann J, Velikanov S, Cipele H, Goren E, Siegel YI. Ureteral stents: morbidity and impact on quality of life. Isr Med Assoc J. 2005;7(8):491–4.
76. Staubli SE, Mordasini L, Engeler DS, Sauter R, Schmid HP, Abt D. Economic aspects of morbidity caused by ureteral stents. Urol Int. 2016;97(1):91–7. https://doi.org/10.1159/000443379.
77. Joshi HB, Stainthorpe A, MacDonagh RP, Keeley FX Jr, Timoney AG, Barry MJ. Indwelling ureteral stents: evaluation of symptoms, quality of life and utility. J Urol. 2003;169(3):1065–9.; ; discussion 1069. https://doi.org/10.1097/01.ju.0000048980.33855.90.
78. Ordonez M, Hwang EC, Borofsky M, Bakker CJ, Gandhi S, Dahm P. Ureteral stent versus no ureteral stent for ureteroscopy in the management of renal and ureteral calculi. Cochrane Database Syst Rev. 2019;2(2):CD012703. https://doi.org/10.1002/14651858.CD012703.pub2.

Disposable Flexible Ureteroscopes

Silvia Proietti, Maria Pia Pavia, Luis Rico,
Yuyi Yeow, Mario Basulto-Martinez,
and Guido Giusti

Abstract

Currently, there are a variety of flexible ureteroscopes available, including fiber-optic and digital flexible ureteroscopes. Despite the technological advancement of flexible ureteroscopes, durability remains a major concern.

Disposable flexible ureteroscopes aim at overcoming the main boundaries of their reusable counterparts.

Herein, we report the characteristics, advantages, and limitations of single-use flexible ureteroscopes, according to the current studies published in literature.

Keywords

Disposable · Single-use · Digital · Flexible ureteroscope · Flexible ureteroscopy

1 Introduction

With the advancement of technology and improved laser lithotripsy, flexible ureteroscopy (fURS) has become an attractive and widespread option among the urology community for surgical management of kidney stones.

In some countries, fURS has become the most utilized surgical treatment modality, exceeding external shock wave lithotripsy by over 30% [1].

The first description of flexible ureteroscope (FU) was provided by Marshall in 1964 (Marshall) and then the technique was promoted by Bagley et al., who first reported their preliminary outcomes of stones treated by means of FUs [2].

Currently, there is a variety of flexible ureteroscopes available, including fiber-optic and digital FUs. Despite the technological advancement of flexible ureteroscopes, durability remains a major concern [3].

Due to the high cost and limited durability, the cost-benefit of these permanent reusable scopes continues to be the most important factor for initiating and maintaining fURS programs worldwide, especially in developing countries.

Therefore, to address these cost-related concerns, manufacturers recently developed disposable FUs.

Herein, we report the characteristics, advantages, and limitations of single-use FUs, according to the current studies published in literature.

S. Proietti (✉) · M. P. Pavia · L. Rico · Y. Yeow
M. Basulto-Martinez · G. Giusti
European Training Center in Endourology,
Department of Urology, San Raffaele Hospital,
IRCCS, Milan, Italy

G. Zeng et al. (eds.), *Flexible Ureteroscopy*, https://doi.org/10.1007/978-981-19-2936-6_18

2 Disposable Flexible Ureteroscopes: From Past to Present

The concept of FUs is not completely new. In fact, some models have reached the market in the past including SemiFlex, Polyscope, and FlexorVue. They might be considered as semidisposable flexible scopes rather than fully single-use FUs.

In 2009, Boylu et al. introduced the SemiFlex Scope characterized by a reusable eyepiece and a SemiFlex shaft and therefore marketed as a "disposable multiuse" scope [4]. The authors compared this device to six different fiber-optic scopes showing slightly inferior results in terms of deflection, visibility, and flow rate. However, no further studies were published after this initial report.

In 2011, Polyscope was introduced in the market; it is composed by a reusable fiber-optic core and disposable actively deflectable multilumen deflectable catheters. Gu et al. showed good results in terms of stone-free rate and an acceptable safety profile [5]. Probably, its complicated and peculiar assembly and functioning of Polyscope together with the fiber-optic vision might be some of the reasons why it did not become a real game changer in endourology.

A concept similar to Polyscope's one was adopted during the manufacturing of FlexorVue (Cook, Bloomington, USA).

However, the large size of 15Fr of this device with the unsatisfactory results in terms of effectiveness [6] led to its withdrawal from the market in 2018.

The real breakthrough in endourology was reached with the introduction in 2015 of the first digital single-use flexible ureteroscope, LithoVue® (Boston Scientific, Marlborough, USA), that has embodied an important step forward.

Proietti et al. published the first study on LithoVue in fresh human cadavers demonstrating that this device was comparable to conventional scopes in terms of visibility and manipulation into the collecting system [7].

Since then several studies have been published in literature on single-use FUs, showing good outcomes in terms of effectiveness and safety [8–10].

To date, more than 15 single FUs are available in the market, albeit, for most of them, data regarding their clinical effectiveness are substantially missing.

3 Image Quality

The image quality of FUs is a fundamental characteristic for a successful management of urinary stones.

Concerning image quality, recent studies have compared disposable and reusable, fiber-optic or digital FUs in terms of image resolution, color reproducibility, contrast, field of view, and distortion.

Dale and colleagues demonstrated in vitro that LithoVue resolution was comparable with Flex-XC and superior to Cobra [11], and furthermore it produced less image distortion than its reusable counterparts.

In another in vitro study, LithoVue resulted having a better evaluation than all fiber-optic scopes and Olympus V2 and Cobra Vision [12].

Dragos et al. compared in vitro 4 single-use FUs versus their digital reusable counterparts and they found that reusable digital FUs had better vision characteristics than single-use FUs [13].

In conclusion, single-use FUs demonstrated superior image quality when compared to fiber-optic FUs and comparable/inferior, depending on the studies, to digital reusable FUs.

It is noteworthy, however, that, to date, no studies have confirmed these findings in vivo.

4 Performance

There are many factors influencing performance status of FUs.

First of all, considering the complex renal anatomy, access to all parts of the renal collecting system, in particular lower-pole calyces, can be challenging [14].

Thus, ureteroscope deflection, maneuverability, flow rate and stone clearance are factors affecting the performance of single-use FUs [6–7, 15–16].

Dale et al. showed that LithoVue maintained full deflection ability with instruments inside the working channel, while Storz Flex-XC and Wolf Cobra lost deflection ranging from 2° to 27°. With the empty channel, LithoVue exhibited the greatest degree of deflection and a flow rate comparable to Flex-XC. Moreover, LithoVue showed better flow rates than both Flex-XC and Wolf Cobra with an empty working channel, as well as with instruments inside [11].

Dragos et al. demonstrated that single-use FUs had superior in vitro deflection characteristics compared to the reusable FUs, in most settings, but at the end of the tests, deflection loss was noted in most of the single-use FUs, while none of the reusable FUs showed any deflection impairment. Irrespective of deflection, the single-use FUs had better irrigation flow than their reusable counterparts [13].

A comprehensive European multicentric study reported that LithoVue maneuverability was rated as very good in 72.5% and good in 17.5% [8]; another multicenter international study showed that the Uscope maneuverability was rated as good and very good in 38 and 52% of cases, respectively [17].

As already mentioned, several other single-use FUs are available on the market but the lack of clinical data does not allow to conclude about their effectiveness and performance.

5 Ergonomics

Ergonomics is the scientific discipline concerned with the understanding of relationships between people and their working environment, especially the equipment they use, in order to optimize human well-being and overall system performance.

Recently, there has been an increased interest on surgeons' occupational health and the ergonomics of FUs has also been exponentially investigated, with a steadily increasing number of studies on hand problems among endourologists [18–19].

With this concept in mind, Ludwig et al. analysed the electrical activity of muscles activated during flexible ureteroscopy [20]; they demonstrated that both single-use and reusable digital FUs had similar ergonomic profiles and better than those of fiber-optic FUs, because they required less significantly less muscle activation and fatigue.

The Authors hypothesized that these findings could be related to the FUs weight.

As a matter of fact, Proietti et al. found that fiber-optic reusable FUs in their integrity, were heavier than their counterparts of digital scopes. Moreover, they demonstrated that LithoVue was the lightest scope among those included in the study [21].

In addition, it should be mentioned that one limitation of the study by Ludwig et al. was that the procedures in a kidney model were relatively short in duration. In real life, fURS are longer and, especially in high-volume centers, can be performed more than one in a single day; therefore, there could surely result in an accumulation of muscular fatigue. As suggested by Moore et al., the disposable FUs have the potential to decrease surgeons' fatigue and, consequently, improve surgical performance [14].

Teplitsky et al. evaluated the forces required to deflect five different ureteroscopes, 2 reusable fiber-optic and three single-use FUs.

The Storz Flex-X2 showed higher forces of deflection compared to the others; the URF-P6 most often required the least force deflection but it was unable to fully deflect with some devices within the working channel.

The single-use FUs reported intermediate results among the aforementioned; these results highlighted the importance of the ureteroscope design and the need of balancing the lightweight and the force for deflection [22].

6 Cost-Effectiveness

To date, the cost-effectiveness of single-use FUs is still an issue of concern.

The procedural cost of reusable FU is based on the initial acquisition, repair costs, maintenance, scope sterilization/disinfection and on the number of procedures performed before it needs to be repaired/replaced, whereas the cost of disposable FU is dependent only on the initial purchase price.

In literature, there are several studies that compare the cost of reusable and disposable FUs, but due to the heterogeneity in cost comparison, it is difficult to analyze costs across the studies.

Nevertheless, it has been shown that the financial viability of fURS is based on case volume, rates of reusable FUs repair and market price of the single-use FUs.

Therefore, relying on this concept, Martin et al. demonstrated, in their cost–benefit analysis conducted in the USA, that single-use FUs may be cost-effective at centers with lower case volumes per year, whereas high-volume centers may find reusable FUs cost beneficial [23].

In addition, the cost of single-use FUs seems to be different across the countries and manufacturers and depending also on the discounts given for the amount of usage; however, these costs seem to vary between $700 and $1500 [24].

Of importance, also, the amount of reimbursement for the procedure by the health care systems and the cost coverage of single-use FU by private insurances.

Another important issue is concerning the direct access to the sterilization unit; the lack of these facilities for some urologists implies higher sterilization costs and administrative work associated with external providers that might favor the use of single-use FUs instead of the reusable ones [25].

In conclusion, the cost-effectiveness of fURS program is based on several aspects and not only on acquisition cost itself.

Single-use FUs represents already a reality and they will progressively become the standard devices for fURS, once the manufacturing price falls.

7 Environmental Impact

Despite the growing interest on environmental health, little attention has been given to the environmental impact of FUs.

Davis and colleagues in a recent study examined the carbon footprint of LithoVue and Olympus URV-F. They collected and analyzed data regarding the carbon cost of ureteroscope manufacturing, sterilization, repairs, replacements, and disposal of both instruments and concluded that LithoVue had slightly lower carbon footprint than Olympus URV-F (4.43 vs. 4.47, respectively) [26].

Undoubtedly, the single-us FUs generate an increase of plastic waste products, but on the other hand, the lack of the sterilization process could be more environmentally friendly.

It is noteworthy that none of the single-use FU manufacturers have created a preferred pathway for waste recycling of these devices [27].

However, in the era of increasing awareness for human-induced climate change, further research is needed to fully establish the real environmental impact of these instruments.

8 Single-Use Flexible Ureteroscopes: Clinical Indications

We still lack official recommendations for the use of disposable FUs, as well as robust clinical data that shows a substantial advantage of single-use over reusable FUs.

Somani et al. suggested some indications for disposable FUs [28].

1. Lower pole kidney stones, greater than 1 cm.
2. Large renal stones (>2 cm).
3. Patients with of urinary diversion or abnormal renal anatomy.
4. Patients with stones and previous urosepsis or multiresistant preoperative urinary culture.

Another indication for disposable FUs may be for the training in fURS, in particular in university hospitals where a residency program is present and unexperienced surgeons might increase the risk of scopes' breakage.

Moreover, single-use FUs could be a reasonable alternative in immunocompromised patients, avoiding the risk of cross-contamination.

Finally, when an hospital cannot afford to acquire and maintain 2 traditional reusable FUs, the availability of disposable FUs in the operating room might be the solution to finish a case when the instrument failure happens during the surgery, avoiding any risk of surgical postponement or any other legal and ethical consequences [29].

In summary, single-use FUs may be appropriate for those procedures that carry an increased risk of instrument breakage or in those hospitals where there is a high rate of FU damage or when there is the need to eliminate any risk of cross-contamination.

9 Conclusion

The main advantages on the use of single-use FUs are embedded into the rationale behind the development of these instruments: immediate availability of an ever-new tool with no risk of cross-contamination.

In the next future, once the price falls down and the quality increases more and more, the single-use FUs will completely replace the reusable counterparts in the endourological armamentarium.

References

1. Ordon M, Urbach D, Mamdani M, et al. The surgical management of kidney stone disease: a population based time series analysis. J Urol. 2014;192(5):1450–6. https://doi.org/10.1016/j.juro.2014.05.095.
2. Bagley DH. Flexible ureteropyeloscopy with modular, "disposable" endoscope. Urology. 1987;29(3):296–300. https://doi.org/10.1016/0090-4295(87)90074-4.
3. Carey RI, Gomez CS, Maurici G, et al. Frequency of ureteroscope damage seen at a tertiary care center. J Urol. 2006;176(2):607–10. https://doi.org/10.1016/j.juro.2006.03.059.
4. Boylu U, Oommen M, Thomas R, et al. In vitro comparison of a disposable flexible ureteroscope and conventional flexible ureteroscopes. J Urol. 2009;182(5):2347–51. https://doi.org/10.1016/j.juro.2009.07.031.
5. Gu SP, Huang YT, You ZY, et al. Clinical effectiveness of the PolyScope™ endoscope system combined with holmium laser lithotripsy in the treatment of upper urinary calculi with a diameter of less than 2 cm. Exp Ther Med Aug. 2013;6(2):591–5. https://doi.org/10.3892/etm.2013.1184.
6. Schlager D, Hein S, Obaid MA, et al. Performance of Single-Use FlexorVue vs Reusable BoaVision Ureteroscope for Visualization of Calices and Stone Extraction in an Artificial Kidney Model. J Endourol. 2017;31(11):1139–44. https://doi.org/10.1089/end.2017.0454.
7. Proietti S, Dragos L, Molina W, et al. Comparison of New Single-Use Digital Flexible Ureteroscope Versus Nondisposable Fiber Optic and Digital Ureteroscope in a Cadaveric Model. J Endourol. 2016;30(6):655–9. https://doi.org/10.1089/end.2016.0051.
8. Doizi S, Kamphuis G, Giusti G, et al. First clinical evaluation of a new single-use flexible ureteroscope (LithoVue™): a European prospective multicentric feasibility study. World J Urol. 2017;35(5):809–18. https://doi.org/10.1007/s00345-016-1936-x.
9. Usawachintachit M, Isaacson DS, Taguchi K, et al. A Prospective Case-Control Study Comparing LithoVue, a Single-Use, Flexible Disposable Ureteroscope, with Flexible, Reusable Fiber-Optic Ureteroscopes. J Endourol. 2017;31(5):468–75. https://doi.org/10.1089/end.2017.0027.
10. Ozimek T, Schneider MH, Hupe MC, et al. Retrospective Cost Analysis of a Single-Center Reusable Flexible Ureterorenoscopy Program: A Comparative Cost Simulation of Disposable fURS as an Alternative. J Endourol. 2017;31(12):1226–30. https://doi.org/10.1089/end.2017.0427.
11. Dale J, Kaplan AG, Radvak D, et al. Evaluation of a Novel Single-Use Flexible Ureteroscope. J Endourol. 2017;35(6):903–7. https://doi.org/10.1089/end.2016.0237.
12. Talso M, Proietti S, Emiliani E, et al. Comparison of flexible ureterorenoscope quality of vision: an in vitro study. J Endourol. 2018;32(6):523–8. https://doi.org/10.1089/end.2017.0838.
13. Dragos LB, Somani BK, Keller EX, et al. Characteristics of current digital single-use flexible ureteroscopes versus their reusable counterparts: an in-vitro comparative analysis. Transl Androl Urol. 2019;8(Suppl 4):S359–70. https://doi.org/10.21037/tau.2019.09.17.
14. Moore B, Proietti S, Giusti G, et al. Single-Use Ureteroscopes. Urol Clin North Am. 2019;46(2):165–74. https://doi.org/10.1016/j.ucl.2018.12.002.
15. Tom WR, Wollin DA, Jiang R, et al. Next-generation single-use ureteroscopes: an in vitro compari-

son. J Endourol. 2017;31(12):1301–6. https://doi.org/10.1089/end.2017.0447.
16. Leveillee RJ, Kelly EF. Impressive performance: new disposable digital ureteroscope allows for extreme lower pole access and use of 365 μm Holmium laser fiber. J Endourol Case Rep. 2016;2(1):114–6. https://doi.org/10.1089/cren.2016.0051.
17. Johnston TJ, Baard J, de la Rosette J, et al. A clinical evaluation of the new digital single-use flexible ureteroscope (UscopePU3022): an international prospective multicentered study. Cent European J Urol. 2018;71(4):453–61. https://doi.org/10.5173/ceju.2018.1787.
18. Memon AG, Naeem Z, Zaman A, et al. Occupational health related concerns among surgeons. Int J Health Sci (Qassim). 2016;10(2):279–91.
19. Healy KA, Pak RW, Cleary RC, et al. Hand problems among endourologists. J Endourol. 2011;25(12):1915–20. https://doi.org/10.1089/end.2011.0128.
20. Ludwig WW, Lee G, Ziemba JB, et al. Evaluating the Ergonomics of Flexible Ureteroscopy. J Endourol. 2017;31(10):1062–6.
21. Proietti S, Somani B, Sofer M, et al. The "Body Mass Index" of flexible ureteroscopes. J Endourol. 2017;31(10):1090–5. https://doi.org/10.1089/end.2017.0438.
22. Teplitsky SL, Leong JY, Calio B, et al. Ergonomics in endourology: measurement of force for deflection in contemporary ureteroscopes. J Endourol. 2021;35(2):215–20. https://doi.org/10.1089/end.2020.0369.
23. Martin CJ, McAdams SB, Abdul-Mushin H, et al. The economic implications of a reusable flexible digital ureteroscope: A Cost-benefit analysis. J Urol. 2017;197:730–5. https://doi.org/10.1016/j.juro.2016.09.085.
24. Davis NF, Quinlan MR, Browne C, et al. Single-use flexible ureteropyeloscopy: a systematic review. World J Urol. 2018;36(4):529–36. https://doi.org/10.1007/s00345-017-2131-4.
25. Marchini GS, Torricelli FC, Batagello CA, et al. A comprehensive literature-based equation to compare cost-effectiveness of a flexible ureteroscopy program with single-use versus reusable devices. Int Braz J Urol. 2019;45(4):658–70. https://doi.org/10.1590/S1677-5538.IBJU.2018.0880.
26. Davis NF, McGrath S, Quinlan M, et al. Carbon Footprint in Flexible Ureteroscopy: A Comparative Study on the Environmental Impact of Reusable and Single-Use Ureteroscopes. J Endourol. 2018;32(3):214–7. https://doi.org/10.1089/end.2018.0001.
27. Ventimiglia E, Somani BK, Traxer O. Flexible ureteroscopy: reuse? Or is single use the new direction? Curr Opin Urol. 2020;30(2):113–9. https://doi.org/10.1097/MOU.0000000000000700.
28. Somani BK, Talso M, Bres-Niewada E. Current role of single-use flexible ureteroscopes in the management of upper tract stone disease. Cent European J Urol. 2019;72(2):183–4. https://doi.org/10.5173/ceju.2019.1937.
29. Proietti S, Somani BK, Pietropaolo A, et al. Italian endourological panorama: results from a national survey. Cent European J Urol. 2018;71(2):190–5. https://doi.org/10.5173/ceju.2018.1623.

Robotic Flexible Ureteroscopy (Robotic fURS)

Nida Zafer Tokatli and Kemal Sarica

Abstract

With the technical advancements in endoscopic procedures and armamentarium, and the increase in surgical skills majority of the practicing urologists began to manage even relatively larger and also multiple upper tract stones with fURS. The suboptimal ergonomic posture and the long-standing position may have a negative impact on the performance of fURS, especially in cases of larger stones that require longer operations, and may add up to increased need of secondary treatment. Moreover, radiation exposure of the surgeon and operating staff is another crucial factor to be kept in mind. Robotic master-slave systems could overcome these limitations; mainly ergonomic restrictions. Robotic-assisted fURS was first reportedly designed for interventional cardiology, using the Sensei-Magellan system in 2008. Avicenna Roboflex (ELMED) was specifically designed for fURS and introduced in clinical practice after CE certification in 2013. This robotic system consists of a robotic manipulator for docking with all commercially available flexible fiber and video ureterorenoscopy and a console for the surgeon. Avicenna Roboflex provides a significant improvement of ergonomics for a suitable and safe platform for robotic fURS.

Keywords

Robotics · Master-slave systems · Urolithiasis · Ureterorenoscopy · Retrograde intrarenal surgery

1 Introduction

Contemporary management of stones faced dramatic alterations in the last decade. On one hand, the popularity of shock wave lithotripsy (SWL) and "standard" percutaneous nephrolithotomy (PNL) began to lose their popularity to some extent (either due to less efficacy with a certain need for repeated procedures or evident invasiveness), and on the other hand relatively less invasive endoscopic procedures namely flexible ureterorenoscopy (fURS) began to gain more acceptance among the endourologists.

Related to this issue, parallel to the significant increase in the acceptance and applications of endourological procedures applied for the removal of stones [1], flexible ureteroscopic stone management (fURS) increased by 86% in the UK [2], use of SWL decreased by 26%. This significant increase in the effective performance of URS has followed the introduction of flexible

N. Z. Tokatli (✉)
Department of Urology, Medicana International Ankara Hospital, Ankara, Turkey

K. Sarica
Department of Urology, Biruni University, Medical School, Istanbul, Turkey

G. Zeng et al. (eds.), *Flexible Ureteroscopy*, https://doi.org/10.1007/978-981-19-2936-6_19

endoscopes which gave rise to these applications in a successful manner. In addition to these advancements, the clinical introduction of the "Holmium YAG laser" for the effective stone disintegration of the calculi with different compositions has led the endourologists to use fURS more commonly than ever [3]. Although the performance of percutaneous nephrolithotomy (PCNL) also increased, considering the total number of treatments, it remained rather stable when compared to the rest of the available treatment options.

Following its clinical introduction in the 1990s, rigid ureteroscopic stone removal has been well performed in all parts of the world with great efficacy and safety. In the light of the huge experience obtained with this technique, flexible ureteroscopy (fURS) applications began to gain more and more popularity by enabling the endourologists to reach every part of the upper urinary tract and treat stones located in different parts of the renal collecting system. Increasing experience after two decades of evolution and obtained successful outcomes (based on rational indications), has clearly shown that fURS is currently, the most preferred endourological stone treatment modality overall. Based on all these achievements and accumulated experience so far, for the first time, fURS began to challenge the highly common worldwide application of PCNL treatment of relatively larger (20–30 mm) renal calculi [4–8].

In summary, as a result of the technical advancements in endoscopic procedures, relevant equipment systems (development of smaller diameter fine scopes, increased scope flexibility, improvement of accessories, and holmium laser technology), and the increase in surgical skills [4, 9, 10], majority of the practicing urologists began to manage even relatively larger and also multiple upper tract stones with fURS. The success rates obtained in terms of stone-free status were found to be acceptable and comparable with PCNL in experienced hands [5, 9, 11].

However, despite its successful outcomes and relatively practical applications, reported data so far has clearly indicated that the learning curve, as well as effective performance of fURS, is somehow longer and more demanding compared to the semirigid approach. Additionally, as the application of fURS gained popularity around the world, in addition to its advantages; certain limitations and mainly ergonomic restrictions, were also clearly demonstrated. Regarding this issue, despite the successful use of ureteral access sheaths (UAS) for easy access and complete laser-fragmentation of the stones in an efficient manner, stone-free status rates after a single session of fURS seemed to be limited depending on the well-established surgeon (experience, physical performance), stone (size, location, hardness, and location) and anatomy (collecting system) related factors. Additionally, the current design of different flexible scopes, management of a moving stone during laser fragmentation were the other limitations observed particularly during the treatment of large as well as multiple stones. These factors coupled with the applications in inadequately experienced hands have resulted in ≥50% secondary procedure rates to reach a completely stone-free rate after this procedure. There are however some other facts which may not let the endourologists perform the fURS procedure in ideal, optimum conditions. Regarding this issue, it is obvious that as the single person operating, the surgeon needs assistance to operate the laser system (open the system and adjust the energy-rate settings), manipulate nitinol baskets, catch the disintegrated fragments, and deal with the irrigation fluid (manipulate, adjust the rate) during all steps of the procedure while holding and keeping the ureterorenoscope tip at the desired position. Additionally, digital endoscopes with "chip-on-the-tip" technology may prove difficult in orienting the renal collecting system in comparison to standard systems with a pendulum camera attached to an eyepiece. Thus, as mentioned above, the surgeon has to deal with and manipulate, activate several accessorial devices by using the foot pedal including fluoroscopy, laser system, or irrigation, and most endourologists do perform all these activities in a "somehow fixed" standing position. This position has been stated to be a suboptimal ergonomic posture which may eventually cause certain orthopedic complaints [12, 13]. Based on these complaints and possible fatigue that may arise during long-lasting procedures for relatively challenging (large, multiple, located in lower calyceal position) stones, such a position may also induce a negative impact on the effective performance of the fURS procedure. Even the presence of an experienced team may overcome some of these problems, the team may be hindered by space limitations in the working field. Prolonged operative times may cause an increased risk of infection, higher secondary treatment rates, and less stone-free rates. However, having a computer and robot functioning as a follower to the urologist's commands, the procedure itself may simply become a matter of advancing or rotating a controller and deciding where to go. Lastly but more importantly exposure of the surgeon and all members of participating staff as well to radiation for a definite period of time (range of 1.7–56 μSv) is another crucial factor to be kept in mind [14–16].

In the light of all the facts mentioned above, it is clear that performing the fURS procedure in a comfortable sitting position (e.g., using a saddle or a chair) may compensate for some of these drawbacks, similar to the use of an ergonomic chair during laparoscopy [17]. This brought the need of developing a robotic device into the agenda of endourologists to improve the performance of the procedure in a successful and effective manner.

Related to this issue, it has been well noted that robotic-assisted surgery has opened a new era in the history of surgery with a very fast acceptance and adoption among surgeons. It has reshaped oncological and reconstructive interventions throughout all surgical specialties. Robotic-assisted surgery has dramatically influenced minimally invasive surgery with the introduction of console-based manipulators, such as the da Vinci robot (Intuitive Surgical, Sunnyvale, CA, USA) or the Hansen device (Hansen Medical, Mountain View, CA, USA) [18–21]. The use of robotic systems has brought many certain advantages for effective and practical applications [22]. (Use of robotics in these fields has rendered practical advantages and effectiveness. And based on the rapid adoption and increasing experience in this field, the use of robotic surgery, especially for oncologic problems like radical prostatectomy and partial nephrectomy became nearly a standard in daily practice [23]. Currently, the use of robotic systems in endourological procedures particularly for stone removal is another rapidly growing area in minimal invasive stone management [24–26]. In other words, despite the common and effective application of robotic-assisted surgery in the field of pelvic urological pathologies and upper tract oncology, a strong desire has been emerged for establishing such a system for stone management of upper tract stones in the last two decades [27, 28].

Additionally, as mentioned above, technical challenges with a flexible ureteroscopy (fURS) were the main factors leading to the development of robotic-assisted flexible ureteroscopes [24].

To accomplish the abovementioned tasks several robotic systems have been developed and clinically used in the management of upper urinary tract stones with some certain theoretical advantages. Regarding the use of robotic systems with this aim, although Desai and colleagues used the Hansen device, designed for cardiovascular interventions, to perform robot-assisted flexible ureterorenoscopy; this project has been discontinued. Following this short-lasting experience, the Sensei-Magellan system flexi fURS was described in 2008 [20]. Desai et al. reported a 94% technical success rate for stone disintegration and a complete stone-clearance rate of 89% in 18 patients undergoing fURS with this system [21]. There was no conversion to manual URS or intraoperative complications in this study. The Sensei-Magellan system project encountered difficulties with scope design development and consequently, the endeavor was abandoned.

Based on this limited experience by Desai M. et al., and as a result of further studies on this issue as well, since 2012, ELMED (Ankara, Turkey) launched the Avicenna Roboflex System in 2011. In 2013 and 2015, new prototypes followed. The first feasibility reports were published in 2014 [24]. After CE certification in 2013, the robot was introduced in clinical practice and tweaked for intraoperative use. As one of the first robots used for ureteroscopy, Avicenna Roboflex

(ELMED) utilized a robotic control and interface that interfaced and docked with all commercially available flexible fiber and video ureteroscopes. The system gained CE approval for use in Europe in 2013 but FDA approval is still pending.

2 The "Avicenna Roboflex" Robotic System

Avicenna Roboflex consists of two main parts. The first is a control console for the surgeon can sit and control all movements and necessary functions. The second is a robotic manipulator for docking with all commercially available flexible fiber and video ureterorenoscopes. The robotic manipulator has the capability of rotation (±220°), advancement (210 mm), deflection (±270°). In addition to the movements of fURS, the irrigation and laser fiber movement operations can be controlled by the surgeon at the console. That robotic system is compatible with a wide range of digital or fiber flexible ureterorenoscopes, access sheaths, laser fibers, and baskets. Saglam R. et al. reported their first experience in 81 patients undergoing robotic-assisted fURS with the Roboflex Avicenna system (prototype 2) [24]. They concluded that the console time and procedure time were within acceptable limits, with only one technical failure requiring manual fURS. The overall success of stone disintegration was recorded at 96% in this study. Geavlete P. et al. published a prospective comparative study between Roboflex Avicenna system (prototype 2) and classical fURS. The study reported similar safety profile and 3-month stone-free rates for the two approaches (89.4% in conventional FURS vs. 92.4% robotic-assisted FURS) [29]. In their prospective multicenter study again Klein E. et al. reported a 97% technical success in stone disintegration and a device failure in only 2 patients (0.7%) for renal stones with an average size of 14 mm [30]. Based on all these preliminary data one may suggest that stone-free rates with robotic-assisted fURS are noninferior to manual fURS.

One of hinderances of fURS performance may be the suboptimal ergonomics resulting in the patients' need for secondary operations and the frequent repair of the endoscopes. Carey et al. [31] reported an 8.1% damage rate at a single tertiary center with 40–48 uses before the initial repair of new flexible ureteroscopes. The main reasons for repair were errant laser firing (36%) and excessive torque (28%). Theoretically, the functions included in Roboflex Avicenna, such as insertion of the laser fiber only in a straight position of the scope using a memory function, stepwise motorized advancement of the laser fiber, and force-controlled deflection of the scope, should contribute to longer life of these precise, smaller, and fine scopes. In their original study, Saglam R. et al. observed one malfunction of the ureterorenoscopes during case 42 (damage of the digital video system); however, the endoscope has been used 25 times or classic fURS. Exact figures can be evaluated only by the planned randomized trial (IDEAL stage 3) [24].

The robotic fURS system has many advantages as stated above but possible limitations of the device may be expressed as the lack of tactile feedback and problems with the use of baskets for extraction of larger stone fragments. Similar to our experiences with the da Vinci robot, lack of tactile feedback did not prove to be a problematic issue during the performance of robotic fURS, mainly due to the superior image quality of the digital endoscope used. Avicenna Roboflex robotic system was found to enable precise movements of the endoscope in deflection, rotation, and advancement which may overcome the lack of tactile feedback well. In addition, displaying the parameters and animated vision of the tip of fURS will help the surgeon for better orientation and control. It is still debatable whether fURS should aim at complete ablation by pulverization of the stone or whether larger fragments should be retrieved using a Dormia basket via the access sheath [32, 33]. One of the arguments in question suggests that, since the robotic fURS requires occasional undocking of the device, aiming and performing these maneuvers may be cumbersome as well as time-consuming if the surgeon in charge is not well accustomed to the device. This issue brings the idea of "pulverization concept" to the fore, and suggests that future robotic fURS studies should focus on overcoming the stated problem. Avicenna Roboflex system is designed to follow up on this argument, by using a combination of high-frequency laser systems, especially Thulium Fiber Lasers (TFL). Last of all, the cost of the device may prove to be an issue of significance, especially regarding the financial restrictions of healthcare systems. Following the IDEAL framework, in order to provide further commentary about the advantages of robot assisted over the classical fURS, a multicenter randomized trial is required. A study as such must include all of the aspects discussed earlier, based on the state-of-the-art definition of primary and secondary outcomes, an example being stone-free rates based on computed tomography rather than on ultrasound and an additional X-ray [34].

3 Current Evidence of the Roboflex

The evidence comparing the Roboflex System to the classical fURS procedure is still limited. (Comparisons of the Roboflex System to the classical fURS system remain insufficient) Geavlete P. et al. [29] reported their first experience in a matched-pair analysis (n = 132) showing no significant difference in terms of clinical parameters and outcome between the two management options. However, they were able to demonstrate a lower retreatment rate and a better stone-free rate at 3 months as well in the robotic treatment group. The study group mentioned some secondary advantages of this approach, mainly ergonomic improvements, for the surgeon as particularly noted in long-lasting surgeries due to difficult stone parameters or a large stone volume to treat [29].

The precision of the system has been investigated by Proietti S. et al. in a K-box Simulator. There was no significant difference between the performance of the robotic fURS group and the manual fURS group, with a slight advantage in the speed for the manual fURS group and a slight significant advantage for the robotic fURS group in terms of stability, centering of the picture, tissue respect, and maneuverability at least in one of the two exercises [35].

In a recent meta-analysis, ample evidence shows serious health risks of prolonged standing, including lower back pain, physical fatigue, muscle pain, tiredness, and body part discomfort. Prolonged standing affects the cardiovascular system as well [24, 36]. The wearing of a protective lead gown can amplify posture-related health problems. Sitting in a personalized position with an armrest at the console reduces physical stress and improves the endurance of the surgeon [24].

4 Future

The robotic systems have no tactile feedback, which is the typical drawback of using master-slave systems. Different companies trying to overcome the limitation of tactile feedback and technical developments show promising early results but a definite solution is not yet on the market [37].

Force sensors could be utilized so that the ureteroscope cannot perforate the renal pelvis by increasing the safety profile. If 3D vision is applied to future ureteroscopy robots, it could also further enhance manipulation and visualization. Furthermore, with the placement of instruments in the kidney, electromagnetic sensors (EM) could be correlated with the preoperative CT images and therefore a 3D GPS-like map could be displayed without using the ionizing radiation with less fluoroscopy time. EM sensing positioning technology used in bronchoscopy systems could be beneficial with this aim. If a real-time ultrasound modality could be added to the robotic systems, this may also help guide surgeons to any remaining stones or fragments that have been displaced during the procedure.

Ultimately, a robot could theoretically control the ureteroscope and synchronize it with respiration during laser lithotripsy to increase the efficiency of fragmentation. Baskets could be controlled by a robotic system and be used to pull the ureteroscope out of the access sheath, drop the stone, and then return to the exact previous spot since it will remember the location in all vectors.

The obvious safety concern with this use is pulling out a stone that does not fit the sheath and avulsing the ureter. The robot could address this in two ways. First, endoscopic measurements of the stone fragments could be made to ensure that the pieces are small enough to fit through the access sheath. Second, force sensors could be incorporated into the system to prevent ureteral avulsion; it would simply stop retracting and the surgeon would be able to further fragment the stone before extraction.

Laser settings could also be programmed into the robot, and instead of the surgeon stopping to alter the settings, the robot could constantly monitor the types of dust or fragment being produced and the amount of retropulsion or stone movement, then alter the settings as lithotripsy is taking place and the stone is decreasing in mass.

Once synchronization of respiratory movements can be accounted for, this may make lithotripsy very fast and efficient. Ultimately, it is conceivable that the surgeon would place a target on the stone in question, hit a "start" button, and then the robot would control the laser, ureteroscope, fluid irrigation, and laser settings to reduce retropulsion and adjust for respiratory movements to break up the stone into dust. This would all take place while the surgeon stands by at the console.

5 Conclusions

Robot-assisted techniques in the minimal invasive management of upper urinary tract stones are still in the early stages of implementation. However, although limited, available data clearly shows that new robotic technologies will provide excellent treatment of renal stones as a result of the improved ability of experts to target stones with better surgeon ergonomics and more importantly reduced ionizing radiation from fluoroscopy. Relatively larger stones and multiple calyceal stones can be successfully treated with robotic systems. The use of robotic technology maintains the performance of the surgeon during long-lasting surgeries due to optimal ergonomic working conditions. However, we believe that further evaluation with long-term follow-up and cost-analysis, multicenter, randomized controlled studies are certainly needed to define the place of robotic surgery in renal tract calculi management. Last but not least, the robotic-assisted fURS procedure could provide some certain potential benefits in the Covid-19 era in the effective minimal invasive management of large as well as multiple renal stones with well-preserved physical distance between the operating room staff and the case.

References

1. Geraghty RM, Jones P, Somani BK. Worldwide trends of urinary stone disease treatment over the last two decades: a systematic review. J Endourol. 2017;31(6):547–56. https://doi.org/10.1089/end.2016.0895.
2. Rukin NJ, Siddiqui ZA, Chedgy ECP, Somani BK. Trends in upper tract stone disease in England: evidence from the hospital episodes statistics database. Urol Int. 2017;98(4):391–6. https://doi.org/10.1159/000449510. Epub 2016 Oct 1
3. Pietropaolo A, Proietti S, Geraghty R, Skolarikos A, Papatsoris A, Liatsikos E, Somani BK. Trends of "urolithiasis: interventions, simulation, and laser technology" over the last 16 years (2000–2015) as published in the literature (PubMed): a systematic review from European section of Uro-technology (ESUT). World J Urol. 2017;35(11):1651–8. https://doi.org/10.1007/s00345-017-2055-z. Epub 2017 Jun 7. PMID: 28593477; PMCID: PMC5649597
4. Breda A, Ogunyemi O, Leppert JT, Lam JS, Schulam PG. Flexible ureteroscopy and laser lithotripsy for single intrarenal stones 2 cm or greater--is this the new frontier? J Urol. 2008;179(3):981–4. https://doi.org/10.1016/j.juro.2007.10.083. Epub 2008 Jan 22
5. Grasso M, Conlin M, Bagley D. Retrograde ureteropyeloscopic treatment of 2 cm. Or greater upper urinary tract and minor staghorn calculi. J Urol. 1998;160(2):346–51.
6. Bader MJ, Gratzke C, Walther S, Weidlich P, Staehler M, Seitz M, Sroka R, Reich O, Stief CG, Schlenker B. Efficacy of retrograde ureteropyeloscopic holmium laser lithotripsy for intrarenal calculi >2 cm. Urol Res. 2010;38(5):397–402. https://doi.org/10.1007/s00240-010-0258-5. Epub 2010 Mar 4
7. Breda A, Ogunyemi O, Leppert JT, Schulam PG. Flexible ureteroscopy and laser lithotripsy for multiple unilateral intrarenal stones. Eur Urol. 2009;55(5):1190–6. https://doi.org/10.1016/j.eururo.2008.06.019. Epub 2008 Jun 13

8. El-Anany FG, Hammouda HM, Maghraby HA, Elakkad MA. Retrograde ureteropyeloscopic holmium laser lithotripsy for large renal calculi. BJU Int. 2001;88(9):850–3. https://doi.org/10.1046/j.1464-4096.2001.01248.x.
9. Wiesenthal JD, Ghiculete D, D'A Honey RJ, Pace KT. A comparison of treatment modalities for renal calculi between 100 and 300 mm^2: are shockwave lithotripsy, ureteroscopy, and percutaneous nephrolithotomy equivalent? J Endourol. 2011;25(3):481–5. https://doi.org/10.1089/end.2010.0208. Epub 2011 Feb 25
10. Riley JM, Stearman L, Troxel S. Retrograde ureteroscopy for renal stones larger than 2.5 cm. J Endourol. 2009;23:1395–8.
11. Al-Qahtani SM, Gil-Deiz-de-Medina S, Traxer O. Predictors of clinical outcomes of flexible ureterorenoscopy with holmium laser for renal stone greater than 2 cm, Adv Urol. 2012;2012:543537. https://doi.org/10.1155/2012/543537. Epub 2011 Jun 9. PMID: 21738531; PMCID: PMC3113263
12. Elkoushy MA, Andonian S. Prevalence of orthopedic complaints among endourologists and their compliance with radiation safety measures. J Endourol. 2011;25(10):1609–13. https://doi.org/10.1089/end.2011.0109. Epub 2011 Aug 5
13. Healy KA, Pak RW, Cleary RC, Colon-Herdman A, Bagley DH. Hand problems among endourologists. J Endourol. 2011;25(12):1915–20. https://doi.org/10.1089/end.2011.0128. Epub 2011 Oct 17
14. Bagley DH, Cubler-Goodman A. Radiation exposure during ureteroscopy. J Urol. 1990;144(6):1356–8. https://doi.org/10.1016/s0022-5347(17)39739-2.
15. Hellawell GO, Mutch SJ, Thevendran G, Wells E, Morgan RJ. Radiation exposure and the urologist: what are the risks? J Urol. 2005;174(3):948–52; ; discussion 952. https://doi.org/10.1097/01.ju.0000170232.58930.8f.
16. Kim KP, Miller DL, Berrington de Gonzalez A, Balter S, Kleinerman RA, Ostroumova E, Simon SL, Linet MS. Occupational radiation doses to operators performing fluoroscopically-guided procedures. Health Phys. 2012;103(1):80–99. https://doi.org/10.1097/HP.0b013e31824dae76. PMID: 22647920; PMCID: PMC3951010
17. Rassweiler JJ, Goezen AS, Jalal AA, Schulze M, Pansadoro V, Pini G, Kim F, Turner C. A new platform improving the ergonomics of laparoscopic surgery: initial clinical evaluation of the prototype. Eur Urol. 2012;61(1):226–9. https://doi.org/10.1016/j.eururo.2011.09.018. Epub 2011 Sep 28
18. Rassweiler J, Safi KC, Subotic S, Teber D, Frede T. Robotics and telesurgery--an update on their position in laparoscopic radical prostatectomy. Minim Invasive Ther Allied Technol. 2005;14(2):109–22. https://doi.org/10.1080/13645700510010908.
19. Aron M, Haber GP, Desai MM, Gill IS. Flexible robotics: a new paradigm. Curr Opin Urol. 2007;17(3):151–5. https://doi.org/10.1097/MOU.0b013e3280e126ab.
20. Desai MM, Aron M, Gill IS, Pascal-Haber G, Ukimura O, Kaouk JH, Stahler G, Barbagli F, Carlson C, Moll F. Flexible robotic retrograde renoscopy: description of novel robotic device and preliminary laboratory experience. Urology. 2008;72(1):42–6. https://doi.org/10.1016/j.urology.2008.01.076. Epub 2008 Apr 18
21. Desai MM, Grover R, Aron M, Ganpule A, Joshi SS, Desai MR, Gill IS. Robotic flexible ureteroscopy for renal calculi: initial clinical experience. J Urol. 2011;186(2):563–8. https://doi.org/10.1016/j.juro.2011.03.128. Epub 2011 Jun 16
22. Peters BS, Armijo PR, Krause C, Choudhury SA, Oleynikov D. Review of emerging surgical robotic technology. Surg Endosc. 2018;32(4):1636–55. https://doi.org/10.1007/s00464-018-6079-2. Epub 2018 Feb 13
23. Khosla A, Wagner AA. Robotic surgery of the kidney, bladder, and prostate. Surg Clin North Am. 2016;96(3):615–36. https://doi.org/10.1016/j.suc.2016.02.015.
24. Saglam R, Muslumanoglu AY, Tokatlı Z, Caşkurlu T, Sarica K, Taşçi Aİ, Erkurt B, Süer E, Kabakci AS, Preminger G, Traxer O, Rassweiler JJ. A new robot for flexible ureteroscopy: development and early clinical results (IDEAL stage 1-2b). Eur Urol. 2014;66(6):1092–100. https://doi.org/10.1016/j.eururo.2014.06.047. Epub 2014 Jul 21
25. Autorino R, Zargar H, Kaouk JH. Robotic-assisted laparoscopic surgery: recent advances in urology. Fertil Steril. 2014;102(4):939–49. https://doi.org/10.1016/j.fertnstert.2014.05.033. Epub 2014 Jun 30
26. Khosla A, Wagner AA. Robotic surgery of the kidney, bladder, and prostate. Surg Clin North Am. 2016;96(3):615–36. https://doi.org/10.1016/j.suc.2016.02.015.
27. McGuinness LA, Prasad RB. Robotics in urology. Ann R Coll Surg Engl. 2018;100(6_sup):38–44. https://doi.org/10.1308/rcsann.supp1.38. PMID: 29717888; PMCID: PMC5956576
28. Rai BP, Jones P, Tait C, Amitharaj R, Gowda R, Bhatti A, Adshead J, Somani B. Is cryotherapy a genuine rival to robotic-assisted partial nephrectomy in the Management of Suspected Renal Malignancy? A systematic review and meta-analysis. Urology. 2018;118:6–11. https://doi.org/10.1016/j.urology.2017.09.008. Epub 2017 Sep 28
29. Geavlete P, Saglam R, Georgescu D, Mulţescu R, Iordache V, Kabakci AS, Ene C, Geavlete B. Robotic flexible ureteroscopy versus classic flexible ureteroscopy in renal stones: the initial Romanian experience. Chirurgia (Bucur). 2016;111(4):326–9.
30. Klein J-T, Fiedler M, Kabuki AS, Sağlam R, Rassweiler J. 1032 prospective European multicentre clinical results of kidney stone treatment using the Avicenna Roboflex URS robot. Eur Urol Suppl. 2016;15:e1032. https://doi.org/10.1016/S1569-9056(16)61033-3.
31. Carey RI, Gomez CS, Maurici G, Lynne CM, Leveillee RJ, Bird VG. Frequency of uretero-

scope damage seen at a tertiary care center. J Urol. 2006;176(2):607–10; discussion 610. https://doi.org/10.1016/j.juro.2006.03.059.
32. Rebuck DA, Macejko A, Bhalani V, Ramos P, Nadler RB. The natural history of renal stone fragments following ureteroscopy. Urology. 2011;77(3):564–8. https://doi.org/10.1016/j.urology.2010.06.056. Epub 2010 Dec 15
33. Kronenberg P, Traxer O. In vitro fragmentation efficiency of holmium: yttrium-aluminum-garnet (YAG) laser lithotripsy--a comprehensive study encompassing different frequencies, pulse energies, total power levels and laser fibre diameters. BJU Int. 2014;114(2):261–7. https://doi.org/10.1111/bju.12567. Epub 2014 Apr 16
34. Macejko A, Okotie OT, Zhao LC, Liu J, Perry K, Nadler RB. Computed tomography-determined stone-free rates for ureteroscopy of upper-tract stones. J Endourol. 2009;23(3):379–82. https://doi.org/10.1089/end.2008.0240.
35. Proietti S, Dragos L, Emiliani E, Butticeè S, Talso M, Baghdadi M, Villa L, Doizi S, Giusti G, Traxer O. Ureteroscopic skills with and without Roboflex Avicenna in the K-box® simulator. Cent European J Urol. 2017;70(1):76–80. https://doi.org/10.5173/ceju.2017.1180. Epub 2017 Mar 14. PMID: 28461993; PMCID: PMC5407341
36. Waters TR, Dick RB. Evidence of health risks associated with prolonged standing at work and intervention effectiveness. Rehabil Nurs. 2015;40(3):148–65. https://doi.org/10.1002/rnj.166. Epub 2014 Jul 7. PMID: 25041875; PMCID: PMC4591921
37. Brodie A, Vasdev N. The future of robotic surgery. Ann R Coll Surg Engl. 2018;100(Suppl 7):4–13. https://doi.org/10.1308/rcsann.supp2.4. PMID: 30179048; PMCID: PMC6216754

Diagnostic Flexible Ureteroscopy

Brian H. Eisner, Jason J. Lee, and Christina Kottooran

Abstract

Since its introduction in the 1980s and popularization in the 1990s, flexible ureteroscopy has become an invaluable diagnostic tool for the urologist. Improvements in equipment and technique have enabled urologists to diagnose conditions with efficiency and accuracy. Today, flexible ureteroscopy plays a central role in the evaluation of various upper tract pathologies, ranging from hematuria of unknown origin to upper tract urothelial tumors. In the following chapter, we review the current state of diagnostic flexible ureteroscopy and its role in the diagnosis of various urologic conditions.

Keywords

Diagnostic · Flexible ureteroscopy Ureteroscopy

1 Introduction

Ureteroscopy is a procedure performed by inserting an endoscope through the urethra to visualize the lower or upper urinary tracts [1]. The use of a rigid or semirigid ureteroscope is commonly used to evaluate the distal ureter for both genders and can be advanced as proximal as the upper pole of the kidney in females and the upper ureter/ureteropelvic junction in males. However, with the development of agile flexible ureteroscopes, many clinicians prefer to utilize flexible ureteroscopy (fURS) for the evaluation of the proximal ureter and the intrarenal collecting system. The advantage of fURS is its ability to maneuver through the tortuous path of the upper urinary tract, which is the main limitation of a nonflexible endoscope [2].

There are three main components of a flexible ureteroscope: optical system, deflection mechanism, and working channel [3]. Recent efforts have focused on advancing the optical and illumination system of the flexible ureteroscope, leading to improvements of the early fiber-optic technology and more recently digital flexible ureteroscopes. Historically, fURS has been utilized for the evaluation of benign and malignant upper urinary tract pathologies as well as therapeutic interventions including ablation of upper tract urothelial carcinoma (UTUC) and laser lithotripsy with stone extraction [4]. Over the past several decades, innovations in the design of fURS have transformed the field of urology. In this chapter, we explore the role of fURS in the diagnosis of upper urinary tract pathologies.

B. H. Eisner (✉) · J. J. Lee · C. Kottooran
Department of Urology, Massachusetts General Hospital, Boston, MA, USA
e-mail: beisner@partners.org

G. Zeng et al. (eds.), *Flexible Ureteroscopy*, https://doi.org/10.1007/978-981-19-2936-6_20

2 Indications

While fURS is utilized for both diagnostic and therapeutic modalities, in this chapter we will primarily focus on the diagnostic indications for fURS. The main indications for diagnostic fURS are unilateral hematuria, positive cytology with normal cystoscopy, radiographic filling defect of the upper urinary tract, obstruction of the upper urinary tract, and follow-up or treatment of low-grade UTUC in the appropriately selected patients. The primary objective during the diagnostic stage is to establish whether the symptomatic lesion is benign or malignant [5]. A complete evaluation of the upper urinary tract can be achieved using fURS in approximately 71–100% of cases, which is dependent on several factors such as anatomical complexity, performance of the flexible ureteroscope used, accessory instruments used for biopsy, visibility, and image quality [6]. With improvements in structural design and maneuverability, fURS has improved accessibility and visualization of the upper urinary tract in a retrograde fashion making it an optimal diagnostic tool. fURS is the first step in the evaluation of the aforementioned upper urinary tract pathologies due to its minimally invasive nature. In a majority of cases, a diagnosis can be achieved by fURS, avoiding more invasive approaches such as percutaneous endoscopy and open, laparoscopic, or robotic surgery.

2.1 Unilateral Hematuria

Patients who present with unilateral hematuria are advised to undergo a diagnostic workup to determine whether the hematuria is a direct symptom caused by a condition such as a neoplasm (benign or malignant) or stone or caused by an isolated event of idiopathic etiology. Furthermore, unilateral essential hematuria, also known as benign essential hematuria or chronic unilateral hematuria, is a diagnosis of exclusion defined as gross unilateral hematuria that is endoscopically demonstrated to lateralize to one upper collecting system. In such cases, patients undergo a diagnostic workup, which includes hematological studies, cytology, and contrast-enhanced imaging of the genitourinary tract (e.g., intravenous pyelography, CT, or MR urography) [7]. Several studies have demonstrated the diagnostic effectiveness of fURS for this condition to vary between 78% and 83% in diagnosing the etiology of unilateral hematuria [6]. Nakada et al. conducted a retrospective review of 17 patients with lateralizing essential hematuria who underwent a diagnostic fURS. Though the study was limited by a small sample size, suggestive lesions were identified in 14 (82%) of 17 patients, specifically 11 (64%) patients with discrete lesions and 3 (18%) patients with diffuse lesions [8]. Similarly, Bagley et al. studied 32 patients undergoing retrograde flexible ureteropyeloscopy for benign essential hematuria. Successful visualization of the entire ureter and pelvicalyceal system was possible in a total of 30 (94%) patients, of which discrete lesions were detected in 16 (50%) patients, diffuse lesions were detected in 9 (28%) patients, and no lesions were detected in 5 (16%) patients [7].

2.2 Upper Tract Urothelial Carcinoma (UTUC)

fURS is the gold standard for establishing the diagnosis of UTUC and is indicated in patients with a positive cytology despite a normal cystoscopy or a "filling defect" suspicious for a neoplastic lesion on CT or MR urography. While urinary cytology can be useful for characterizing the pathological features of urothelial cancer in the bladder, its use is less well-defined for UTUC [9]. Potretzke et al. was the first to perform a meta-analysis along with a pooled analysis of the literature that studied the diagnostic capacity of selective cytology. This study determined that upper urinary tract cytology had an overall sensitivity based on final pathology of 55.3% and specificity based on biopsy pathology of 90.7% when patients with bladder cancer were excluded [10]. Therefore, diagnostic ureteroscopy is recommended in these situations in order to more accurately evaluate the upper urinary tract with direct endoscopic vision and rule out UTUC or other pathologies. Furthermore, cases with an unremarkable CT urography and positive upper urinary tract cytology may require a diagnostic ureteroscopy and subsequent biopsy given the high specificity of selective cytology [10].

A filling defect of the upper urinary tract on radiological imaging is another common indication for diagnostic ureteroscopy. A filling defect may be caused by the presence of UTUCs, calculus, vasculitis, or other tumors—however, CT urography or other imaging modalities will often distinguish the cause of the filling defect as "stone" or "non-stone." fURS is commonly used in the evaluation of upper urinary tract filling defects given its high diagnostic accuracy compared to more historical standard diagnostic regimens, which consists of cystoscopy, retrograde pyelography, urinary cytology, and in some cases ultrasonography or CT [11]. Bagley et al. prospectively studied 59 patients presenting with various symptoms or indications for fURS and successfully diagnosed every patient with a radiological filling defect [12]. In addition, Puppo et al. performed fURS on 23 patients for purely diagnostic indications, radiologic filling defects and/or hematuria, of which 22 (96%) patients were successfully diagnosed [13].

Over the past several decades, ureteroscopic ablation of UTUC and surveillance has played an increasing role in the management of UTUC. While a radical nephroureterectomy (RNU) is the preferred choice for patients with high-risk nonmetastatic or metastatic disease, endoscopic resection via fURS is commonly utilized for low-risk nonmetastatic disease [9]. Endoscopic resection in comparison to RNU is associated with higher tumor recurrence rates ranging from 15% to 90% [14], with additional contributing factors such as tumor size >2 cm, high tumor grade, or history of bladder tumor. Proietti et al. demonstrated that with strict postoperative surveillance, recurrence-free survival (RFS) rates measured between initial treatment and tumor recurrence were 31.7% [15]. In addition, Cutress et al. found that tumor recurrence rate was as high as 52% after ureteroscopic ablation of a UTUC [16]. Given such high recurrence rates, it is recommended that patients who undergo endoscopic ablation comply with a strict surveillance regimen with an earlier second-look URS within 60 days of their first URS [17]. Regardless, the low complication rates, maintenance of a closed-loop system, reduced risk of tumor seeding, and low progression to RNU renders ureteroscopy an acceptable method in managing low-risk UTUC, especially in patients who are poor candidates for RNU.

3 Diagnostic Findings

3.1 Upper Urinary Tract Tumors

UTUC is a relatively uncommon condition, accounting for 5% of urothelial cancers. The incidence of UTUC is difficult to approximate because tumors of the renal pelvis and ureter are reported collectively with renal cell carcinoma, classifying all renal tumors into one category. However, the annual incidence of UTUC in Western countries is about 2 cases per 100,000 patients [18]. Although a rare primary condition, a majority are invasive at the time of diagnosis, 60% for UTUC versus 20–25% for bladder tumors [19]. The most common presenting symptoms of UTUC are gross or microscopic hematuria with or without flank pain. Brant et al. conducted a retrospective study of 168 patients with upper urinary tract tumors and found that hematuria and flank pain were seen in over 70% and 30% patients respectively. Generally, constitutional symptoms such as fever, weight loss, and night sweats indicate worsened prognosis that require further investigation for potential metastases [20].

There are three major steps to definitively diagnose UTUC.

- Imaging.
- Cystoscopy with urinary cytology.
- Diagnostic fURS.

Cross-sectional abdominal imaging is often the first step in the diagnosis of a patient with UTUC. CT urography has the highest diagnostic accuracy of all available imaging techniques and thus remains the gold standard imaging modality [21]. CT urography consists of the intravenous administration of contrast and CT imaging during the excretory phase, approximately 10 min after the injection of contrast, to optimize distension and opacification of the upper and lower urinary tracts [22]. A recent meta-analysis of 1233 patients demonstrated the diagnostic value of multidetector CT urography with a pooled sensitivity and specificity of 92% and 95% respectively. MT urography is utilized for patients with contraindications to radiation or iodinated contrast agents. However, overall, CT urography is superior to MR urography for the diagnosis and staging of UTUC. Prior to curative treatment, a CT scan of the chest, abdomen, and pelvis is required to assess for metastasis [23].

Diagnostic ureteroscopy is recommended for the evaluation of patients who demonstrate a filling defect on CT or MR urography. Evaluation of the bladder can be performed at the time of ureteroscopy or is occasionally performed prior to this as an outpatient office evaluation. The introduction of fURS in the diagnostic workup of UTUC has reduced the misdiagnosis rate from 15.5% to 2.1% compared to multidetector CT urography [24]. Wang et al. conducted a study in which the sensitivity of fURS compared to multidetector CT urography in the diagnosis of upper urinary tract tumors was 78.4% versus 54.5% respectively [25]. Moreover, fURS has demonstrated its multifunctionality in the clinical setting. For example, fURS may guide the sampling of the upper urinary tract for patients referred for selective cytology. In addition, fURS allows for the characterization of tumor size and appearance, biopsy of suspicious tissue, and obtention of information that can aid risk stratification of UTUC.

While fURS has demonstrated adequate results in terms of the presence or absence of tumor and the ability to biopsy a lesion to achieve a definitive diagnosis of UTUC, accurate tumor staging is not always possible [9]. Several studies have questioned whether ureteroscopic biopsy can accurately determine the grade and stage of a UTUC lesion [26]. Roja et al. demonstrated that the histologic grade of the biopsy sample accurately predicted the final histologic grade of the nephroureterectomy specimens at a high concordance rate of 92.6%, even if the biopsy volume was small. While concordance of tumor grade was high between the biopsy and resected specimens, concordance of tumor stage was lower at 43% emphasizing the need for other diagnostic tools to improve tumor staging [27]. Overall, the preoperative evaluation of hydronephrosis with imaging, ureteroscopic biopsy and grade, and urinary cytology can identify patients at risk for advanced UTUC and guide the decision of surgical removal, either by endoscopic resection or RNU [28].

Despite the added diagnostic value fURS provides for the diagnosis of UTUC, concerns about its role in the development of intravesical recurrence exist. Marchioni et al. conducted a pooled analysis of 2372 patients and found a statistically significant association between fURS performed prior to RNU and intravesical tumor recurrence. The rate of intravesical recurrence ranged from 39.2–60.7% versus 16.7–46% in patients who did and did not undergo a diagnostic ureteroscopy respectively [29]. Guo et al. conducted a meta-analysis that similarly conducted a higher risk of intravesical recurrence in the same scenario, regardless of the patient's prior history of bladder tumors [30]. Conversely, Nison et al. found no significant difference of intravesical recurrence rates between patients who did or did not undergo preoperative diagnostic fURS, 27.5% versus 28.3% respectively [31].

3.2 Benign Upper Tract Lesions

Ureteral tumors are a historically uncommon diagnosis that has increased in incidence over the past several years, occurring in about 1 in every 3600–10,000 cases. In a clinical setting, malignant lesions are more common than benign lesions of the ureter [32]. Benign ureteral tumors are classified based on embryological origin with a majority derived from the epithelium. However, approximately 20% are nonepithelial in origin, specifically derived from the mesoderm [33].

The most common benign lesion of the ureter is a fibroepithelial polyp [34]. Fibroepithelial polyps are benign mucosal projections composed of fibrous tissue and lined by a normal layer of surface epithelium [35]. The location varies along the urinary tract, including the urethra, bladder, ureters, and renal pelvis [36]. Historically, fibroepithelial polyps were a rare pathologic diagnosis, that have recently increased in incidence due to improvements in diagnostic endoscopic tools. Preoperative evaluation with various imaging modalities such as contrast-enhanced CT or MR cannot distinguish benign filling defects from UTUC; therefore, the gold standard for diagnosis is retrograde ureteroscopy [34, 37]. One of the benefits of retrograde ureteroscopy is its ability to rule out malignancy as fibroepithelial polyps can clinically mimic malignancy. Georgescu et al. demonstrated that in all 11 patients who underwent an investigative retrograde ureteroscopy for various clinical symptoms, the presumed benign aspects of the lesion identified during semirigid or fURS was confirmed by a final pathologic diagnosis of fibroepithelial polyp. The most common presenting symptom is flank pain, followed by hematuria, suprapubic discomfort, and urinary frequency [34]. An open approach had been historically used for surgical resection of a fibroepithelial polyp, however more recently, endoscopic therapy with a percutaneous or ureteroscopic approach has become more commonly utilized [38].

Hemangiomas are benign vascular tumors that are embryologically derived from unipotent angioblasts that develop in an atypical manner within blood vessels [39]. They generally grow by endothelial hyperplasia. The most common types of hemangiomas are capillary and cavernous, which are classified primarily based on the size of the vascular channel. Capillary hemangiomas have a small diameter, while cavernous hemangiomas have a large vascular channel diameter [40]. Hemangiomas of the genitourinary tract are an extremely rare pathological entity, with only eight cases reported worldwide, and are more commonly found on the liver or skin. Interestingly, almost all cases are diagnosed postoperatively based on pathologic examination. The most common presenting symptom is chronic intermittent unilateral hematuria due to erosion of the urothelial lining, which may be accompanied by lower urinary tract symptoms and colicky flank pain due to ureteral obstruction. However, it is also common for patients to experience no symptoms [41]. Patients undergo a routine diagnostic workup, including imaging, cytology, cystoscopy, and diagnostic fURS, for a malignant etiology such as UTUC given its difficulty to preoperatively identify the pathologic cause. The choice of RNU versus endoscopic management is based on tumor size and location as well as preoperative factors indicating the benign nature of the mass seen with a diagnostic fURS and biopsy margins [41, 42].

There are several other rare benign lesions such as fibromas, leiomyomas, granulomas, endometriomas, and neurofibromas that may occur throughout the urinary tract. The rising incidence of these lesions coincide with the advent of improved endoscopic technique which not only has improved diagnostic capability but also patient mortality through an endoscopic versus open approach to surgical resection [33].

4 Others

There are several other causes for the clinical presentation of hematuria or radiologic filling defects that require the diagnostic efforts of fURS. Bagley et al. conducted a prospective study in which flexible ureteropyeloscopy was performed on 59 patients with various presenting symptoms. An anatomical variant was found in 5 of 23 patients evaluated for a filling defect and/or hematuria. Anatomical variants of the upper urinary tract that may cause a filling defect on imaging or hematuria can include aberrant papillae, compound renal calyces, and renal infundibular septum. Interestingly, in cases where a vascular anatomical variant is located near the renal pelvis causing a filling defect on imaging, diagnostic fURS is able to detect pulsations from blood flowing through the vessel and subsequently diagnose the lesion [12].

Lateralizing hematuria can be distressing for patients, especially when an etiology is not readily identified. As described above, fURS has shown utility in visualizing and determining the source of bleeding. Kumon et al. evaluated 12 patients with unilateral gross hematuria and was able to endoscopically identify the bleeding source in 10 patients. 9 patients had localized bleeding sites: 1 patient with a papillary mass, 4 patients with a hemangioma, and 4 patients with minute venous rupture [43]. A minute venous rupture is ultimately bleeding without a clear abnormality that can appear as a stream of blood from the papillary tip, with an adherent clot at times [12]. Bagley et al. used fURS to diagnose clots within the intrarenal collecting system in 10 of 32 patients who experienced intermittent colic [7]. If bleeding is truly benign, patients may be followed without therapy [44]. However, if the clot induces colic pain, urgent diagnosis and treatment are warranted [7].

5 Guidelines

5.1 Microhematuria

The primary objective during the evaluation of hematuria or a radiologic filling defect is to rule out urologic malignancy. The European Association of Urology 2020 guidelines have updates the recommendations for the diagnostic and treatment modalities for UTUCs. The diagnostic workup for UTUC includes imaging, cystoscopy with urine cytology, and diagnostic ureteroscopy. The initial and preferred imaging technique is CT urography. For patients with contraindications to CT urography, MR urography is often used. The next step in the diagnostic workup of UTUC is cystoscopy and urine cytology, which are important to rule out concomitant bladder cancer. However, urine cytology is less sensitive for UTUC than for bladder tumors, and therefore selective cytology should be performed for patients suspected to have UTUC. Patients with a normal cystoscopy and abnormal cytology results have a greater likelihood of being diagnosed with a high-grade UTUC.

The final approach in the diagnostic workup is fURS to access the upper urinary tract, specifically the ureters and pyelocalyceal and intrarenal collecting systems. In addition to visualization and attainment of tissue biopsy, fURS conveniently allows for the collection of selective cytology samples. However, it is not uncommon for ureteroscopic biopsy to lead to pathologic undergrading and inaccurate assessment of staging. This emphasizes the utility of guiding management with information obtained from both ureteroscopic biopsy and selective cytology and the importance of strict surveillance in patients who elect a conservative treatment approach. Several technical advancements have been made to improve visualization and diagnostic techniques of fURS [9].

The American Urological Association has also published guidelines for the evaluation of microscopic hematuria [45]. While the role of ureteroscopy is less well defined in the investigative workup of microhematuria, for cases with high suspicion of an upper tract malignancy, endoscopic exploration is recommended to better visualize the upper urinary tract and characterize suspicious lesions via biopsy.

6 Novel Technologies and Future Directions

The urologic community has aimed to improve ureteroscopic technique over the past several decades to reliably select patients for a less invasive treatment approach, such as endoscopic therapy. Recent technological advancements have allowed for improved optics when access the upper urinary tract using fURS [46].

6.1 Photodynamic Diagnosis

Traditionally, flexible ureteroscopes utilized white light (WL) to capture endoscopic images. However, the use of WL has posed challenges in obtaining a high-resolution image that provides optimal visualization of upper urinary tract lesions. Photodynamic diagnosis (PDD) is a technique that uses fluorescent contrast agents to better visualize malignant tissue [47]. Both of the commonly used fluorochrome agents, 5-aminolevulinic acid (5-ALA) and hexaminolevulinate hydrochloride (HAL), induce the accumulation of protoporphyrin IX in cells. When tissues are exposed to a blue light at a range of wavelengths between 375 nm to 440 nm, neoplastic cells tend to absorb more light, thus enhancing the excretion of protoporphyrin compared to normal tissue. As such, malignant cells will appear red against normal cells that appear blue, allowing for discrimination between tissues [48].

The role of PDD in the diagnosis of bladder cancer has been well established, but its role in UTUC has only recently been investigated [49]. Several studies demonstrate the added diagnostic value of PDD [49–54]. Recently, Liu et al. conducted a meta-analysis including 289 cases to determine the efficacy of PDD-assisted ureteroscopy in diagnosing UTUCs. Pooled analysis concluded that PDD can differentiate between UTUC and benign upper urinary tract lesions with a high sensitivity of 96% and specificity of 86%. Furthermore, the use of PDD in comparison to WL improves UTUC detection rate [50]. Similarly, Osman et al. conducted a systematic review of 194 patients to determine the sensitivity of 95.8% versus 53.5% respectively and specificity of 96.6% versus 95.2% respectively, leading to the conclusion that PDD is more accurate than WL ureteroscopy for the diagnosis of UTUC [51]. Compared to other novel optical technologies, more studies have been conducted and have demonstrated the additional diagnostic utility that PDD provides with fURS. It is a promising endoscopic technique for the upper urinary tract and requires further studies on larger sample sizes to exemplify its advantages and reduce its limitations.

6.2 Narrow-Band Imaging

Narrow-band imaging (NBI) is an optical enhancement technique that utilizes higher wavelengths such as blue t 415 nm and green at 540 nm to better penetrate the tissue and enhance contrast between mucosa and microvasculature. Both wavelengths of light are strongly absorbed by hemoglobin. On imaging, the vasculature will appear either dark brown or green against the mucosa that appears light pink or white [47].

Several studies have investigated the diagnostic role of NBI-assisted digital fURS. Traxer et al. performed fURS using both WL and NBI to assess whether detection of malignancy was increased. A total of 27 patients underwent examination of the entire renal collecting system first with WL followed by NBI, and images obtained during both were compared to the final pathologic diagnosis. Not only did NBI produce improved endoscopic visualization, but it also detected five additional tumors in 4 patients and three tumors with extended margins in 3 patients. Overall, NBI-assisted fURS improved tumor detection rate by 22.7% [55]. Hao et al. performed a similar study of 54 cases of UTUC. The study demonstrated that NBI-assisted fURS improved tumor diagnosis by 20% and provided better image quality especially in areas near the border between normal tissue and tumor [56]. Iordache et al. also performed a similar prospective analysis of 87 patients with similar results illustrating an improved tumor detection rate for NBI-assisted fURS than standard fURS, 98.4% versus 91.7% respectively. However, interestingly NBI in comparison to WL was associated with a higher false-positive rate, 17.5% versus 10.1% respectively [57]. NBI has demonstrated its value as an addition to a diagnostic modality exploring the upper urinary tract. However, it is important to study its use in larger sample sizes to gain a better understanding of its benefits and limitations.

6.3 Optical Coherence Tomography

Optical coherence tomography (OCT), also referred to as optical biopsy or light ultrasound, is a noninvasive imaging technology that uses signal interference between the tissue sample under observation and a local reference signal to generate a cross-sectional image of tissue while capturing individual layers of the tissue in real time [58, 59]. This diagnostic technique has been widely used in ophthalmology, but only a few studies have explored its use in urology, specifically in diagnostic fURS. OCT has been shown to obtain high resolution images, grade, and stage UTUC as a real-time, intraoperative diagnostic modality. For tumor grading, OCT had a sensitivity of 87% and specificity of 90%. For tumor staging, OCT had a sensitivity of 100% and specificity of 92% [60]. Furthermore, various studies have investigated the optical attenuation coefficient, μ_{OCT}, which measures how quickly light penetrates the medium under investigation, allowing for quantitative analysis of tissue from OCT signals [61]. Bus et al. reported that for low and high-grade lesions, the median μ_{OCT} was 2.1 mm^{-1} and 3.0 mm^{-1} respectively [60]. Similarly, Freund et al. calculated a median μ_{OCT} for low-grade and high-grade UTUC of 3.3 mm^{-1} and 4.9 mm^{-1} respectively. This study also identified an μ_{OCT} cut-off value of 4.0 mm^{-1} to discriminate between high-grade and low-grade papillary UTUC [62]. Further studies are required to accurately extract and optimize the optical attenuation coefficient to be used more extensively in the clinical setting.

6.4 Confocal Laser Endomicroscopy

Confocal laser endomicroscopy (CLE) is a probe-based optical technology that captures real-time images of sectioned tissue and provides a high-resolution dynamic evaluation of tissue microarchitecture and morphology. A confocal microscope is packaged into the small probe utilized in this optical technique, which is compatible with standard endoscopes [63]. Similar to PDD, CLE requires either the topical or intravenous administration of a fluorescent agent, most commonly fluorescein dye [64]. After the tissue is stained with fluorescent dye and molecules of the dye have been excited, the dye emits light that is filtered through a pinhole so that the photodetector measures in-focus light and rejects out-of-focus light. This process ultimately creates optical sectioning of the tissue of interest. Through direct contact between the probe inserted through the endoscope and tissue, images are obtained at a rate of 12 frames per second as a video sequence [63]. CLE was first used to study histopathologic changes in bronchial and colonic tissue [65, 66]. More recently, however, CLE has been utilized during fURS and a few studies have reported favorable experiences. Breda et al. found CLE with fURS to be a reliable real-time histologic characterization of UTUC lesions and the clinical use may be especially useful in patients who are potential candidates for conservative management [67]. Villa et al. demonstrated that CLE was able to recognize distorted microarchitecture and tortuous vasculature more clearly in patients with confirmed high-grade UTUC [68]. Limitations include susceptibility to motion artefact [47] and the inability to determine the sensitivity and specificity of this optical technique [68]. Further studies are required to further determine the diagnostic accuracy of CLE, understand its limitations, and identify its tole in the clinical setting.

7 Conclusion

In conclusion, fURS is a key diagnostic tool in the workup of UTUC and other upper urinary tract pathologies. Several advancements that have been made in diagnostic technique, including optics and image processing, have shown promising results and require further research to better understand their potential use in the clinical setting as well as rectify its shortcomings.

References

1. Rajamahanty S, Grasso M. Flexible ureteroscopy update: indications, instrumentation and technical advances. Indian J Urol. 2008;24(4):532–7. https://doi.org/10.4103/0970-1591.44263.
2. Wason SE, Monfared S, Ionson A, Leslie SW. Ureteroscopy. Treasure Island (FL): StatPearls Publishing; 2021.
3. Bird VG, Shields JM. Smith's Textbook of Endourology. 4th ed. Hoboken, New Jersey: John Wiley & Sons; 2019. Chapter 40, Flexible Ureteroscopes; p. 475–485

4. Ridyard D, Dagrosa L, Pais VM Jr. From novelty to the every-day: the evolution of ureteroscopy. Minerva Urol Nefrol. 2016;68(6):469–78. Epub 2016 Sep 1
5. Geavlete P, Multescu R, Geavlete B. Retrograde flexible ureteroscopy: reshaping the upper urinary tract endourology. Arch Esp Urol. 2011;64(1):3–13.
6. Geavlete P, Multescu R, Georgescu D, Geavlete B. VID-03.08: Indications and limitations of diagnostic flexible ureteroscopy. Urology. 2007;70:178–9. https://doi.org/10.1016/j.urology.2007.06.611.
7. Bagley DH, Allen J. Flexible ureteropyeloscopy in the diagnosis of benign essential hematuria. J Urol. 1990;143(3):549–53. https://doi.org/10.1016/s0022-5347(17)40016-4.
8. Nakada SY, Elashry OM, Picus D, Clayman RV. Long-term outcome of flexible ureterorenoscopy in the diagnosis and treatment of lateralizing essential hematuria. J Urol. 1997;157(3):776–9.
9. Rouprêt M, Babjuk M, Burger M, Capoun O, Cohen D, Compérat EM, Cowan NC, Dominguez-Escrig JL, Gontero P, Hugh Mostafid A, Palou J, Peyronnet B, Seisen T, Soukup V, Sylvester RJ, Rhijn BWGV, Zigeuner R, Shariat SF. European Association of Urology guidelines on upper urinary tract urothelial carcinoma: 2020 update. Eur Urol. 2021;79(1):62–79. https://doi.org/10.1016/j.eururo.2020.05.042. Epub 2020 Jun 24
10. Potretzke AM, Knight BA, Vetter JM, Anderson BG, Hardi AC, Bhayani SB, Figenshau RS. Diagnostic utility of selective upper tract urinary cytology: A systematic review and meta-analysis of the literature. Urology. 2016;96:35–43. https://doi.org/10.1016/j.urology.2016.04.030. Epub 2016 May 2
11. Streem SB, Pontes JE, Novick AC, Montie JE. Ureteropyeloscopy in the evaluation of upper tract filling defects. J Urol. 1986;136(2):383–5. https://doi.org/10.1016/s0022-5347(17)44875-0.
12. Bagley DH, Huffman JL, Lyon ES. Flexible ureteropyeloscopy: diagnosis and treatment in the upper urinary tract. J Urol. 1987;138(2):280–5. https://doi.org/10.1016/s0022-5347(17)43119-3.
13. Puppo P, Ricciotti G, Bottino P, Germinale F, Perachino M. Exploración del sistema colector intrarrenal a través de fibroscopia flexible [exploration of the intra-renal collecting system using flexible fibroscopy]. Arch Esp Urol. 1991;44(5):541–5.
14. Raman JD, Park R. Endoscopic management of upper-tract urothelial carcinoma. Expert Rev Anticancer Ther. 2017;17(6):545–54. https://doi.org/10.1080/14737140.2017.1326823. Epub 2017 May 15
15. Proietti S, Marchioni M, Eisner BH, Lucianò R, Saitta G, Rodríguez-Socarrás ME, D'orta C, Bellinzoni P, Schips L, Gaboardi F, Giusti G. Conservative treatment of upper urinary tract carcinoma in patients with imperative indications. Minerva Urol Nephrol. 2020;73(2):245–52. https://doi.org/10.23736/S0393-2249.20.03710-8. Epub ahead of print
16. Cutress ML, Stewart GD, Zakikhani P, Phipps S, Thomas BG, Tolley DA. Ureteroscopic and percutaneous management of upper tract urothelial carcinoma (UTUC): systematic review. BJU Int. 2012;110(5):614–28. https://doi.org/10.1111/j.1464-410X.2012.11068.x. Epub 2012 Apr 3
17. Villa L, Cloutier J, Letendre J, Ploumidis A, Salonia A, Cornu JN, Montorsi F, Traxer O. Early repeated ureteroscopy within 6-8 weeks after a primary endoscopic treatment in patients with upper tract urothelial cell carcinoma: preliminary findings. World J Urol. 2016;34(9):1201–6. https://doi.org/10.1007/s00345-015-1753-7. Epub 2015 Dec 23
18. Siegel RL, Miller KD, Jemal A. Cancer statistics, 2019. CA Cancer J Clin. 2019;69(1):7–34. https://doi.org/10.3322/caac.21551. Epub 2019 Jan 8
19. Margulis V, Shariat SF, Matin SF, Kamat AM, Zigeuner R, Kikuchi E, Lotan Y, Weizer A, Raman JD, Wood CG. The upper tract urothelial carcinoma collaboration. Outcomes of radical nephroureterectomy: a series from the upper tract urothelial carcinoma collaboration. Cancer. 2009;115(6):1224–33. https://doi.org/10.1002/cncr.24135.
20. Inman BA, Tran VT, Fradet Y, Lacombe L. Carcinoma of the upper urinary tract: predictors of survival and competing causes of mortality. Cancer. 2009;115(13):2853–62. https://doi.org/10.1002/cncr.24339.
21. Cowan NC, Turney BW, Taylor NJ, McCarthy CL, Crew JP. Multidetector computed tomography urography for diagnosing upper urinary tract urothelial tumour. BJU Int. 2007;99(6):1363–70. https://doi.org/10.1111/j.1464-410X.2007.06766.x. Epub 2007 Apr 8
22. Cheng K, Cassidy F, Aganovic L, Taddonio M, Vahdat N. CT urography: how to optimize the technique. Abdom Radiol (NY). 2019;44(12):3786–99. https://doi.org/10.1007/s00261-019-02111-2.
23. Janisch F, Shariat SF, Baltzer P, Fajkovic H, Kimura S, Iwata T, Korn P, Yang L, Glybochko PV, Rink M, Abufaraj M. Diagnostic performance of multidetector computed tomographic (MDCTU) in upper tract urothelial carcinoma (UTUC): a systematic review and meta-analysis. World J Urol. 2020;38(5):1165–75. https://doi.org/10.1007/s00345-019-02875-8. Epub 2019 Jul 18
24. Soria F, Shariat SF, Lerner SP, Fritsche HM, Rink M, Kassouf W, Spiess PE, Lotan Y, Ye D, Fernández MI, Kikuchi E, Chade DC, Babjuk M, Grollman AP, Thalmann GN. Epidemiology, diagnosis, preoperative evaluation and prognostic assessment of upper-tract urothelial carcinoma (UTUC). World J Urol. 2017;35(3):379–87. https://doi.org/10.1007/s00345-016-1928-x. Epub 2016 Sep 7
25. Wang KY, Hu JS, Fang L, Zhang DX, Li Q, Ng DM, Haleem M, Xie GH, Ma Q. Advantages of retrograde flexible ureteroscopy in determining the etiology of painless hematuria originating from the upper urinary tract. Exp Ther Med. 2020;19(4):2627–31. https://doi.org/10.3892/etm.2020.8482. Epub 2020 Jan 31
26. Foerster B, Shariat SF, Klein JT, Bolenz C. Biopsietechniken im oberen Harntrakt zur Diagnostik des Urothelkarzinoms: systematische

Übersicht [Biopsy techniques in the upper urinary tract for the diagnosis of urothelial carcinoma: systematic review]. Urologe A. 2019;58(1):14–21. https://doi.org/10.1007/s00120-018-0829-6.
27. Rojas CP, Castle SM, Llanos CA, Santos Cortes JA, Bird V, Rodriguez S, Reis IM, Zhao W, Gomez-Fernandez C, Leveillee RJ, Jorda M. Low biopsy volume in ureteroscopy does not affect tumor biopsy grading in upper tract urothelial carcinoma. Urol Oncol. 2013;31(8):1696–700. https://doi.org/10.1016/j.urolonc.2012.05.010. Epub 2012 Jul 21
28. Brien JC, Shariat SF, Herman MP, Ng CK, Scherr DS, Scoll B, Uzzo RG, Wille M, Eggener SE, Terrell JD, Lucas SM, Lotan Y, Boorjian SA, Raman JD. Preoperative hydronephrosis, ureteroscopic biopsy grade and urinary cytology can improve prediction of advanced upper tract urothelial carcinoma. J Urol. 2010;184(1):69–73. https://doi.org/10.1016/j.juro.2010.03.030. Epub 2010 May 15
29. Marchioni M, Primiceri G, Cindolo L, Hampton LJ, Grob MB, Guruli G, Schips L, Shariat SF, Autorino R. Impact of diagnostic ureteroscopy on intravesical recurrence in patients undergoing radical nephroureterectomy for upper tract urothelial cancer: a systematic review and meta-analysis. BJU Int. 2017;120(3):313–9. https://doi.org/10.1111/bju.13935. Epub 2017 Jul 19
30. Guo RQ, Hong P, Xiong GY, Zhang L, Fang D, Li XS, Zhang K, Zhou LQ. Impact of ureteroscopy before radical nephroureterectomy for upper tract urothelial carcinomas on oncological outcomes: a meta-analysis. BJU Int. 2018;121(2):184–93. https://doi.org/10.1111/bju.14053. Epub 2017 Nov 1
31. Nison L, Rouprêt M, Bozzini G, Ouzzane A, Audenet F, Pignot G, Ruffion A, Cornu JN, Hurel S, Valeri A, Roumiguie M, Polguer T, Hoarau N, Mérigot de Treigny O, Xylinas E, Matte A, Droupy S, Fais PO, Descazeaud A, Colin P, MD for the French Collaborative National Database on UUT-UC. The oncologic impact of a delay between diagnosis and radical nephroureterectomy due to diagnostic ureteroscopy in upper urinary tract urothelial carcinomas: results from a large collaborative database. World J Urol. 2013;31(1):69–76. https://doi.org/10.1007/s00345-012-0959-1. Epub 2012 Oct 16
32. Brenez J, Hawotte P. Les tumeurs primitives de l'uretère et du bassinet [primary neoplasms of the ureter and pelvis]. Acta Urol Belg. 1972;40(3):505–32.
33. Kiel H, Ullrich T, Roessler W, Wieland WF, Knuechel-Clarke R. Benign ureteral tumors. Four case reports and a review of the literature. Urol Int. 1999;63(3):201–5. https://doi.org/10.1159/000030448.
34. Georgescu D, Mulţescu R, Geavlete BF, Geavlete P, Vrabie CD, Drăghici IM, Stănescu C, Enescu A. Fibroepithelial polyps - a rare pathology of the upper urinary tract. Romanian J Morphol Embryol. 2014;55(4):1325–30.
35. Adey GS, Vargas SO, Retik AB, Borer JG, Mandell J, Hendren WH, Lebowitz RL, Bauer SB. Fibroepithelial polyps causing ureteropelvic junction obstruction in children. J Urol. 2003;169(5):1834–6. https://doi.org/10.1097/01.ju.0000061966.21966.94.
36. Dolan R, Morton S, Granitsiotis P. Presentation of a benign fibroepithelial polyp with frank haematuria: an unusual diagnosis. Scott Med J. 2015;60(1):e24–6. https://doi.org/10.1177/0036933014563891. Epub 2014 Dec 12
37. Manuel M, Nadeem S, Moredock E, Rakheja D, Scott S. Fibroepithelial polyp: an unusual cause of acute urinary retention in a 5-year-old boy. Consultant. 2021;61(7):E30–2 . Published online November 5, 2020. https://doi.org/10.25270/con.2020.11.00007.
38. Lam JS, Bingham JB, Gupta M. Endoscopic treatment of fibroepithelial polyps of the renal pelvis and ureter. Urology. 2003;62(5):810–3. https://doi.org/10.1016/s0090-4295(03)00691-5.
39. Sajitha K, Kishan Prasad HL, Pradeep A, Rajeev TP, Mathias M, Shetty KJ. Cavernous hemangioma of ureter masquerading as malignancy – A rare case report. Urol Sci. 2020;31:139–41. https://doi.org/10.4103/UROS.UROS_15_20.
40. George A, Mani V, Noufal A. Update on the classification of hemangioma. J Oral Maxillofac Pathol. 2014;18(Suppl 1):S117–20. https://doi.org/10.4103/0973-029X.141321.
41. Tak GR, Agrawal S, Desai MR, Ganpule AP, Singh AG, Sabnis RB. Hemangioma of ureter: A diagnostic dilemma-managed surgically using robotic platform. J Endourol Case Rep. 2020;6(3):128–31. https://doi.org/10.1089/cren.2019.0148.
42. Araki M, Uehara S, Sasaki K, Monden K, Tsugawa M, Watanabe T, Monga M, Nasu Y, Kumon H. Ureteroscopic management of chronic unilateral hematuria: a single-center experience over 22 years. PLoS One. 2012;7(6):e36729. https://doi.org/10.1371/journal.pone.0036729. Epub 2012 Jun 8
43. Kumon H, Tsugawa M, Matsumura Y, Ohmori H. Endoscopic diagnosis and treatment of chronic unilateral hematuria of uncertain etiology. J Urol. 1990;143(3):554–8. https://doi.org/10.1016/s0022-5347(17)40017-6.
44. Lano MD, Wagoner RD, Leary FJ. Unilateral essential hematuria. Mayo Clin Proc. 1979;54(2):88–90.
45. Barocas DA, Boorjian SA, Alvarez RD, Downs TM, Gross CP, Hamilton BD, Kobashi KC, Lipman RR, Lotan Y, Ng CK, Nielsen ME, Peterson AC, Raman JD, Smith-Bindman R, Souter LH. Microhematuria: AUA/SUFU Guideline. J Urol. 2020;204(4):778–86. https://doi.org/10.1097/JU.0000000000001297. Epub 2020 Jul 23
46. Bus MT, de Bruin DM, Kamphuis GM, Zondervan PJ, Laguna Pes MP, de Reijke TM, van Leeuwen TG, de la Rosette JJ. Current position of diagnostics and surgical treatment for upper tract urothelial carcinoma. Minerva Urol Nefrol. 2017;69(2):159–65. https://doi.org/10.23736/S0393-2249.16.02720-X. Epub 2016 Oct 21
47. Bus MT, de Bruin DM, Faber DJ, Kamphuis GM, Zondervan PJ, Laguna Pes MP, de Reijke TM, Traxer O, van Leeuwen TG, de la Rosette JJ. Optical

diagnostics for upper urinary tract urothelial cancer: technology, thresholds, and clinical applications. J Endourol. 2015;29(2):113–23. https://doi.org/10.1089/end.2014.0551. Epub 2014 Oct 16
48. Cauberg EC, de Bruin DM, Faber DJ, van Leeuwen TG, de la Rosette JJ, de Reijke TM. A new generation of optical diagnostics for bladder cancer: technology, diagnostic accuracy, and future applications. Eur Urol. 2009;56(2):287–96. https://doi.org/10.1016/j.eururo.2009.02.033. Epub 2009 Mar 6
49. Knoedler JJ, Raman JD. Advances in the management of upper tract urothelial carcinoma: improved endoscopic management through better diagnostics. Ther Adv Urol. 2018;10(12):421–9. https://doi.org/10.1177/1756287218805334.
50. Liu Q, Zhang X, Zhou F, Lian Q, Lv H, Guo B, Xi X. Diagnostic accuracy of photodynamic diagnosis for upper urinary tract urothelial carcinoma: A systematic review and meta-analysis. Photodiagnosis Photodyn Ther. 2020;32:102067. https://doi.org/10.1016/j.pdpdt.2020.102067. Epub 2020 Oct 20
51. Osman E, Alnaib Z, Kumar N. Photodynamic diagnosis in upper urinary tract urothelial carcinoma: A systematic review. Arab J Urol. 2017;15(2):100–9. https://doi.org/10.1016/j.aju.2017.01.003.
52. Kata SG, Aboumarzouk OM, Zreik A, Somani B, Ahmad S, Nabi G, Buist R, Goodman C, Chlosta P, Golabek T, Moseley H. Photodynamic diagnostic ureterorenoscopy: A valuable tool in the detection of upper urinary tract tumour. Photodiagn Photodyn Ther. 2016;13:255–60. https://doi.org/10.1016/j.pdpdt.2015.08.002. Epub 2015 Aug 6
53. Aboumarzouk OM, Mains E, Moseley H, Kata SG. Diagnosis of upper urinary tract tumours: is photodynamic diagnosis assisted ureterorenoscopy required as an addition to modern imaging and ureterorenoscopy? Photodiagn Photodyn Ther. 2013;10(2):127–33. https://doi.org/10.1016/j.pdpdt.2012.11.008. Epub 2012 Dec 11
54. Aboumarzouk OM, Ahmad S, Moseley H, Kata SG. Accuracy of photodynamic diagnosis in the detection and follow-up of patients with upper urinary tract lesions: initial 3-year experience. Arab J Urol. 2012;10(2):138–42. https://doi.org/10.1016/j.aju.2012.01.006. Epub 2012 Feb 28
55. Traxer O, Geavlete B, de Medina SG, Sibony M, Al-Qahtani SM. Narrow-band imaging digital flexible ureteroscopy in detection of upper urinary tract transitional-cell carcinoma: initial experience. J Endourol. 2011;25(1):19–23. https://doi.org/10.1089/end.2009.0593.
56. Hao YC, Xiao CL, Liu K, Liu YQ, Ma LL. Application of narrow-band imaging flexible ureteroscopy in the diagnosis, treatment and follow-up of upper tract urothelial carcinomas. Zhonghua Wai Ke Za Zhi. 2018;56(3):222–6. https://doi.org/10.3760/cma.j.issn.0529-5815.2018.03.011.
57. Iordache VF, Geavlete PA, Georgescu DA, Ene CV, Păunescu MA, Niculae A, Peride I, Neagu TP, Bulai CA, Bălan GX, Geavlete BF, Lascăr I. NBI-assisted digital flexible ureteroscopy in transitional renal cell carcinoma - an evidence-based assessment "through the looking glass" of the pathological analysis. Romanian J Morphol Embryol. 2018;59(4):1091–6.
58. Podoleanu AG. Optical coherence tomography. J Microsc. 2012;247(3):209–19. https://doi.org/10.1111/j.1365-2818.2012.03619.x. Epub 2012 Jun 18
59. Kriegmair MC, Hein S, Schoeb DS, Zappe H, Suárez-Ibarrola R, Waldbillig F, Gruene B, Pohlmann PF, Praus F, Wilhelm K, Gratzke C, Miernik A, Bolenz C. Erweiterte Bildgebung in der urologischen Endoskopie [Enhanced imaging in urological endoscopy]. Urologe A. 2021;60(1):8–18. https://doi.org/10.1007/s00120-020-01400-9. Epub 2020 Dec 10
60. Bus MT, de Bruin DM, Faber DJ, Kamphuis GM, Zondervan PJ, Laguna-Pes MP, van Leeuwen TG, de Reijke TM, de la Rosette JJ. Optical coherence tomography as a tool for in vivo staging and grading of upper urinary tract urothelial carcinoma: A study of diagnostic accuracy. J Urol. 2016;196(6):1749–55. https://doi.org/10.1016/j.juro.2016.04.117. Epub 2016 Jul 27
61. Chang S, Bowden AK. Review of methods and applications of attenuation coefficient measurements with optical coherence tomography. J Biomed Opt. 2019;24(9):1–17. https://doi.org/10.1117/1.JBO.24.9.090901.
62. Freund JE, Faber DJ, Bus MT, van Leeuwen TG, de Bruin DM. Grading upper tract urothelial carcinoma with the attenuation coefficient of in-vivo optical coherence tomography. Lasers Surg Med. 2019; https://doi.org/10.1002/lsm.23079. Epub ahead of print
63. Chen SP, Liao JC. Confocal laser endomicroscopy of bladder and upper tract urothelial carcinoma: a new era of optical diagnosis? Curr Urol Rep. 2014;15(9):437. https://doi.org/10.1007/s11934-014-0437-y.
64. Liem EI, Freund JE, Baard J, de Bruin DM, Laguna Pes MP, Savci-Heijink CD, van Leeuwen TG, de Reijke TM, de la Rosette JJ. Confocal laser endomicroscopy for the diagnosis of urothelial carcinoma in the bladder and the upper urinary tract: protocols for two prospective explorative studies. JMIR Res Protoc. 2018;7(2):e34. https://doi.org/10.2196/resprot.8862.
65. Thiberville L, Moreno-Swirc S, Vercauteren T, Peltier E, Cavé C, Bourg HG. In vivo imaging of the bronchial wall microstructure using fibered confocal fluorescence microscopy. Am J Respir Crit Care Med. 2007;175(1):22–31. https://doi.org/10.1164/rccm.200605-684OC. Epub 2006 Oct 5
66. Wang TD, Friedland S, Sahbaie P, Soetikno R, Hsiung PL, Liu JT, Crawford JM, Contag CH. Functional imaging of colonic mucosa with a fibered confocal microscope for real-time in vivo pathology. Clin Gastroenterol Hepatol. 2007;5(11):1300–5. https://doi.org/10.1016/j.cgh.2007.07.013. Epub 2007 Oct 23
67. Breda A, Territo A, Guttilla A, Sanguedolce F, Manfredi M, Quaresima L, Gaya JM, Algaba F, Palou

J, Villavicencio H. Correlation between confocal laser endomicroscopy (Cellvizio®) and histological grading of upper tract urothelial carcinoma: A step forward for a better selection of patients suitable for conservative management. Eur Urol Focus. 2018;4(6):954–9. https://doi.org/10.1016/j.euf.2017.05.008. Epub 2017 Jun 4

68. Villa L, Cloutier J, Cotè JF, Salonia A, Montorsi F, Traxer O. Confocal laser endomicroscopy in the Management of endoscopically treated upper urinary tract transitional cell carcinoma: preliminary data. J Endourol. 2016;30(2):237–42. https://doi.org/10.1089/end.2015.0644. Epub 2015 Dec 30

Flexible Ureteroscopy in UPJ and Ureteral Stenosis

Yongda Liu

Abstract

Flexible ureteroscopy is a treatment for UPJ and ureteral stenosis. This method is applied for the length of stricture is less than 2 cm and the semirigid retrograde approach is difficult or impossible. It has minimal trauma and a definite short-term effect, but its long-term effect still need to be improved.

Keywords

Flexible ureteroscopy · UPJO · Ureteral stenosis

A ureteral stricture is a constriction of the ureter that causes a functional obstruction. The most common form of ureteral stricture is UPJ stricture.

Ureteroscopic treatment of ureteropelvic junction (UPJ) obstruction was first reported in 1986 by Ingis and Tolley [1]. Numerous improvements and optimizations have been achieved since then, the most prominent of which being the invention of compact, high optical-quality ureteroscopes and flexible ureteroscopes.

Rigid ureteroscopy is used to treat the majority of UPJ or ureteral strictures. However, flexible ureteroscopy is beneficial in the treatment of ureteral pathology when rigid or semirigid retrograde approach is problematic or impossible, such as in patients with urinary diversions, upper urinary tract anatomic abnormalities, musculoskeletal deformities, and so on.

The initial reports of a ureteroscopic approach described using electcautery for the endopeylotomy incision. More recently, however, the holmium laser has been recognized as having ideal qualities for cutting tissue, namely, precision and minimal thermal spread.

Y. Liu (✉)
Department of Urology and Guangdong Key Laboratory of Urology, The First Affiliated Hospital of Guangzhou Medical University, Guangzhou, Guangdong, China

G. Zeng et al. (eds.), *Flexible Ureteroscopy*, https://doi.org/10.1007/978-981-19-2936-6_21

1 Etiology

These strictures can be congenital, acquired, or iatrogenic.

> **Box 1. Iatrogenic Causes of Ureteral Strictures**
>
> *Urology*
> - Rigid or flexible ureteroscopy (perforation, dehiscence, ischemia)
> - Percutaneous stone extraction
> - Open pyeloplasty
> - Open ureterolithotomy
> - Transureteral surgery
> - Prostatectomy
> - Bladder neck surgery
>
> *General surgery*
> - Colorectal surgery
> - Aortic abdominal aneurysm grafting
> - Aortobifemoral grafting
> - Renal transplant (ureterneocystotomy)
>
> *Gynecology*
> - Hysterectomy
> - Bladder surgery
> - Vaginal surgery
>
> *Radiation therapy*
> - Pevic malignancy
> - Retroperioneal treatment

2 Indications

At present, The acknowledged indication for the treatment of UPJ or ureteral stricture with flexible ureteroscope includes the length of stricture is less than 2 cm and the semirigid retrograde approach is difficult or impossible. Patients ureteral stenosis greater than 2 cm may benefit from open surgery or laparoscopy.

3 Methods

Endoscopic procedures for ureteral stricture have been introduced based on Davis' 1943 theory that "the ureteral wall regenerates on a tutor probe in 6 weeks following a longitudinal incision" [2].

3.1 Preparation

Ultrasonography, intravenous pyelography, and a CT scan were performed on all of the patients. The topography and length of the stenosis were determined by retrograde ureteropyelography, which was performed in all patients. In selected patients of urographic hypofunctional kidney, renal scintigraphy was recommended to assess the kidney in greater detail.

3.2 Technique

The procedure carried out under the supervision of a fluoroscope. A retrograde pyelogram was acquired as a baseline. The image intensifier is turned obliquely to both sides during the operation in order to determine the exact length and location of the obstruction. A guidewire was inserted into the renal pelvis and coiled. When substantial kinking of the ureter prevents safe passage into the renal pelvis, a second wire may be necessary. The two guidewires together effectively straightened the ureter. The flexible ureteroscope was passed along the stenotic ureter alongside the guidewire. Once the stenotic ureter was reached, a 200-μm holmium laser fibre was employed using the flexible ureteroscope.

The stenotic ureter was incised either laterally or posterolaterally under direct vision at a setting of 1.5–2.5 J and a frequency of 10–15 Hz. The laser power was initially set to 1.5 J, then altered according to the patient's tissue penetrability different in each case.

Under video and fluoroscopy guidance, the incision was made until the perinephric fat was mostly exposed and the ureter was wide enough for the ureteroscope to penetrate into the renal pelvis. A successful incision was confirmed by eruption of the contrast fluid. Endoureterotomy was necessary both proximally and distally to encompass some normal ureteral tissue. The incision was made anteromedially for those strictures that involved the distal ureter. Finally, an 8/12F pyelostent was inserted for an 8-week period.

All cases were evaluated at 6, 12, and 18 month post procedure, through clinical examination, gray-scale and Doppler ultrasonography, and IVP.

4 Results

Endoscopic treatment of ureteral stricture or UPJ has been proven to be reasonable. Within strictures < 2 cm, good outcomes rates have been reported after endoscopic treatment, up to 85.7% of success rates for intrinsic stenosis and 89% of symptoms resolution [3, 4]. Postoperative double J stenting for 4–8 weeks may improve surgical outcomes. Open or laparoscopic salvage procedures allow adaptation to intraoperative findings, transposition of crossing vessels, and mobilization of kidney and ureter to create a primary anastomosis.

Significant expertise in the context of a salvage procedure is required in both of the above approaches, since the fibrosis and scarring subsequent to the initial operation makes this technically more challenging. Although the laparoscopic method was less invasive and with shorter hospital stay, the associated operating times (mean, 254 and 310 min) were prolonged, as reported in [5, 6].

5 Complications

During or after flexible endopyelotomy, there is low morbidity and no significant bleeding. Aside from ureteroscopic and ureter incision-related risks, reported complications include hemorrhage, guide fragmentation during endopyelotomy, stent migration through the incision, proximal stent migration, subcapsular hematoma, and urinary infections.

References

1. Inglis JA, Tolley DA. Ureteroscopic pyelolysis for pelviureteric junction obstruction. Br J Urol. 1986;58:250–2.
2. Davis DM. Intubated ureterotomy: a new operation for ureteral and ureteropelvic strictures. Surg Gynecol Obestet. 1943;76:513.
3. Rassweiler JJ, Subotic S, Feist-Schwenk M, et al. Minimally invasive treatment of ureteropelvic junction obstruction: long-term experience with an algorithm for laser endopyelotomy and laparoscopic retroperitoneal pyeloplasty. J Urol. 2007;177:1000–5.
4. Stilling NM, Jung H, Nørby B, et al. Retrograde ureteroscopic holmium laser endopyelotomy in a selected population of patients with ureteropelvic junction obstruction. Scand J Urol Nephrol. 2009;43:68–72.
5. Levin BM, Herrell SD. Salvage laparoscopic pyeloplasty in the worst case scenario: after both failed open repair and endoscopic salvage. J Endourol. 2006;20:808–12.
6. Basiri A, Behjati S, Zand S, Moghaddam SMH. Laparoscopic pyeloplasty in secondary ureteropelvic junction obstruction after failed open surgery. J Endourol. 2007;21:1045–51; discussion 1051

Flexible Ureteroscopy for Upper Tract Urothelial Carcinoma

Francesco Soria, Paolo Gontero, Maria del Pilar Laguna Pes, and Jean de la Rosette

Abstract

Flexible ureteroscopy (fURS) is an essential tool for the diagnosis, risk stratification, and treatment of upper tract urothelial carcinoma (UTUC). fURS should actually be performed in case of uncertainty, for kidney-sparing surgery (KSS), and even before radical surgery being able to provide important information for decision-making regarding perioperative systemic treatments. Flexible diagnostic URS is a stepwise procedure, starting with bladder cystoscopy and urine sampling for selective cytology and eventually ending with tumor ablation. Ureteral access sheaths can be used to allow for multiple biopsies, thereby diminishing the risk of inadequate tumor sampling. While the advent of digital scopes and that of enhanced technology imaging has dramatically improved the quality of the visualization of the upper urinary tract, a demonstration of their clinical utility over fiber-optic scopes is, to date, missing. Meanwhile, the experience of the surgeon and strict adherence to the guidelines recommendations remain the cornerstones of diagnostic fURS and KSS.

Keywords

Flexible ureteroscopy · UTUC · Digital · NBI Image 1-S · Laser · Ablation · Biopsy

1 Flexible Ureteroscopy for UTUC: When to Perform It

Diagnostic ureteroscopy has to be performed in any case in which a kidney-sparing surgery (KSS) may be feasible, mainly depending on tumor size and location, and in case of diagnostic uncertainty. Diagnostic URS allows for the assessment of tumor focality and the performance of tumor biopsy, therefore being essential for UTUC risk stratification and subsequent treatment decision-making. Conversely, diagnostic URS may theoretically be skipped if radical surgery is already planned due to the presence of a high-risk tumor on CT scan and/or urinary cytology (i.e., tumor size >2 cm, multifocal tumor, invasive aspect at imaging).

Nonetheless, diagnostic fURS may provide useful information even when RNU is already planned. Currently, to improve long-term oncological outcomes, adjuvant chemotherapy after RNU is the standard treatment for pT3-T4 and/or N+ disease [1]. Adjuvant chemotherapy has shown to be able to significantly improve disease-

F. Soria (✉) · P. Gontero
Division of Urology, Department of Surgical Sciences, San Giovanni Battista Hospital, University of Studies of Torino, Turin, Italy
e-mail: francesco.soria@unito.it

M. del Pilar Laguna Pes · J. de la Rosette
Department of Urology, Istanbul Medipol Mega University Hospital, Istanbul Medipol University, Istanbul, Turkey

G. Zeng et al. (eds.), *Flexible Ureteroscopy*, https://doi.org/10.1007/978-981-19-2936-6_22

free survival (3-year recurrence-free rate of 71% vs. 46% for patients receiving therapy vs. surveillance, respectively) in the recently published POUT trial [2]. However, the administration of adjuvant chemotherapy after RNU may be compromised by several factors, first among all the impaired renal function after surgery. A retrospective analysis of patients who underwent RNU for UTUC found a median decrease in eGFR by 8–12% after surgery; in details, patients with eGFR ≥60 ml/min decreased from 37% preoperatively to 16% postoperatively, while those with eGFR ≥45 ml/min decreased from 72% to 52%, respectively [3]. Based on this data, only 16% of patients may be eligible for cisplatin-based adjuvant chemotherapy. To overcome this important limitation, the role of neoadjuvant chemotherapy is currently under investigation in several randomized controlled trials (NCT02876861, NCT04574960, NCT02969083). However, one of the main concerns with neoadjuvant chemotherapy is related to patients' selection. The majority of published series about neoadjuvant chemotherapy include patients with cT3-T4 and/or cN1 tumor stage, high-grade pathology at biopsy, and sessile architecture [4–6]. Similarly, ongoing RCTs require histologically confirmed high-grade UTUC to enter the study. Therefore, if the activity of neoadjuvant chemotherapy before RNU will be demonstrated, diagnostic fURS will become essential even in this clinical scenario.

Finally, diagnostic URS before RNU may provide important information for decision-making regarding the need and extent of lymph node dissection (LND). Template-based and complete LND has been demonstrated to improve cancer-specific survival in patients with high-stage (≥pT2) UTUC and to reduce the risk of local recurrence [7]. The combination of imaging and ureteroscopic information could help to predict muscle-invasive and non–organ-confined disease at the time of surgery [8]. Margulis et al. developed and internally validated a nomogram for the prediction of non–organ-confined UTUC based on preoperative variables such as tumor grade, architecture, and location [9]. The nomogram achieved a predictive accuracy of 76.6%. Similarly, Brien et al. by combining the presence of preoperative hydronephrosis with biopsy tumor high grade and positive urinary cytology reached a positive predictive value for muscle-invasive and non-organ-confined disease of 89% [10]. Interestingly, when all the three variables were absent, the negative predictive value was 100%.

In conclusion, preoperative diagnostic fURS is not only mandatory for risk-stratification when a KSS is taken into consideration but provides essential information regarding surgery and perioperative treatment even in patients undergoing radical nephroureterectomy. Single-dose postoperative instillation of chemotherapy may be considered.

2 Flexible Ureteroscopy for UTUC: The Risk of Delayed Treatment and Intravesical Recurrence

Some controversies still exist regarding the possible detrimental impact of diagnostic fURS before RNU on delaying definitive treatment and on bladder recurrence rate. Nison et al. evaluated the long-term oncological outcomes of 512 patients who had RNU [11]; of these, 170 underwent diagnostic fURS before surgery. Median treatment time, calculated from the time of diagnosis to definitive treatment, was significantly longer in patients receiving fURS (80 vs. 45 days). However, this did not translate into worse oncological outcomes (5-years recurrence-free, metastasis-free and cancer-specific survival rates did not differ between groups). Conversely, diagnostic fURS has been shown to increase the risk of intravesical recurrence after RNU. Firstly, Sung et al. retrospectively analyzed a cohort of 630 patients who received RNU, of whom 282 underwent diagnostic fURS before surgery and demonstrated a significantly worse 5-year intravesical recurrence-free survival rate among the fURS group (42.6% vs. 63.6%) [12]. Moreover, it has been shown that the timing of diagnostic fURS plays an important role in the probability of developing intravesical recurrence; while immediate pre-RNU diagnostic fURS seems to not affect the probability of recurrence, a time interval of 5 days between fURS and RNU increases the risk of intravesical recurrence of about 1.5 to 4 times [13]. To overcome this important limitation a postoperative single-dose intravesical instillation of chemotherapy may be proposed. A single postoperative dose of chemotherapy 2–10 days after RNU has proven to reduce the risk of bladder recurrence within the initial years after surgery in two different prospective randomized trials and is currently recommended from international guidelines [14, 15]. Based on this data, a single postoperative instillation may be a reasonable option after diagnostic fURS, even if evidence about its efficacy in this setting is still lacking.

3 Flexible Ureteroscopy for UTUC: How to Perform It

The incidence of concomitant bladder cancer at the time of UTUC diagnosis is around 17% [16]. Therefore, when approaching a case of suspicious UTUC, it is imperative to start the procedure with a formal cystoscopy in which a complete investigation of the urethra and bladder wall is conducted. In case of bladder tumor, the resection should be delayed at the end of the procedure unless the tumor covers the ureteral orifice, thereby preventing the access to the upper urinary tract. Subsequently, a cone-tipped catheter is inserted in the ureteral orifice and may serve both for selective cytology and for retrograde pyelography, able to provide imaging of the upper urinary tract and identify filling defects [17]. At this point, semi-rigid ureteroscopy should be performed with a "no-touch" technique whenever feasible. The avoidance of a guide wire may actually prevent the scraping of small tumors as well as the occurrence of unnecessary bleeding that could compromise the endoscopic view of the upper urinary tract. After having ruled out the presence of ureteral cancer, a guide wire is inserted and flexible URS performed to allow the visualization of the renal collecting system. A ureteral access sheath may be used, as described below.

4 Selective Urine Cytology During Ureteroscopy: Yes or No

Urine cytology represents one of the cornerstones for UTUC diagnosis and risk-assessment, being one of the items used to distinguish between low- and high-risk UTUC cancer, with subsequent implications on decision-making regarding treatment approach. Therefore, it should be performed in any case of suspected UTUC. Positive urine cytology may indicate the presence of high-grade UTUC when cystoscopy is normal and a CIS of bladder/prostatic urethra has been ruled out [1, 8]. The overall sensitivity of voided urine cytology is lower for UTUC compared to bladder cancer. Messer et al., reviewing urinary cytology results from 326 patients with UTUC, found an overall sensitivity and positive predictive value of 56% and 54% for high-grade tumors, and of 62% and 44% for muscle-invasive disease [18].

To improve the accuracy of voided urine cytologic for the UTUC diagnosis, the use of selective cytology has been proposed and subsequently validated. In the above-mentioned Messer study, when restricting the analysis to patients who had cytology obtained by selective catheterization only, the sensitivity of the test improved from 56% to 71% and from 62% to 78% for high-grade tumors and muscle-invasive disease, respectively [18]. A systematic review and meta-analysis of the literature of 33 articles comparing selective cytology to either final pathology (21) or tissue biopsy (12) found an overall sensitivity and specificity of 53% and 90%, respectively [19]. As expected, sensitivity rates were significantly higher for high-grade tumors (70%) compared to low-grade cancers (46%).

The accuracy of selective cytology may be also lowered by the manipulation of the upper tract. The collection of urine before manipulation ensures that all collected cellular material is exfoliated and avoids the difficulties related to the distinction between low-grade tumor and traumatically detached hyperplastic epithelium [20]. To avoid erroneous sample collection, a stepwise procedure has been proposed and may be integrated into clinical practice to increase the accuracy of urine cytology [21]. Malm et al. showed that a protocol comprising bladder barbotage before manipulation, nontouch URS, renal pelvis barbotage, and collection of fluid from the bladder after URS to detect ureteral tumors led to an impressive sensitivity rate of 91%. Interestingly, urine cytology collected following the described protocol was as effective as final pathology to identify UTUC and to assess tumor grade.

5 Ureteral Access Sheath to Optimize Biopsy Sampling: Yes or No

One of the main issues in the UTUC diagnostic algorithm regards the accuracy of ureteroscopic biopsy, essential for risk-stratification and subsequent treatment decision-making. The accuracy of ureteroscopic biopsy for tumor grade assessment is lower than expected when compared to final pathology. Guarnizo et al., by evaluating 40 patients with UTUC who underwent URS with biopsy and the RNU, found an upstaging and upgrading rates at final pathology of 45% and 22%, respectively [22]. These preliminary results were successively confirmed by Smith and colleagues who retrospectively evaluated a series of 56 patients who underwent two or more consecutive biopsies or biopsy followed by surgical resection [23]. A change in grade or stage was found in more than one-third of patients; because of the short time interval between biopsies, this finding is likely representative of high variability in tumor sampling on biopsy rather than of a biologic evolution of the tumor. Upgrading occurs more often than downgrading, as demonstrated by the group of Wang who compared the final pathologic grade at RNU to that of ureteroscopic biopsy among 184 patients with UTUC [24]. Upgrading from G1 to either G2 or G3 occurred in almost the totality of patients (96%) while only 4% of patients were found to have a lower tumor grade on the final pathologic examination.

The main reason for biopsy inaccuracy relies on the inability of performing a good tissue sampling for pathologic examination at the time of URS. This is mainly the consequence of the miniaturization needed for performing tissue biopsy in the upper tract. A good quality tissue sampling for pathologic examination has been reported in only 75% of cases [25]. The use of ureteral access sheaths (UAS) allows for multiple passages of the ureteroscope into the upper urinary tract, thus allowing for multiple biopsies, and contributes to lower the intrarenal pressure, thereby theoretically minimizing the risk of cancer dissemination. The first and only description of the utility of UAS in the setting of UTUC dates back to 2011 when the group of Gorin reported their experience with UAS during 235 procedures in 125 patients [26]. The use of UAS facilitated the acquisition of multiple biopsy specimens adequate for histopathologic evaluation, thus preventing the need for repeat ureteroscopy to establish a diagnosis. A pathologic specimen adequate for diagnosis was obtained in 90% of the procedures. Moreover, among 35 patients who finally received RNU, concordant pathologic grade was observed in 31 cases (89%). No complications related to UAS use were reported. However, it has to be underlined that the use of UAS has been related to ureteral trauma in an impressively high percentage of cases in animal models and that the extension and severity of the lesion may be often underestimated during endoscopy when compared to the subsequent histopathological evaluation [27]. Therefore, the use of UAS may be suggested only after a "no-touch" ureteroscopy assessing the absence of ureteral stenosis and the compliance of the ureter itself.

6 Digital vs. Fiber-Optic Ureteroscopy

The advent of digital technology has dramatically improved the endoscopic view of the upper urinary tract, thus facilitating both the diagnosis and the treatment of patients with UTUC. An accurate visualization of the entire urinary tract is essential for the assessment of tumor focality, the performance of tumor biopsy as well as tumor ablation in case of KSS. In vitro studies have demonstrated superior image quality in favor of digital URS compared to fiber optic URS, and most authors agree that digital technology is superior for the detection of UTUC [28]. The major advantage of digital URS over fiber optic relies on lower image quality losses and higher image resolution [29]. In stone treatment, this translates into digital shorter operative time but comparable stone-free rates compared to fiber-optic URS [30]. In the management of UTUC, despite most authors agree that digital technology is superior in detecting urothelial carcinoma, to date, a direct comparison between fiber-optic and digital for the diagnosis and treatment of UTUC in terms of oncological outcomes is lacking.

7 Enhanced Imaging Technology: Sense or Nonsense

The diagnostic accuracy of flexible URS for UTUC is of paramount importance for risk-stratification, treatment planning, and in case of KSS. Diagnostic URS may allow an accurate evaluation of tumor size and focality as well as the performance of adequate tissue sampling for the assessment of tumor grade. Despite the continuous improvement in the visualization of the upper urinary tract thanks to the advent of digital imaging, the accuracy of flexible URS is far to be perfect, especially concerning the diagnosis of carcinoma in situ (CIS) and that of small lesions, with a nonnegligible detrimental impact on the risk-stratification accuracy. Yamani et al., in a retrospective study of 76 patients who underwent URS and subsequent RNU, quite surprisingly showed that diagnostic fURS missed a lesion in one out of four patients and that nearly 50% of these patients had a missed CIS lesion at final pathology [31]. The underdetection of CIS at prenephroureterectomy URS was subsequently confirmed by comparing final pathology at RNU of 106 patients previously evaluated with diagnostic fURS [32]. The presence of CIS was reported in 39 patients (37%) at final pathology; prenephroureterectomy fURS failed to diagnose CIS in 29 out of 39 patients (75%).

To overcome these limitations, and similarly to what happened for bladder cancer, enhanced imaging technologies have been tested also during diagnostic URS. The feasibility of photodynamic diagnosis (PDD) technology in the upper urinary tract has been firstly demonstrated in 2010 in 4 patients who underwent white light and PDD URS: all areas with fluorescence suspicious for urothelial cancer were biopsied and subsequently confirmed to be localizations of transitional cell carcinoma [33]. Since then, the feasibility and effectiveness of PDD have been confirmed in other small retrospective series [34, 35]. More recently, the same research group aimed to report the sensitivity, specificity, and detection rates of PDD vs white light URS in 54 patients (106 urinary tract units) with suspicious UTUC [36]. PDD-guided URS significantly detected more lesions and, especially, more CIS tumors compared to white light, with reported sensitivity and specificity rates of 96% and 97% (compared to 54% and 95% of white light). However, several obstacles have to date hindered the widespread of PDD-guided URS. Among these, the most relevant concern the difficulty of administering fluorochrome instillation into the upper urinary tract and the longitudinal illumination of the urothelium that may lower the specificity of the technique leading to a higher rate of unnecessary biopsies.

Both narrow-band imaging (NBI) and Image 1S have been tested in fURS and are nowadays incorporated in the last generation of flexible scopes (NBI in Olympus URF-V, URF-V2, and URF-V3 while Image 1S in the Storz Flex X^c). While no data regarding Image 1S in UTUC have been reported so far, NBI has been shown to improve the diagnostic accuracy of UTUC over white light. The group of Traxer performed NBI and white light URS in 27 patients with either previously conservatively treated UTUC or with first suspicion of cancer [37]. Biopsies were taken in case of suspects and laser ablation was performed for all apparent lesions. NBI was able to find 5 additional tumors (14%) in four patients, leading to a diagnostic advantage of 22.7% over white light; interestingly, NBI extended the limits of three tumors in three different patients, thereby improving the efficacy of KSS to potentially reduce the risk of in-site recurrence. However, external validations of these data are missing.

In conclusion, while enhanced imaging technology may improve the visualization of the upper urinary tract, a demonstration of its clinical utility during URS for UTUC is, to date, missing, and its use should be considered experimental.

8 Guidelines Recommendations about Flexible Ureteroscopy in UTUC

European Urology Association (EAU) Guidelines recommend the use of diagnostic fURS whenever the combination of urinary cytology and imaging is not sufficient for diagnosis and/or risk stratification. Moreover, it is underlined that diagnostic fURS facilitates selective ureteral sampling for in situ cytology. Despite the low level of evidence, a single postoperative intravesical instillation of chemotherapy may be used after diagnostic/therapeutic fURS to prevent intravesical recurrences. Finally, fURS is essential for KSS, and patients undergoing conservative management of UTUC should be informed and counseled about the need for an early second-look fURS (at three months) and subsequent stringent surveillance.

9 Highlights

- *Flexible diagnostic URS is a fundamental procedure for the diagnosis, risk stratification, and treatment of UTUC and should probably be performed even when radical surgery is planned.*
- *Diagnostic URS is a stepwise procedure that should be performed by expert surgeons following a strict protocol.*
- *During diagnostic fURS, selective cytology should be collected since it has demonstrated a superior accuracy compared to voided urinary cytology.*
- *Ureteral access sheaths can be used to allow multiple biopsies, thereby reducing the risk of inadequate tissue sampling.*
- *Digital fURS has improved the visualization of the urinary tract, but to date, this has not translated into better diagnostic accuracy nor in improved oncological outcomes.*
- *Enhanced technology imaging such as PDD, NBI, and Image 1-S is feasible and seems to improve the diagnostic accuracy over white light fURS. However, to date, a demonstration of their clinical utility in a real-world scenario is missing.*

References

1. Rouprêt M, Babjuk M, Burger M, Capoun O, Cohen D, Compérat EM, et al. European Association of Urology Guidelines on Upper Urinary Tract Urothelial Carcinoma: 2020 Update. Eur Urol. 2020;79(1):62–79. https://doi.org/10.1016/j.eururo.2020.05.042.
2. Birtle AJ, Chester JD, Jones RJ, Johnson M, Hill M, Bryan RT, et al. Results of POUT: a phase III randomised trial of perioperative chemotherapy versus surveillance in upper tract urothelial cancer (UTUC). J Clin Oncol. 2018; https://doi.org/10.1200/JCO.2018.36.6_suppl.407.
3. Xylinas E, Rink M, Margulis V, Clozel T, Lee RK, Comploj E, et al. Impact of renal function on eligibility for chemotherapy and survival in patients who have undergone radical nephroureterectomy. BJU Int. 2013;112:453–61. https://doi.org/10.1111/j.1464-410X.2012.11649.x.
4. Matin SF, Margulis V, Kamat A, Wood CG, Grossman HB, Brown GA, et al. Incidence of downstaging and complete remission after neoadjuvant chemotherapy for high-risk upper tract transitional cell carcinoma. Cancer. 2010;116:3127–34. https://doi.org/10.1002/cncr.25050.
5. Margulis V, Puligandla M, Trabulsi EJ, Plimack ER, Kessler ER, Matin SF, et al. Phase II trial of neoadjuvant systemic chemotherapy followed by extirpative surgery in patients with high grade upper tract urothelial carcinoma. J Urol. 2020;203:690–8. https://doi.org/10.1097/JU.0000000000000644.
6. Foerster B, Abufaraj M, Petros F, Azizi M, Gupta M, Schweitzer D, et al. Efficacy of preoperative chemotherapy for high risk upper tract urothelial carcinoma. J Urol. 2020;203:1101–8. https://doi.org/10.1097/JU.0000000000000737.
7. Dominguez-Escrig JL, Peyronnet B, Seisen T, Bruins HM, Yuan CY, Babjuk M, et al. Potential benefit of

lymph node dissection during radical nephroureterectomy for upper tract urothelial carcinoma: a systematic review by the European Association of Urology guidelines panel on non–muscle-invasive bladder cancer. Eur Urol Focus. 2019;5:224–41. https://doi.org/10.1016/j.euf.2017.09.015.

8. Soria F, Shariat SF, Lerner SP, Fritsche H-M, Rink M, Kassouf W, et al. Epidemiology, diagnosis, preoperative evaluation and prognostic assessment of upper-tract urothelial carcinoma (UTUC). World J Urol. 2017;35:379–87. https://doi.org/10.1007/s00345-016-1928-x.
9. Margulis V, Youssef RF, Karakiewicz PI, Lotan Y, Wood CG, Zigeuner R, et al. Preoperative multivariable prognostic model for prediction of nonorgan confined urothelial carcinoma of the upper urinary tract. J Urol. 2010;184:453–8. https://doi.org/10.1016/j.juro.2010.03.142.
10. Brien JC, Shariat SF, Herman MP, Ng CK, Scherr DS, Scoll B, et al. Preoperative hydronephrosis, ureteroscopic biopsy grade and urinary cytology can improve prediction of advanced upper tract urothelial carcinoma. J Urol. 2010;184:69–73. https://doi.org/10.1016/j.juro.2010.03.030.
11. Nison L, Rouprêt M, Bozzini G, Ouzzane A, Audenet F, Pignot G, et al. The oncologic impact of a delay between diagnosis and radical nephroureterectomy due to diagnostic ureteroscopy in upper urinary tract urothelial carcinomas: results from a large collaborative database. World J Urol. 2013;31:69–76. https://doi.org/10.1007/s00345-012-0959-1.
12. Sung HH, Jeon HG, Han DH, Jeong BC, Seo S II, Lee HM, et al. Diagnostic Ureterorenoscopy Is Associated with Increased Intravesical Recurrence following Radical Nephroureterectomy in Upper Tract Urothelial Carcinoma. PLoS One. 2015;10:e0139976. https://doi.org/10.1371/journal.pone.0139976.
13. Lee JK, Kim KB, Park YH, Oh JJ, Lee S, Jeong CW, et al. Correlation between the timing of diagnostic ureteroscopy and intravesical recurrence in upper tract urothelial cancer. Clin Genitourin Cancer. 2016;14:e37–41. https://doi.org/10.1016/j.clgc.2015.07.008.
14. O'Brien T, Ray E, Singh R, Coker B, Beard R, et al. British Association of Urological Surgeons Section of oncology. Prevention of bladder tumours after nephroureterectomy for primary upper urinary tract urothelial carcinoma: a prospective, multicentre, randomised clinical trial of a single postoperative intravesical dose of mitomycin C (the ODMIT-C trial). Eur Urol. 2011;60:703–10. https://doi.org/10.1016/j.eururo.2011.05.064.
15. Ito A, Shintaku I, Satoh M, Ioritani N, Aizawa M, Tochigi T, et al. Prospective randomized phase II trial of a single early intravesical instillation of pirarubicin (THP) in the prevention of bladder recurrence after nephroureterectomy for upper urinary tract urothelial carcinoma: the THP monotherapy study group trial. J Clin Oncol. 2013;31:1422–7. https://doi.org/10.1200/JCO.2012.45.2128.
16. van Doeveren T, van de Werken HJG, van Riet J, Aben KKH, van Leeuwen PJ, Zwarthoff EC, et al. Synchronous and metachronous urothelial carcinoma of the upper urinary tract and the bladder: are they clonally related? A systematic review. Urol Oncol Semin Orig Investig. 2020;38:590–8. https://doi.org/10.1016/j.urolonc.2020.01.008.
17. Shvero A, Zilberman DE, Dotan ZA, Laufer M, Fridman E, Winkler H, et al. Endoscopic management of upper tract urothelial carcinoma—tips and tricks. Transl Androl Urol. 2020;9:1815–20. https://doi.org/10.21037/tau.2020.01.07.
18. Messer J, Shariat SF, Brien JC, Herman MP, Ng CK, Scherr DS, et al. Urinary cytology has a poor performance for predicting invasive or high-grade upper-tract urothelial carcinoma. BJU Int. 2011;108:701–5. https://doi.org/10.1111/j.1464-410X.2010.09899.x.
19. Potretzke AM, Knight BA, Vetter JM, Anderson BG, Hardi AC, Bhayani SB, et al. Diagnostic utility of selective upper tract urinary cytology: a systematic review and meta-analysis of the literature. Urology. 2016;96:35–43. https://doi.org/10.1016/j.urology.2016.04.030.
20. Highman WJ. Transitional carcinoma of the-upper urinary tract: a histological and cytopathological study. J Clin Pathol. 1986;39:297–305. https://doi.org/10.1136/jcp.39.3.297.
21. Malm C, Grahn A, Jaremko G, Tribukait B, Brehmer M. Diagnostic accuracy of upper tract urothelial carcinoma: how samples are collected matters Diagnostic accuracy of upper tract urothelial carcinoma: how samples are collected matters. Scand J Urol. 2017;51(2):137–45. https://doi.org/10.1080/21681805.2017.1295102.
22. Guarnizo E, Pavlovich CP, Seiba M, Carlson DL, Vaughan ED, Sosa RE. Ureteroscopic biopsy of upper tract urothelial carcinoma: improved diagnostic accuracy and histopathological considerations using a multi-biopsy approach. J Urol. 2000;163:52–5. https://doi.org/10.1016/S0022-5347(05)67970-0.
23. Smith AK, Stephenson AJ, Lane BR, Larson BT, Thomas AA, Gong MC, et al. Inadequacy of biopsy for diagnosis of upper tract urothelial carcinoma: implications for conservative management. Urology. 2011;78:82–6. https://doi.org/10.1016/j.urology.2011.02.038.
24. Wang JK, Tollefson MK, Krambeck AE, Trost LW, Thompson RH. High rate of pathologic upgrading at nephroureterectomy for upper tract urothelial carcinoma. Urology. 2012;79:615–9. https://doi.org/10.1016/j.urology.2011.11.049.
25. Tavora F, Fajardo DA, Lee TK, Lotan T, Miller JS, Miyamoto H, et al. Small endoscopic biopsies of the ureter and renal pelvis: pathologic pitfalls. Am J Surg Pathol. 2009;33:1540–6. https://doi.org/10.1097/PAS.0b013e31817aec42a.
26. Gorin MA, Santos Cortes JA, Kyle CC, Carey RI, Bird VG. Initial clinical experience with use of ureteral access sheaths in the diagnosis and treatment of upper

tract urothelial carcinoma. Urology. 2011;78:523–7. https://doi.org/10.1016/j.urology.2011.01.048.

27. Lildal SK, Sørensen FB, Andreassen KH, Christiansen FE, Jung H, Pedersen MR, et al. Histopathological correlations to ureteral lesions visualized during ureteroscopy. World J Urol. 2017;35:1489–96. https://doi.org/10.1007/s00345-017-2035-3.
28. Talso M, Proietti S, Emiliani E, Gallioli A, Dragos L, Orosa A, et al. Comparison of flexible Ureterorenoscope quality of vision: an in vitro study. J Endourol. 2018;32:523–8. https://doi.org/10.1089/end.2017.0838.
29. Keller EX, Doizi S, Villa L, Traxer O. Which flexible ureteroscope is the best for upper tract urothelial carcinoma treatment? World J Urol. 2019;37:2325–33. https://doi.org/10.1007/s00345-019-02675-0.
30. Somani BK, Al-Qahtani SM, Gil De Medina SD, Traxer O. Outcomes of flexible ureterorenoscopy and laser fragmentation for renal stones: comparison between digital and conventional ureteroscope. Urology. 2013;82:1017–9. https://doi.org/10.1016/j.urology.2013.07.017.
31. Yamany T, Van Batavia J, Ahn J, Shapiro E, Gupta M. Ureterorenoscopy for upper tract urothelial carcinoma: how often are we missing lesions? Urology. 2015;85:311–5. https://doi.org/10.1016/j.urology.2014.08.030.
32. Gillan A, El-Mokadem I, Rai B, Lang S, Alcorn J, Shams Ud Din A, et al. Carcinoma in situ is significantly underdetected by prenephroureterectomy ureteroscopy in the management of upper tract urothelial cancers. Biomed Res Int. 2015;2015:547586. https://doi.org/10.1155/2015/547586.
33. Somani BK, Moseley H, Eljamel MS, Nabi G, Kata SG. Photodynamic diagnosis (PDD) for upper urinary tract transitional cell carcinoma (UT-TCC): evolution of a new technique. Photodiagn Photodyn Ther. 2010;7:39–43. https://doi.org/10.1016/j.pdpdt.2009.12.005.
34. Aboumarzouk OM, Mains E, Moseley H, Kata SG. Diagnosis of upper urinary tract tumours: is photodynamic diagnosis assisted ureterorenoscopy required as an addition to modern imaging and ureterorenoscopy? Photodiagn Photodyn Ther. 2013;10:127–33. https://doi.org/10.1016/j.pdpdt.2012.11.008.
35. Ahmad S, Aboumarzouk O, Somani B, Nabi G, Kata SG. Oral 5-aminolevulinic acid in simultaneous photodynamic diagnosis of upper and lower urinary tract transitional cell carcinoma—a prospective audit. BJU Int. 2012;110(11 Pt B):E596–600. https://doi.org/10.1111/j.1464-410X.2012.11326.x.
36. Kata SG, Aboumarzouk OM, Zreik A, Somani B, Ahmad S, Nabi G, et al. Photodynamic diagnostic ureterorenoscopy: a valuable tool in the detection of upper urinary tract tumour. Photodiagn Photodyn Ther. 2016;13:255–60. https://doi.org/10.1016/j.pdpdt.2015.08.002.
37. Traxer O, Geavlete B, de Medina SGD, Sibony M, Al-Qahtani SM. Narrow-band imaging digital flexible ureteroscopy in detection of upper urinary tract transitional-cell carcinoma: initial experience. J Endourol. 2011;25:19–23. https://doi.org/10.1089/end.2009.0593.

Training

Ramandeep Chalokia, Satyendra Persaud, and Azhar Khan

Abstract

Flexible ureterorenoscopy (FURS) or retrograde intrarenal surgery is performed universally for both diagnostic and therapeutic indications. Although a minimally invasive and relatively safe procedure, it is not without complications. The urologist needs to be competent in this procedure to be able to effectively manage the patient with urolithiasis. Beginning with the initial phase of a learning curve and culminating as an expert user entails regular training and mentoring. With a change in the training conditions due to several factors such as limited working hours, ethical issues, and patient expectations, there is a need for different and innovative ways of training. Novel learning platforms like e-learning are useful to the trainee to gain theoretical knowledge. Simulation has been proven without a doubt to shorten the learning curve of this procedure and should be incorporated into the training curriculum of the residents. Various models are available and have been validated in numerous studies. Nontechnical skills are an integral prerequisite of surgical training and should also form part of the training. Assessment of competence in this procedure should be more objective and nonbiased and to overcome the traditional, more subjective means of assessment, a global rating scale is attractive. Following the completion of the training and to achieve proficiency, a fellowship in a large stone center to learn the nuanced skills required for managing complex patients is recommended.

Keywords

Training · Flexible ureterorenoscopy Retrograde intrarenal surgery · E-learning Simulation · Urolithiasis · Fidelity · Assessment Nontechnical skills · Fellowship

1 Introduction

Advances in technology and innovation have expanded the role of flexible ureterorenoscopy (FURS) or retrograde intrarenal surgery (RIRS) in the diagnosis and management of upper uri-

R. Chalokia
Department of Urology, Warrington and Halton Teaching Hospitals NHS Foundation Trust, Cheshire, UK

S. Persaud
Department of Urology, University of the West Indies, St. Augustine, Trinidad and Tobago

A. Khan (✉)
Department of Urology, King's College Hospital NHS Foundation Trust, London, UK
e-mail: azharkhan1@nhs.net

G. Zeng et al. (eds.), *Flexible Ureteroscopy*, https://doi.org/10.1007/978-981-19-2936-6_23

nary tract conditions such as urolithiasis, uretero-pelvic obstruction, ureteric stricture, and urothelial cancers [1]. The procedure has now found utility in a range of challenging patient populations including those with bleeding diatheses, obesity, pregnancy, calyceal diverticula, and anatomical malformations [2]. A low complication profile coupled with a high degree of effectiveness has resulted in the widespread adoption of this technique into clinical practice worldwide [3]. This increased demand has led to a proportional increase in the need for training for the residents and the urologists alike.

Training is essential not only for safety and optimum clinical outcomes but perhaps equally as crucial for recognizing the importance of careful handling of this sensitive and costly piece of equipment. The lifespan of the flexible ureteroscope depends on the method of handling which in turn relates to the experience of the operator, with damage more likely to occur early in the initial learning curve [4]. Flexible ureterorenoscopy demands a high degree of expertise and thorough knowledge of anatomy to enable this procedure to be done with minimal risk of complication. Efforts should therefore be made to improve the training for this procedure and reduce the learning curve [5].

2 Concept of Learning Curve and Its Implications

Although this term in surgical parlance is bereft of scientific definition, it is generally considered an improvement of surgeon's skills over a period culminating in a reasonable outcome of that specific procedure during the plateau phase of the curve. During the initial stages of the learning curve, a surgeon would encounter difficulty, longer operating time, and associated higher risk of complications. The importance of learning curve in surgical practice assumed great significance after the General.

Medical Council inquiry into the Bristol Pediatrics Surgical Unit where, following fatalities above the national figures, it was recommended that patients should not be subject to a surgeon in the initial stages of the learning curve [6].

In urologic surgery, much of the research on the learning curve of stone-related surgery has been conducted on percutaneous nephrolithotomy and rigid ureteroscopy. Increased surgical experience is correlated with improved patient outcomes in patients undergoing semirigid ureteroscopy in different studies. One could well argue that this may be extrapolated to patients undergoing flexible ureterorenoscopy but few studies have explored this relationship [7]. Lu et al. have contested that prior experience in Semirigid URS does not necessarily transfer to FURS expertise and that it requires a specific skill set [8]. Cruz et al. in their qualitative analyses concluded that a minimum performance of 60 cases is required to reach a plateau of the learning curve for FURS [9].

Although there is a relative paucity of discussion surrounding the learning curve in FURS, available data support the influence of increased operator experience on improved patient safety and outcome. It is essential to acknowledge the importance of the learning curve for FURS to tailor the training and also to ratify the training methods and forms of assessment for the trainee [6]. The introduction of the European Working Time Directive legislation a few years ago along with several factors such as economic constraints, service provision, legal and ethical issues, patient expectations of experienced surgeons operating on them have all had a negative impact on training time. This reduction in training hours has caused a significant impact with a deleterious effect on trainee surgical education [10].

The historical surgical training model based on" learning by doing" is no longer sustainable and this has led to the development of innovative surgical platforms to meet training demand. Taking a cue from the airline industry where it plays an integral role and has a proven safety record, simulation has emerged as a powerful tool in surgical education [11]. Benchtop and virtual reality models and cadaveric models are all viable options in surgical simulation.

3 Importance of Structured Training and Recommendations for Training

It has been well demonstrated that structured training positively affects the acquisition of skill and that a good framework enhances learning. Simply having access to a training material is unlikely to be as beneficial. If one were to extrapolate data from general surgery, Palter and colleagues assessed the impact of a surgical training and assessment curriculum (STAC) on technical proficiency at laparoscopic cholecystectomy. In this small randomized controlled trial, the authors noted improved performance among residents in the STAC arm versus those who were conventionally trained [12]. Of greater relevance, Matsumoto noted similar effects of a structured program among residents undergoing training in ureteroscopy [13]. Ruiz and colleagues developed a curriculum involving didactic classes and operating room (OR) exposure, successfully introducing ureteroscopy to their unit safely and practically [14]. The SIMULATE (Simulation in Urological Training and Education) trial is a recently published randomised controlled trial (RCT) evaluating whether there was improved proficiency among inexperienced residents undergoing a structured simulation-based training curriculum [15]. The program was rated as having high educational value by participants, who felt that it provided skills that were transferrable to the OR. There was statistically significant improvement noted throughout the curriculum as well as with the first performance in the operating theatre. The authors intend to perform a follow-up compared to those with no simulation experience. Taken together, these data suggest that a well-organized and multimodal curriculum seems to confer the most benefit.

A panel of experts from across Europe has recommended a guide to future training in urolithiasis. The body has recommended e-learning as the first step in the training pathway [16]. E-learning will be the starting platform for training with the knowledge of these modules essential before further progression to hands-on training. The modules would be designed by the experts and consist of interactive sessions with the use of multimedia and assessment of cognitive learning (Fig. 1).

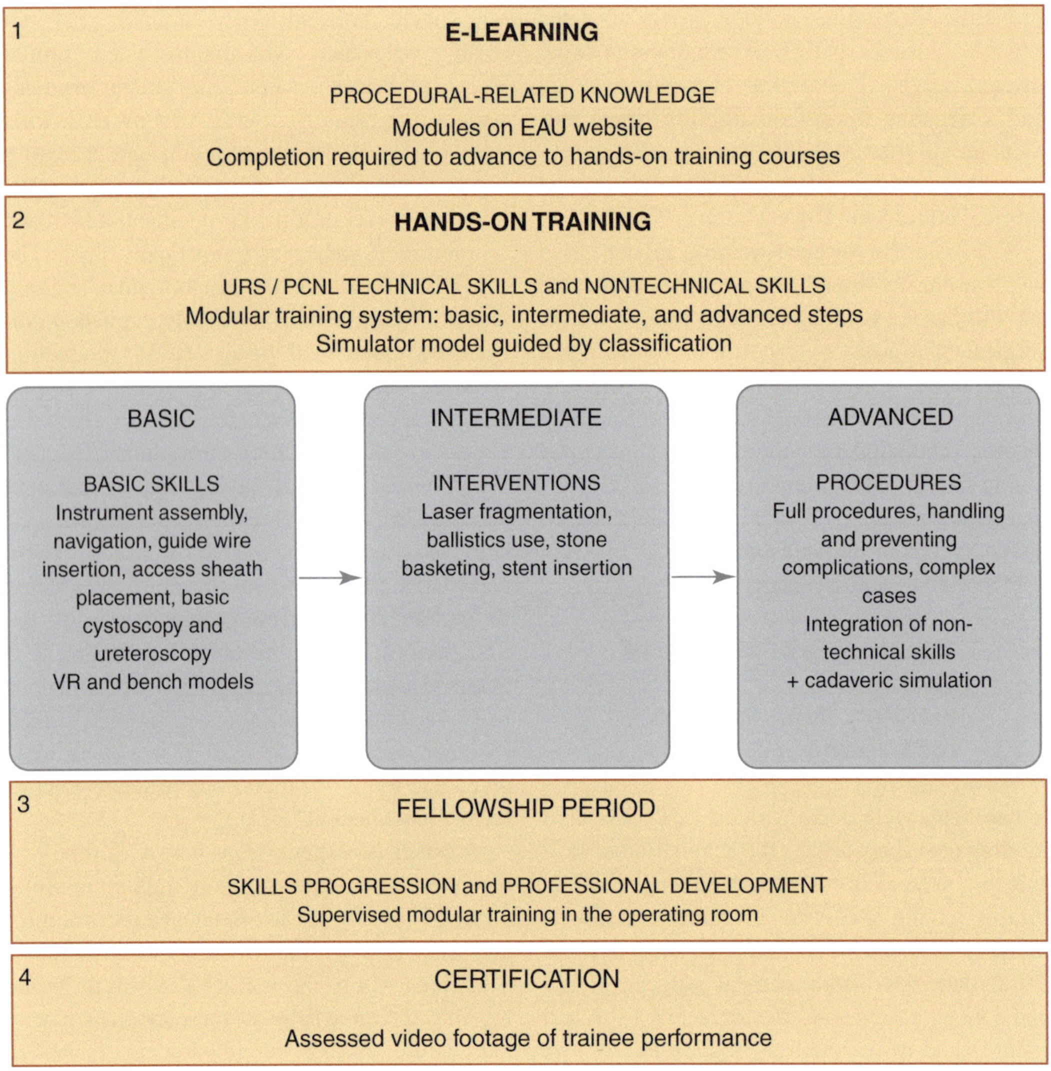

Fig. 1 A proposed algorithm of training in urolithiasis, (permission from Kamran et al. [16])

4 E-Learning

Time constraints in the surgical curriculum due to the above-outlined factors have led to the development of a unique platform for acquiring theoretical knowledge employing e-learning. E-learning comprises online educational modules such as tutorials, surgical skills modules and virtual case discussions. It can be of two types, "spaced learning," where the same course is repeated at least once for retention and "blended learning," which includes online learning supplemented with traditional teaching methods. [17] E-learning as a tool for learning has been practised widely in the USA. The Surgical Council on Resident Education (SCORE), an organization that delivers e-learning to General surgery residents, has comprehensive content meant for the trainee. Klingensmith et al. found a small statistically significant difference in the pass rate in favour of the residents using the SCORE website as compared to those not subscribing to it [18]. Similar websites can be designed for e-learning for training in urolithiasis.

Few studies have also demonstrated the cost-effectiveness, flexibility and applicability of this novel platform. Once initiated in a curriculum it needs regular updates to the content [17].

5 Simulation in Training

Simulation-based training offers an attractive option where the training can occur safely and cost-effectively. It should be performance based to enable the trainee to achieve the desired level of competence and should be integrated into the curriculum. The past few years have witnessed rapid developments in simulation-based training and scientific evidence borne out of randomized trials have established the positive impact it has on the performance of the trainee surgeon [19].

A range of simulators is available for training in FURS and which will be discussed in the chapter. It is important to be aware of the validation of the respective simulator tool for education and clinical practice. They are broadly classified into subjective and objective methods of validation. The subjective methods include face and content and the objective methods comprise construct, criterion and predictive validity [19] (Fig. 2) [10, 20, 21] Fidelity or "model" realism is a term often used to describe a simulator tool and a high fidelity mimicking more real-life scenario [22].

6 Benchtop Models

6.1 K-Box

Developed by Porges-Coloplast (France) the K-Box is a low fidelity-training model for flexible ureterorenoscopy. It consists of four independent boxes made of polyurethane and each box depicting a different training model with three separate entry and exit points. It also contains a "tool tray" for different training activities. To practice on the trainer, one requires all the equipment one would use in the real OR. This includes a camera system and the screen, endoscope, light source, and disposables such as guidewires, access sheath, baskets, and stents (Fig. 3).

This trainer provides an opportunity for the trainees to practice the different maneuvers of the flexible ureterorenoscopy, simulating a real renal collecting system (Fig. 4). It also provides provision for guidewire and sheath insertion and laser fragmentation of stones. The training task is performed with the box closed and the trainee can watch it on the screen, but one has the option of opening the box to review if lost or unsure.

Face Validity - Opinions, including non-experts, regarding the realism of the simulator
Content Validity - Opinions of experts about the simulator and its appropriateness of training
Construct Validity

- Within one group- Ability of the simulator to assess and differentiate between the level of experience of an individual or group measured over time
- Between groups – Ability of the simulator to distinguish between levels of experience

Concurrent Validity – Comparison of the new model against the older and gold standard, usually by OSATS
Predictive Validity – Correlation of performance with operating room performance, usually measured by OSATS

Fig. 2 Definitions of validity, based on definitions by Mc Dougall et al. [20] and van Nortwick et al. [21] OSATS Objective Structured Assessment of Technical Skills and permission to use the figure from Aydin et al. [10]

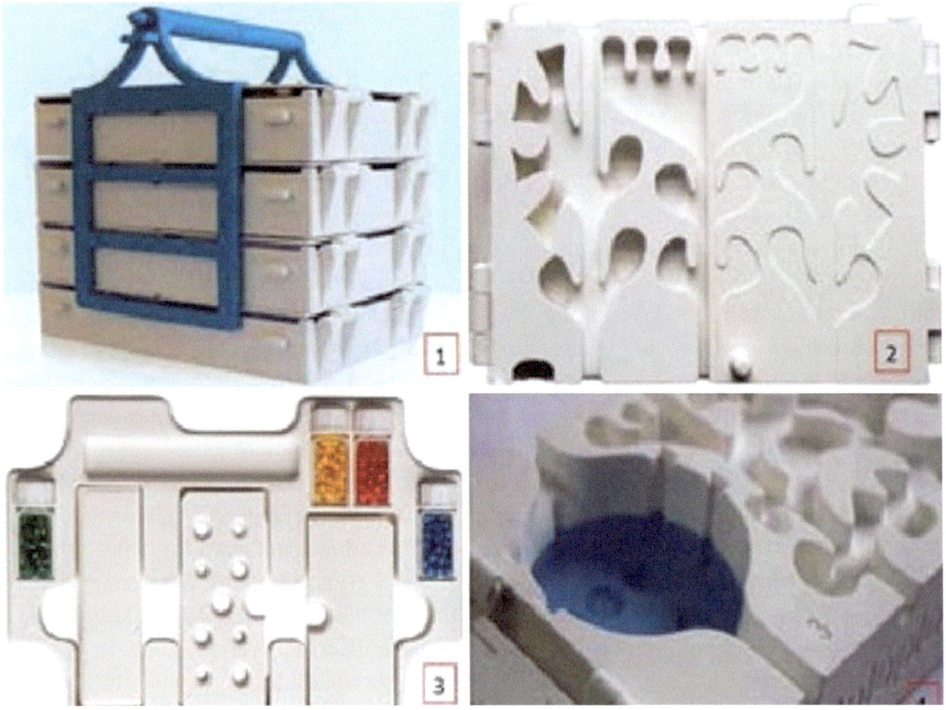

Fig. 3 K-box and its components (1.1—portable K-box, 1.2—box open (left) and closed (right), 1.3—tool tray, 1.4—K-box with water to use with laser for stone fragmentation [23] (With permission from O. Traxer).

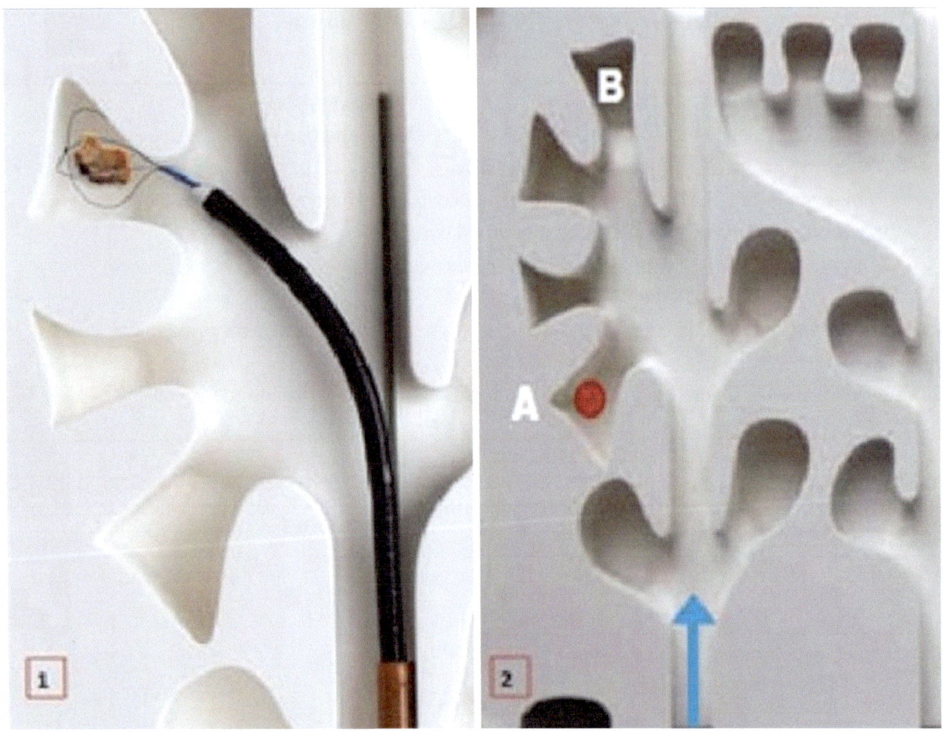

Fig. 4 Manipulation in the pelvicalyceal system (4.1—stone basketing with a flexible ureteroscope via the access sheath, 4.2—the movement of an object from A to B) [23]. (With permission from O. Traxer)

Villa et al. conducted a randomized study on medical students with no prior experience on flexible ureteroscopy to evaluate the content validity of this low fidelity model [23]. A global rating scale developed by Matsumoto et al. [13] was used to assess each student on different domains. They found that the trained students' mean scores were significantly higher than the untrained control group in all the domains of the exercise. They concluded that this model, although a low-fidelity one, provided effective basic endourological skills.

Villa et al. have advocated this trainer for training in flexible URS and they recommend this low-cost model for basic training and assessment. They also suggest developing a scoring system based on the completion of specific tasks such as scope handling, stone retrieval, and time taken to complete the procedure, which may improve the skills [24].

6.2 Advanced Scope Trainer (AST)

This simulator was developed by Mediskills Ltd. (Northampton, UK) is a high-fidelity benchtop model. It has a distensible bladder with anatomically appropriate ureteric orifices, both ureters and a thoughtfully designed renal collecting system containing stones and papillary tumors along with enabled functions for fluoroscopy to facilitate flexible URS. One can make this simulator close to reality by placing the model on the operating table with lithotomy stirrups and irrigating fluid next to the model. It utilizes a clear acrylic casing making it transparent for the trainee and the trainer to observe the movements while performing FURS. Besides, it has one large kidney with a tortuous ureter to simulate a potentially difficult real-life situation. Another key characteristic of this trainer is the ability to replace kidney stones via external ports (Fig. 5).

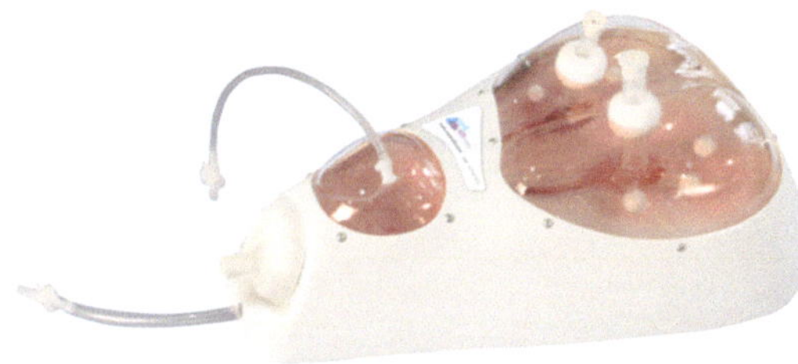

Fig. 5 Advanced Scope Trainer, an image with permission from Mediskills, UK [25]

Al-Jabir et al. conducted a robust study which was prospective, comparative, observational and multinational recruiting 60 participants including medical students, urological trainees and senior urologists [25]. Each participant was required to conduct a diagnostic flexible ureteroscopy followed by laser fragmentation of the stone and basket retrieval of calyceal stones on the model. To establish concurrent validity 14 junior urologists further performed diagnostic FURS on fresh frozen cadavers. The performance was assessed by the validated Objective Structured Assessment of Technical Skills (OSATS) tool [26] with its specific domains for construct validity. Face and content validity, acceptance and feasibility were assessed by anonymous surveys from participants and faculty. The trainer was found to have face, content, construct and concurrent validity for FURS training with participants generally finding the simulator to be realistic. The only weakness of the model was difficulty in ureteric catheterization often requiring expert help before trainees could continue with the task and was reflected in the feedback.

Brehmer et al. had earlier demonstrated on a more basic model of Scope Trainer (Mediskills, Northampton, UK) that there was no statistically significant difference between the consultants and the trainee while performing a task on the bench model and patients. Those who had subspecialist experience in endourology performed better on both patients and the bench model. All the participants found the bench model to be comparable to real surgery [27]. This study was able to confirm concurrent validity.

6.3 Cook URS Trainer

The Cook URS model was designed by Cook Medical (Bloomington IN) and was validated among Canadian residents in a paper by Blankstein et al. [28]. The model itself consists of

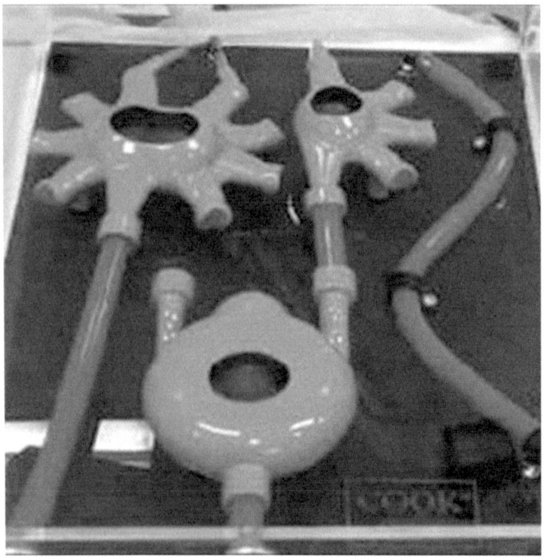

Fig. 6 Cook URS Trainer, Cook Medical, Bloomington, IN, USA [28]

three main parts—a dual calyceal system, a left ureter and kidney, and a tortuous ureter. It is constructed of polyurethane tubing and plastic, and can be filled with water as necessary to simulate the collecting system (Fig. 6). The training model in this case was part of a comprehensive simulator-based training curriculum and residents were allowed independent practice sessions. Of the participants, 80% rated this model as realistic (mean = 4.2/5) and five endourology experts rated it as useful (mean = 4.9/5) demonstrating face and content validity for this model. All the trainees rated this course as valuable and there was a significant improvement in task performance following this course as compared to baseline.

6.4 The Smart Simulator

This is an advanced bench model developed by Olympus (Japan) and has the advantages of being portable and ultrarealistic. It can mimic respiratory movements, consists of model calyces akin to human anatomical type and can simulate a real-life flexible URS field. It also includes an irrigation system and has special features to create a field that is not only clear but can be modified to simulate the field of stone dust and hematuria as one would encounter in real life. The papillae are 4 mm and 3 mm and enable the trainee to get familiar with the concept of removing a fragment through the access sheath before the encounter with the patient in OR (Figs. 7 and 8). Inoue and colleagues found this simulator to be realistic, acceptable, and feasible, meeting all the requisites of the face and content validities and scored significantly as compared to Scope Trainer in all the domains [29].

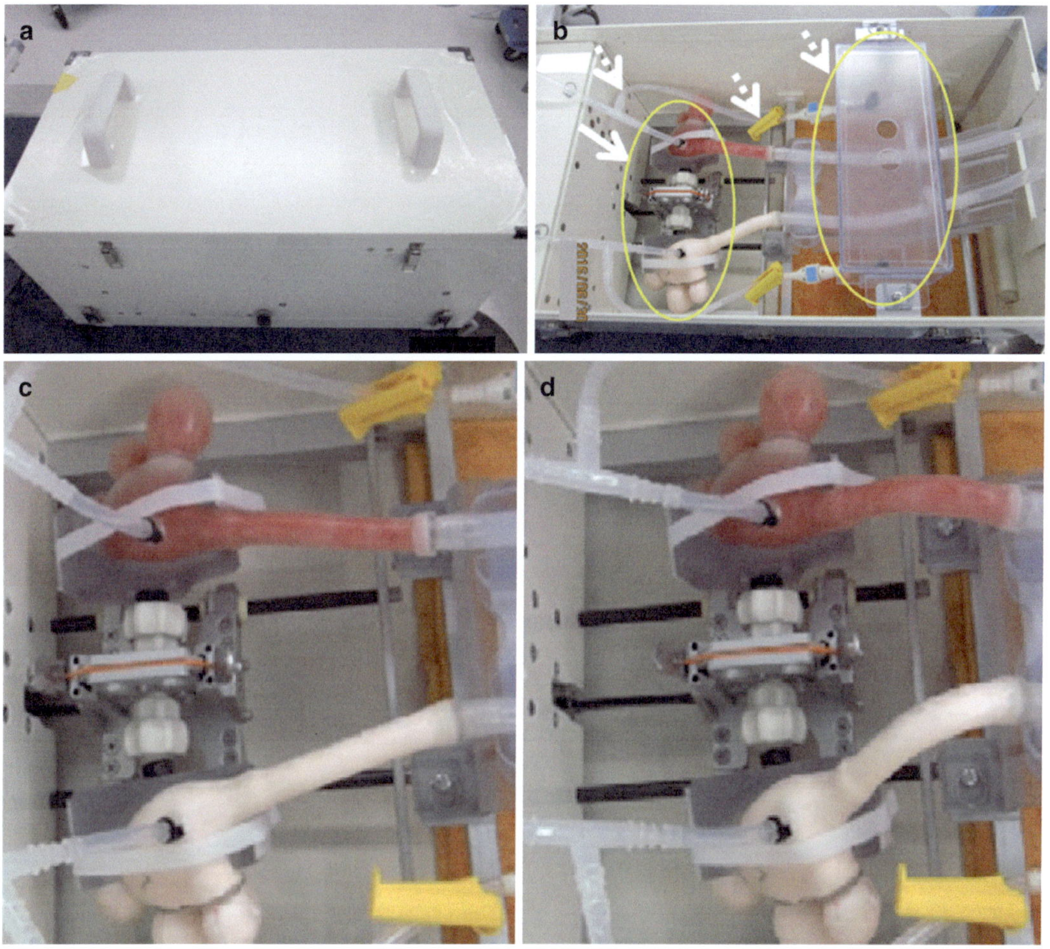

Fig. 7 With permission from Inoue et al. [29]. Smart Simulator and its components: (**a**) Portable box. (**b**) Two components of the system that simulate breathing-induced movement of the kidney (arrow indicates the bilateral pyelocalyceal model) and the irrigation system (dotted arrow indicates the irrigation tube and saline tank) in the opened box. (**c**, **d**) Amplitude of the kidney swing

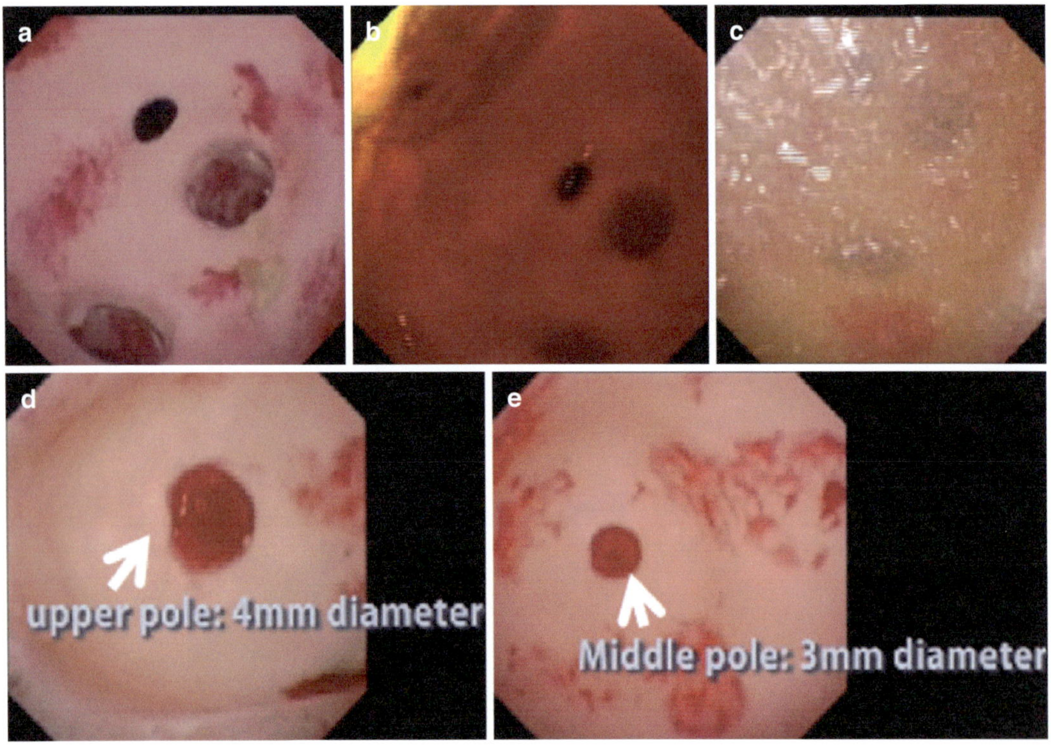

Fig. 8 Simulation showing clear field (**a**) hematuria (**b**) and stone dust (**c**), Papilla size **d** and **e** as shown (with permission from Inoue et al. [29])

6.5 Adult Ureterorenoscopy Trainer (Ideal Anatomic Modelling, Holt, MI)

This was designed as a high-fidelity simulator modelled on a patient's actual upper urinary tract images. The computerized tomography images were used to develop a silicone mold using rapid prototyping and animation modeling software. White et al. used this simulator in a study comprising 46 participants which included attending urologists, urology residents, medical students and biotechnology industry representatives [30]. They found that all of the participants rated the trainer as realistic and easy to use and 98% rated this a good practice model. All the participants felt that it should be used in residency and 96% would or would have used it during training. On a given performance task which was basket extraction of lower pole stone, experienced participants fared significantly better than the novice participants with respect to global rating and checklist scores (mean global rating scale 33.1 vs. 15.0, $p < 0.0001$) and time taken to complete the task (mean 141.2 vs. 447.2, $p = 0.01$). The authors were able to demonstrate face, content, and construct validities but acknowledged that it was a preliminary study with few participants.

7 Virtual-Reality Simulators

The URO Mentor (3D Systems, Simbionix, Tel Aviv, Israel) is a high-fidelity virtual simulator platform that is Windows-based. It has a rich source of virtual training sessions on a wide array of patient case scenarios. It incorporates virtual endourological instruments with the use of fluoroscopy and laser fragmentation facilities. (Fig. 9) Using a mannequin, a computer interface, and a special haptic device offers the trainees a unique opportunity to practice both diagnostic and therapeutic procedures in a low stake environment. Michel et al. described the

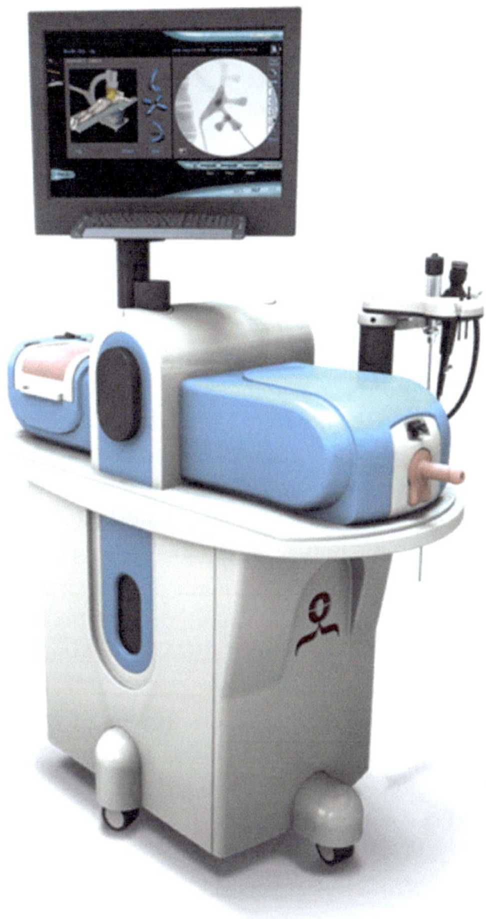

Fig. 9 Uro Mentor—Symbionix, 3D systems [31]

utility of this simulator in seven training courses which included the participation of the trainees and experienced urologists. The trainees reported better training and reduced time to gain experience [31]. Additionally, the experienced urologists felt they were able to manage the complications better which arise in endourology after training with this model. Several studies have validated the performance of the model in training [32, 33].

The advantages of the virtual simulator (VR) have been well proven with immediate virtual expert feedback and the ability to practice on different clinical scenarios with a range of instruments. However, it is not possible to include this training facility in all the centers as the cost of the model can be very high- between $60,000 to $85,000 and this may not be a feasible option when the resources are limited especially in developing countries.

Chou et al. compared the outcome of training of first-year medical students on a high-fidelity bench model (Ureteroscopy training model, TMU, Limbs and Things, UK) and the URO Mentor (Simbionix) [34]. Sixteen first-year medical students were randomized into two groups, the first group trained on the ureteroscopy training model (TMU) and the second group on the VR simulator, URO Mentor. Assessment on a porcine model after 2 months of training and using objective structured assessment of technical skills (OSATS) did not show any difference in the performance of either cohort ($p = 0.38$). The authors feel although high fidelity bench model, TMU, was cheaper to purchase, the sum of the cost of the disposables, flexible URS, fluoroscopy, laser, attendance of supervising expert was perhaps equal to the cost of VR and in the long term, the benefit of VR would be significant once the training objectives are satisfied. The TMU has, however, been discontinued from production for some years now.

Mishra et al. evaluated the training outcomes of 21 urologists with no prior FURS experience on 3 simulators which included 2 high-fidelity and URO Mentor, the VR simulator [35]. After initial training from an expert, these participants rotated among the 3 simulators and the assessment was done using the global rating scale and pass ratings. The results did not show any significant difference in training outcomes between the non-VR and VR simulators although the VR simulator scored significantly with regard to the respiratory movements. The authors concluded that although VR simulator may feel superior due to the construct of respiratory movements, alternative high-fidelity bench models are not inferior in training and practice on these models is the key.

8 Animal or Cadaveric Models

Cadaveric models have been shown to provide a good training experience and fresh frozen cadavers have been used in urologic simulation training before. Embalming offers an advantage in that it improves tissue durability, allowing for the cadaver to be reused. Cadavers prepared by Thiel's method offer particularly realistic training opportunities and have been utilized in several scenarios including laparoscopy and transurethral resection [36]. Mains et al. explored the use of Thiel cadavers in ureteroscopy simulation, noting that it proved to be a high-fidelity training model with good haptic feedback [5]. There are differences in cadaveric specimens to keep in mind while using them for simulations and these include lack of bleeding and peristalsis. Although the porcine urinary tract has been successfully used as a training model for ureteroscopy, [37] animal models are now less popular, perhaps due to ethical issues and the cost [38]. Hu et al., however, used isolated porcine kidneys and ureters instead of experimental pigs to evaluate the training of flexible URS [39]. Arguments in favor of isolated porcine kidneys include that it is cheaper, is easily available, and provides an intuitive model of practice. The authors trained young urologists who had prior rigid ureteroscopy experience but had never performed flexible URS independently. Following the training, the average operation time decreased significantly from 18 ±3.4 min to 11 ± 2.2 min ($p < 0.05$). Significant differences were seen in the posttest scores with regard to the global rating scale and pass/fail rating.

9 Assessment

Ureteroscopy is considered a core urological procedure and as such assessing trainee competency is key, as technical skills are linked to patient outcomes [40]. Several credentialing bodies outline indicative numbers required to certify proficiency in the procedure. For example, in the UK, the Joint Committee on Surgical Training (JCST) lists ureteroscopy among a group of procedures for which a resident is expected to attain a minimum level of competence and the indicative number, in this case, is listed as 50 [41]. Traditionally, competence has been certified via a compilation of logbooks and direct observation of procedures. However, this is rater-dependent and lacks objectivity. The objective structured assessment of technical skills (OSATS) was compiled to mitigate these shortcomings is considered the gold standard in surgical assessment [26]. Contemporary evidence seems to support the utility of simulation-based assessments and one may reasonably use scores derived from these assessments to define competence [42]. Another simple tool that can be utilized to assess the competency of ureteroscopy is the Global Rating Scale (see Fig. 10), described by Matsumoto and colleagues and adapted from the OSATS rubric [13]. These structured instruments may be used in the OR skills lab to provide assessment and feedback.

URETEROSCOPIC GLOBAL RATING SCALE

Please circle the number corresponding to the candidate's performance in each category, irrespective of training level.

	1	2	3	4	5
Respect for Tissue	Scope frequently pushed into urothelial wall. Used unnecessary force with guidewire and/or basket		Scope occasionally pushed into urothelial wal. Careful handling of guidewire and/or basket for the most part.		No trauma to urochelial wall with scope. Consistent and careful handling of guidewire and/or basket.
Time and Motion	Many unnecessary moves.		Made some Unnecessary moves but time more efficient.		No unnecessary moves and time is maximized.
Instrument Handling	Needed to repeatedy attempt guidewire insertion and/or basketing of stone.		Able to insert guidewire and basket stone within first few tries. Occasional awkward maneuver.		Able to insert guidewire and basket with fluid motion and no awkwardness.
Handling of Endoscope	Frequently had scope pointing away from the center of the urethra or ureter. Scope poorly aligned during procedure.		Had scope centered for the most part. Guidewire in view for the most part. Better use of scope angle during procedure.		Scope always centered and guidewire always in view. Scope always set at a good angle throughout procedure.
Flow of Procedure and Forward Planning	Frequently stopped or need advice or assistance from examiner.		Demoratrated the ability to think forward with relatively steady progression of procedure.		Obviously planned procedure from beginning to end with fluid motion.
Use of Assistants	Failed to have assistants help with guidewise insertion and/or stone basketing.		Appropriate use of assistants most of the time		Strategically used assistants to the best advantage at all times
Knowledge of Procedure	Deficient knowledge. Needed specific instruction al most operative steps.		Knew all important aspects of operation		Demonstrated familiarity with all aspects of operation

Pass Rating:

Would you feel confident in allowing this trainee to perform this procedure in the operating room?YES NO

Fig. 10 The Ureteroscopic Global rating Scale, permission from Matsumoto et al. [13]

10 Nontechnical Skills Training

The acquisition of nontechnical skills (NTS) has assumed great significance in the training of the surgical craft. Surprisingly, the majority of the errors in surgery occur not due to technical factors but nontechnical skills such as communication, teamwork and decision making [19]. Interestingly, these skills are not inborn with but with adequate training, these can be cultivated and developed. There is little evidence in the literature exploring the role of NTS in ureteroscopy; however, these skills are universal and intuitively should apply to all surgical fields.

Nontechnical skills are classified into 3 categories: social skills (leadership, communication and teamwork), cognitive skills (decision making and situational awareness) and personal resource factors (ability to cope with stress or fatigue) [43]. In a UK based survey, only 41% of the urology trainees felt the training in NTS was adequate for the first day of practice as compared to 76% of specialists [44]. Interestingly, 90% of trainees and 70% of specialists felt that there is a role of simulation in NTS training in urology. Although several approaches have been suggested to improve NTS, simulation-based team training in NTS has been considered the most suitable to achieve it [19]. Broadly, NTS simulation has been classified into three main categories: full immersion/ distributed simulation (FIDS), high-fidelity OR simulation (HFROS), and crisis resource management (CRM) [45]. FIDS, a commonly used simulation model consists of an inflatable 360-degree "igloo" shell simulating a real OR situation. This simulation has been shown to have face, content and construct validity [43]. Integration of technical skills and NTS in a curriculum is a very effective and relevant educational tool. Aydin and colleagues conducted a study on ureterorenoscopy specific NTS curriculum for junior residents in a full immersion simulation. [46] The junior residents participated in a training session with an expert supervisor on 4 scenarios that involved both technical and NTS skills. The participants felt that the session significantly improved their technical skills (mean:4.1/5) and nontechnical skills (mean:4.6/5) and further added the session was of good educational value and one that would also enable the transfer of skills to OR. It is also crucial to recognize the significance of the NTS outside the OR. Crisis resource management simulation training is a valuable means of reducing mistakes in emergency care [10].

11 Further Aids

The future of training adage of "see one, do one, teach one" as a model for surgical training no longer applies. As technology evolves, so too will our ability to deliver innovative methods of training. Newer and more portable virtual and augmented reality systems are likely to become cheaper, more commonplace and offer an increasingly realistic simulation. Head-mounted displays continue to miniaturize from the clumsy wired devices they once were. The Microsoft HoloLens is a novel HMD that has shown promise in improving ergonomics and even procedural times [47]. Any complex anatomy can now be individually recreated via 3D modeling, enabling procedural rehearsal and training for difficult cases [48]. Along with developments in haptic feedback, these technologies are likely to be integrated for a more immersive training experience. These are likely to be combined with curriculum development and adoption, to improve the overall quality of training.

12 Conclusion

With the extensive use of flexible URS currently for a variety of endourologic indications, it is imperative to develop effective training techniques which are robust, effective, and reproducible [49]. Simulation has largely addressed the constraints arising out of modern surgical training. However, simulation is more suitable for beginners in the procedure but is likely to reduce the learning curve. Development of a comprehensive and well-structured curriculum including e-learning modules, didactics, hands-on/simulation exposure, a minimum number of this procedure as laid out for competence and NTS training is highly recommended by the experts. To achieve a desired level of expertise, fellowship training in a large volume of stone centers may be necessary to deal with complex and challenging stone cases [50]. This would lead to a strong foundation for independent practice in endourology.

References

1. Doizi S, Traxer O. Flexible ureteroscopy: technique, tips and tricks. Urolithiasis. 2018;46(1):47–58.
2. Giusti G, Proietti S, Peschechera R, Taverna G, Sortino G, Cindolo L, et al. Sky is no limit for ureteroscopy: extending the indications and special circumstances. World J Urol. 2015;33(2):257–73.

3. Ozimek T, Kramer MW, Hupe MC, Laturnus JM, Struck JP, Hennig MJP, et al. The impact of endourological experience on flexible ureteroscopy outcomes and performance at different levels of expertise: retrospective multifactorial analysis. Urol Int. 2020;104(5-6):452–8.
4. Karaolides T, Bach C, Kachrilas S, Goyal A, Masood J, Buchholz N. Improving the durability of digital flexible ureteroscopes. Urology. 2013;81(4):717–22.
5. Mains E, Tang B, Golabek T, Wiatr T, Ross G, Duncan A, et al. Ureterorenoscopy training on cadavers embalmed by Thiel's method: simulation or a further step towards reality? Cent Eur J Urol. 2017;70(1):81–7.
6. Quirke K, Aydin A, Brunckhorst O, Bultitude M, Khan MS, Dasgupta P, et al. Learning curves in urolithiasis surgery: a systematic review. J Endourol. 2018;32(11):1008–20.
7. Berardinelli F, Cindolo L, De Francesco P, Proietti S, Hennessey D, Dalpiaz O, et al. The surgical experience influences the safety of retrograde intrarenal surgery for kidney stones: a propensity score analysis. Urolithiasis. 2017;45(4):387–92.
8. Lu J, Thandapani K, Kuo T, Tiong HY. Validation of laparoscopy and flexible ureteroscopy tasks in inanimate simulation training models at a large-scale conference setting. Asian J Urol. 2020;8(2):215–9.
9. Da Cruz JAS, Thiago C, De Queiros BU, De La Roca RLF, Lima JPC, Di Migueli R. The learning curve for retrograde intra-renal surgery (RIRS): how many cases are necessary? J Urol. 2016;1:e443.
10. Aydın A, Al-Jabir A, Smith B, Ahmed K. Training in percutaneous nephrolithotomy. In: Zeng G, Sarica K, editors. Percutaneous nephrolithotomy. New York: Springer; 2020. https://doi.org/10.1007/97-981-15-0575-1_21.
11. Kneebone R. Simulation in surgical training: educational issues and practical implications. Med Educ. 2003;37(3):267–77.
12. Palter VN, Orzech N, Reznick RK, Grantcharov TP. Validation of a structured training and assessment curriculum for technical skill acquisition in minimally invasive surgery: a randomized controlled trial. Ann Surg. 2013;257(2):224–30.
13. Matsumoto ED, Hamstra SJ, Radomski SB, Cusimano MD. A novel approach to endourological training: training at the surgical skills center. J Urol. 2001;166(4):1261–6.
14. Ruiz L, Hyams E, Donderis R, Alvarado A, Persky I, Ruiz S, et al. Implementation of a focused curriculum on flexible ureteroscopic surgery: a multi-institutional collaborative effort. Clin Nephrol. 2013;79(2):132–5.
15. Aydın A, Ahmed K, Baig U, et al. The SIMULATE ureteroscopy training curriculum: educational value and transfer of skills. World J Urol. 2021;39(9):3615–21. https://doi.org/10.1007/s00345-021-03604-w.
16. Ahmed K, et al. European Association of Urology section of urolithiasis (EULIS) consensus statement on simulation, training, and assessment in urolithiasis. Eur Urol Focus. 2017;4(4):614–20. https://doi.org/10.1016/j.euf.2017.03.006.
17. Jayakumar N, Brunckhorst O, Dasgupta P, Khan MS, Ahmed K. E-learning in surgical education: a systematic review. J Surg Educ. 2015;72(6):1145–57. https://doi.org/10.1016/j.jsurg.2015.05.008. Epub 2015 Jun 22
18. Klingensmith ME, Jones AT, Smiley W, Biester TW, Malangoni MA. Subscription to the surgical council on resident education web portal and qualifying examination performance. J Am Coll Surg. 2014;218(4):566–70. https://doi.org/10.1016/j.jamcollsurg.2013.12.015. Epub 2013 Dec 20
19. Brewin J, Ahmed K, Challacombe B. An update and review of simulation in urological training. Int J Surg. 2014;12(2):103–8.
20. McDougall EM. Validation of surgical simulators. J Endourol. 2007;21(3):244–7. https://doi.org/10.1089/end.2007.9985.
21. Van Nortwick SS, Lendvay TS, Jensen AR, Wright AS, Horvath KD, Kim S. Methodologies for establishing valididty in surgical simulation studies. Surgery. 2010;147(5):622–30. https://doi.org/10.1016/j.surg.2009.10.068.
22. Matsumoto ED. Low-fidelity ureteroscopy models. J Endourol. 2007;21(3):248–51.
23. Villa L, Şener TE, Somani BK, Cloutier J, Butticè S, Marson F, et al. Initial content validation results of a new simulation model for flexible ureteroscopy: The key-box. J Endourol. 2017;31(1):72–7.
24. Villa L, Somani BK, Sener TE, Cloutier J, Cloutier J, Butticè F, et al. Comprehensive flexible ureteroscopy (FURS) simulator for training in endourology: the k-box model. Central European. J Urol. 2016;69(1):118–20.
25. Al-Jabir A, Aydin A, Abe T, Raison N, Khan MS, Dasgupta P, et al. Validation of the advanced scope trainer for flexible Ureterorenoscopy training. Urology. 2017;110:45–50.
26. Martin JA, Regehr G, Reznick R, Macrae H, Murnaghan J, Hutchison C, et al. Objective structured assessment of technical skill (OSATS) for surgical residents. Br J Surg. 1997;84(2):273–8.
27. Brehmer M, Tolley DA. Validation of a bench model for endoscopic surgery in the upper urinary tract. Eur Urol. 2002;42(2):175–9.
28. Blankstein U, Lantz AG, D'A Honey RJ, Pace KT, Ordon M, Lee JY. Simulation-based flexible ureteroscopy training using a novel ureteroscopy part-task trainer. J Can Urol Assoc. 2015;9(9-10):331–5.
29. Inoue T, Okada S, Hamamoto S, Matsuda T. New advanced bench model for flexible Ureteroscopic training: the smart simulator. J Endourol. 2018;32(1):22–7.
30. White MA, DeHaan AP, Stephens DD, Maes AA, Maatman TJ. Validation of a high Fidelity adult ureteroscopy and Renoscopy simulator. J Urol. 2010;183(2):673–7.
31. Michel MS, Knoll T, Köhrmann KU, Alken P. The URO Mentor: development and evaluation of a new computer-based interactive training system

for virtual life-like simulation of diagnostic and therapeutic endourological procedures. BJU Int. 2002;89(3):174–7.

32. Knoll T, Trojan L, Haecker A, Alken P, Michel MS. Validation of computer-based training in ureterorenoscopy. BJU Int. 2005;95(9):1276–9.
33. Schout BMA, Ananias HJK, Bemelmans BLH, D'Ancona FCH, Muijtjens AMM, Dolmans VEMG, et al. Transfer of cysto-urethroscopy skills from a virtual-reality simulator to the operating room: a randomized controlled trial. BJU Int. 2010;106(2):226–31.
34. Chou DS, Abdelshehid C, Clayman RV, McDougall EM. Comparison of results of virtual-reality simulator and training model for basic ureteroscopy training. J Endourol. 2006;20(4):266–71.
35. Mishra S, Sharma R, Kumar A, Ganatra P, Sabnis RB, Desai MR. Comparative performance of high-fidelity training models for flexible ureteroscopy: are all models effective. Indian J Urol. 2011;27(4):451–6.
36. Healy SE, Rai BP, Biyani CS, Eisma R, Soames RW, Nabi G. Thiel embalming method for cadaver preservation: a review of new training model for urologic skills training. Urology. 2015;85(3):499–504.
37. Strohmaier WL, Giese A. Porcine urinary tract as a training model for ureteroscopy. Urol Int. 2001;66(1):30–2.
38. Brunckhorst O, Aydin A, Abboudi H, Sahai A, Khan MS, Dasgupta P, et al. Simulation-based ureteroscopy training: a systematic review. J Surg Educ. 2015;72(1):135–43.
39. Hu D, Liu T, Wang X. Flexible ureteroscopy training for surgeons using isolated porcine kidneys in vitro endourology and technology. BMC Urol. 2015;15:71.
40. Fecso AB, Szasz P, Kerezov G, Grantcharov TP. The effect of technical performance on patient outcomes in surgery. Ann Surg. 2017;265(3):492–501.
41. Certification Guidelines and Checklists, JCST, Uroweb. Available at: https://www.jcst.org/qualityassurance/certification-guidelines-and-checklists/. Accessed June 2022.
42. Goldenberg M, Ordon M, Honey JRDA, Andonian S, Lee JY. Objective assessment and standard setting for basic flexible Ureterorenoscopy skills among urology trainees using simulation-based methods. J Endourol. 2021;47(2):462–3.
43. Griffin C, Aydın A, Brunckhorst O, Raison N, Khan MS, Dasgupta P, et al. Non-technical skills: a review of training and evaluation in urology. World J Urol. 2020;38(7):1653–61.
44. Aydin A, Ahmed K, Shafi AMA, Khan MS, Dasgupta P. The role of simulation in urological training – a quantitative study of practice and opinions. Surgeon. 2016;14(6):301–7.
45. Ounounou E, Aydin A, Brunckhorst O, Khan MS, Dasgupta P, Ahmed K. Nontechnical skills in surgery: a systematic review of current training modalities. J Surg Educ. 2019;76(1):14–24.
46. Aydin A, Brunckhorst O, Aya H, Eldred-Evans D, Al-Jabir A, Brewin J, et al. Development and validation of a ureterorenoscopy non-technical skills curriculum. J Urol. 2016;195(4):E323–214.
47. Al Janabi HF, Aydin A, Palaneer S, Macchione N, Al-Jabir A, Khan MS, et al. Effectiveness of the HoloLens mixed-reality headset in minimally invasive surgery: a simulation-based feasibility study. Surg Endosc. 2020;34(3):1143–9.
48. Bendre HH, Rajender A, Barbosa PV, Wason SEL. Robotic dismembered pyeloplasty surgical simulation using a 3D-printed silicone-based model:development, face validation and crowdsourced learning outcomes assessment. J Robot Surg. 2020;14(6):897–902.
49. Seitz C, Fajkovic H. Training in ureteroscopy for urolithiasis. Arab J Urol. 2014;12(1):42–8. https://doi.org/10.1016/j.aju.2013.08.010.
50. Skolarikos A, Gravas S, Laguna M, Traxer O, Preminger G, de la Rosette J. Training in ureteroscopy: a critical appraisal of the literature. BJU Int. 2011;108:798–805.

MIX
Papier aus verantwortungsvollen Quellen
Paper from responsible sources
FSC® C105338

If you have any concerns about our products,
you can contact us on
ProductSafety@springernature.com

In case Publisher is established outside the EU,
the EU authorized representative is:
Springer Nature Customer Service Center GmbH
Europaplatz 3, 69115 Heidelberg, Germany

Printed by Libri Plureos GmbH
in Hamburg, Germany